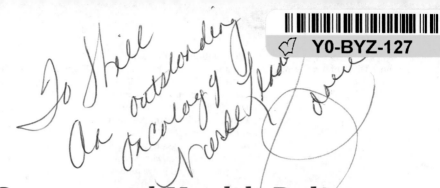

Cancer and Health Policy:
ADVANCEMENTS AND OPPORTUNITIES

Edited by

Janice M. Phillips, PhD, RN, FAAN,
and Barbara Holmes Damron, PhD, RN, FAAN

ONS Publications Department
Executive Director, Professional Practice and Programs: Elizabeth Wertz Evans, PhD, RN, MPM, CPHQ, CPHIMS, FHIMSS, FACMPE
Publisher and Director of Publications: William A. Tony, BA, CQIA
Managing Editor: Lisa M. George, BA
Assistant Managing Editor: Amy Nicoletti, BA, JD
Acquisitions Editor: John Zaphyr, BA, MEd
Copy Editor: Vanessa Kattouf, BA
Graphic Designer: Dany Sjoen
Editorial Assistant: Judy Holmes

Library of Congress Cataloging-in-Publication Data
Cancer and health policy : advancements and opportunities / edited by Janice M. Phillips and Barbar Holmes Damron.
    p. ; cm.
Includes bibliographical references and index.
ISBN 978-1-935864-38-7 (alk. paper)
I. Phillips, Janice Mitchell, editor. II. Damron, Barbara Holmes, editor.
[DNLM: 1. Neoplasms–United States. 2. Health Policy–United States. 3. Legislation, Medical–United States. QZ 200]
RA645.C3
362.19699'400973–dc23
                                                                                    2015002840

Publisher's Note
This book is published by the Oncology Nursing Society (ONS). ONS neither represents nor guarantees that the practices described herein will, if followed, ensure safe and effective patient care. The recommendations contained in this book reflect ONS's judgment regarding the state of general knowledge and practice in the field as of the date of publication. The recommendations may not be appropriate for use in all circumstances. Those who use this book should make their own determinations regarding specific safe and appropriate patient care practices, taking into account the personnel, equipment, and practice available at the hospital or other facility at which they are located. The editor and publisher cannot be held responsible for any liability incurred as a consequence from the use or application of any of the contents of this book. Figures and tables are used as examples only. They are not meant to be all-inclusive, nor do they represent endorsement of any particular institution by ONS. Mention of specific products and opinions related to those products do not indicate or imply endorsement by ONS. Websites mentioned are provided for information only; the hosts are responsible for their own content and availability. Unless otherwise indicated, dollar amounts reflect U.S. dollars.

ONS publications are originally published in English. Publishers wishing to translate ONS publications must contact ONS about licensing arrangements. ONS publications cannot be translated without obtaining written permission from ONS. (Individual tables and figures that are reprinted or adapted require additional permission from the original source.) Because translations from English may not always be accurate or precise, ONS disclaims any responsibility for inaccuracies in words or meaning that may occur as a result of the translation. Readers relying on precise information should check the original English version.

Printed in the United States of America

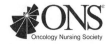

Integrity • Innovation • Stewardship • Advocacy • Excellence • Inclusiveness

This book is dedicated to Sean C. Tenner, BA, the Chicagoland Area Affiliate of Susan G. Komen, and the Metropolitan Chicago Breast Cancer Task Force for their sustained and contagious commitment to eliminating cancer disparities through advocacy and data-driven health policy.

—Janice

This book is dedicated to J.R. Damron, MD, FACR, my husband, best friend, and colleague, whom I met while working on cancer policies decades ago. This is in honor of all the patients with cancer with whom we have worked together and for all the state and federal policies upon which we collaborated.

—Barbara

Contributors

Editors

Janice M. Phillips, PhD, RN, FAAN
Director of Government and Regulatory Affairs
CGFNS International
Philadelphia, Pennsylvania
Chapter 15. Oncology Implications of the Patient Protection and Affordable Care Act

Barbara Holmes Damron, PhD, RN, FAAN
Director, Office of Community Partnerships and Cancer Health Disparities
University of New Mexico Cancer Center
Associate Professor
Robert Wood Johnson Foundation Nursing and Health Policy Collaborative
University of New Mexico College of Nursing
Associate Professor
Department of Family and Community Medicine
University of New Mexico School of Medicine
Albuquerque, New Mexico
Chapter 18. Legislative Topics in Cancer Research and Practice

Authors

David Ansell, MD, MPH
Senior Vice President for System Integration
Rush University Medical Center
Chicago, Illinois
Chapter 12. Creation of a Statewide Mammography Surveillance Program

Brian Bunn, REHS/RS, CPFS-IT, Dual MPH(c)
Graduate Research Fellow
Fairbanks School of Public Health
Indiana University–Purdue University
    Indianapolis
Indianapolis, Indiana
Chapter 4. The Environment and Cancer

Sally S. Cohen, PhD, RN, FAAN
Virginia P. Crenshaw Endowed Chair
Director, Robert Wood Johnson Foundation
Nursing and Health Policy Collaborative
College of Nursing
University of New Mexico
Institute of Medicine AAN/ANF/ANA Distinguished Nurse Scholar
Albuquerque, New Mexico
Chapter 2. Public Policy, Public Health, and Health Policy

Devra Lee Davis, PhD, MPH
Fellow, American College of Epidemiology
President
Environmental Health Trust
Washington, District of Columbia
Chapter 4. The Environment and Cancer

Danielle M. Dupuy, MPH
Consultant
Metropolitan Chicago Breast Cancer Task
 Force
Chicago, Illinois
*Chapter 12. Creation of a Statewide Mammog-
raphy Surveillance Program*

Kimberly R. Enard, PhD, MBA, MSHA
Assistant Professor
Health Management and Policy
College for Public Health and Social Justice
Saint Louis University
St. Louis, Missouri
*Chapter 9. Eliminating Cancer Disparities
Through Legislative Action*

**Valerie Eschiti, PhD, RN, AHN-BC, CHTP,
CTN-A**
Associate Professor
University of Oklahoma Health Sciences
 Center
College of Nursing
Oklahoma City, Oklahoma
*Chapter 11. American Indians and Alaska
Natives and Cancer*

Carol Estwing Ferrans, PhD, RN, FAAN
Professor and Associate Dean for Research
Director, UIC Center of Excellence in Elimi-
 nating Health Disparities
University of Illinois at Chicago College of
 Nursing
Chicago, Illinois
*Chapter 12. Creation of a Statewide Mammog-
raphy Surveillance Program*

Ellen Giarelli, EdD, RN, CRNP
Associate Professor
Interdisciplinary Research Unit
Drexel University College of Nursing and
 Health Professions
Philadelphia, Pennsylvania
*Chapter 7. Biospecimen Collection and
Cancer Genomics*

Barbara Given, PhD, RN, FAAN
University Distinguished Professor; Director
 of PhD Program, College of Nursing
Michigan State University
East Lansing, Michigan
Chapter 17. Using Research to Influence Policy

Emily A. Haozous, PhD, RN
Assistant Professor
University of New Mexico College of Nursing
Albuquerque, New Mexico
*Chapter 11. American Indians and Alaska
Natives and Cancer*

Lovell Jones, PhD
Professor
Director, Center for Research on Minority
 Health, Department of Health Disparities
 Research
The University of Texas MD Anderson
 Cancer Center
Houston, Texas
*Chapter 9. Eliminating Cancer Disparities
Through Legislative Action*

Karen M. Kedrowski, PhD
Dean of Arts and Sciences
Winthrop University
Rock Hill, South Carolina
*Chapter 13. Lessons in Cancer Activism From
the Breast Cancer and Prostate Cancer Move-
ments*

John Lunstroth, LLM, MPH
Research Professor
University of Houston Law Center
Houston, Texas
*Chapter 9. Eliminating Cancer Disparities
Through Legislative Action*

Gail Mallory, PhD, NEA-BC
Director of Research
Oncology Nursing Society
Pittsburgh, Pennsylvania
Chapter 17. Using Research to Influence Policy

Karen McKeown, MSN, RN
State Health Officer and Administrator,
 Division of Public Health
Wisconsin Department of Health Services
Madison, Wisconsin
*Chapter 2. Public Policy, Public Health, and
Health Policy*

Karen Meneses, PhD, RN, FAAN
Professor and Associate Dean for Research,
School of Nursing
Co-Leader, Cancer Control and Population
Sciences Program, Comprehensive Cancer
Center
The University of Alabama at Birmingham
Birmingham, Alabama
*Chapter 6. Contributions of the Federal
Advisory Boards*

Anne Marie Murphy, PhD
Executive Director
Metropolitan Chicago Breast Cancer Task
Force
Chicago, Illinois
*Chapter 12. Creation of a Statewide Mammog-
raphy Surveillance Program*

Brenda Nevidjon, MSN, RN, FAAN
Chief Executive Officer
Oncology Nursing Society
Pittsburgh, Pennsylvania
*Chapter 5. The Role of Professional and Volun-
tary Organizations*

Guadalupe Palos, DrPH, LMSW, RN
Manager, Clinical Protocol Administration
Office of Cancer Survivorship
The University of Texas MD Anderson
Cancer Center
Houston, Texas
Chapter 10. Latinos and Cancer

Ilisa Halpern Paul, MPP
President, District Policy Group
Managing Government Relations Director
Drinker Biddle & Reath LLP
Washington, District of Columbia
*Chapter 3. A Brief History of Major Federal
Cancer Policy—1970s to Present*

Carolyn Phillips, ACNP-BC, MSN, AOCNP®
Oncology Nurse Practitioner
New Mexico Cancer Care Associates
Santa Fe, New Mexico
*Chapter 18. Legislative Topics in Cancer
Research and Practice*

Barbara D. Powe, PhD, RN, FAAN
Former Director, Cancer Communication
Science
American Cancer Society
Atlanta, Georgia
*Chapter 15. Oncology Implications of the
Patient Protection and Affordable Care Act*

Mandi Pratt-Chapman, MA
Director
The George Washington University Cancer
Institute
Washington, District of Columbia
*Chapter 14. The Cancer Survivorship Move-
ment Exemplar of Cancer Activism; Chapter
15. Oncology Implications of the Patient
Protection and Affordable Care Act*

Nancy Ridenour, PhD, APRN, BC, FAAN
Professor and Dean
University of New Mexico College of Nursing
Albuquerque, New Mexico
Chapter 1. Introduction to Health Policy

Marilyn Stine Sarow, PhD
Interim Chair and Professor of Mass Commu-
nication
Winthrop University
Rock Hill, South Carolina
*Chapter 13. Lessons in Cancer Activism From the
Breast Cancer and Prostate Cancer Movements*

Mark H. Smith
Liberty Partners Group
Principal
Washington, District of Columbia
*Chapter 3. A Brief History of Major Federal
Cancer Policy—1970s to Present*

Alec Stone, MA, MPA
Health Policy Director
Oncology Nursing Society
Pittsburgh, Pennsylvania
*Chapter 16. Leading Change in the Health
Policy Arena*

Deborah E. Trautman, PhD, RN
Executive Director
Center for Health Policy and Healthcare
Transformation
Johns Hopkins Medicine
Baltimore, Maryland
Chapter 1. Introduction to Health Policy

Robert Twillman, PhD, FAPM
Executive Director
American Academy of Pain Management
Sonora, California
Clinical Associate Professor of Psychiatry and
  Behavioral Sciences
University of Kansas School of Medicine
Kansas City, Kansas
*Chapter 8. Policy Considerations in Cancer
Pain Management*

Margaret C. Wilmoth, PhD, MSS, RN, FAAN
Professor
Byrdine F. Lewis School of Nursing and
  Health Professions
Georgia State University
Atlanta, Georgia
Major General, U.S. Army Reserve
Deputy Surgeon General for Mobilization,
  Readiness and Army Reserve Affairs
Office of the Surgeon General
United States Army
The Pentagon
*Chapter 16. Leading Change in the Health
Policy Arena*

Disclosure

Editors and authors of books and guidelines provided by the Oncology Nursing Society are expected to disclose to the readers any significant financial interest or other relationships with the manufacturer(s) of any commercial products.

A vested interest may be considered to exist if a contributor is affiliated with or has a financial interest in commercial organizations that may have a direct or indirect interest in the subject matter. A "financial interest" may include, but is not limited to, being a shareholder in the organization; being an employee of the commercial organization; serving on an organization's speakers bureau; or receiving research from the organization. An "affiliation" may be holding a position on an advisory board or some other role of benefit to the commercial organization. Vested interest statements appear in the front matter for each publication.

Contributors are expected to disclose any unlabeled or investigational use of products discussed in their content. This information is acknowledged solely for the information of the readers.

The contributors provided the following disclosure and vested interest information:
Danielle M. Dupuy, MPH: Metropolitan Chicago Breast Cancer Task Force, Rush University Medical Center and Star Institute, consultant or advisory role
Karen Meneses, PhD, RN, FAAN: Women's Breast Health Fund, consultant or advisory role; Community Foundation of Greater Birmingham, research funding
Brenda Nevidjon, MSN, RN, FAAN: Oncology Nursing Society, honoraria
Barbara D. Powe, PhD, RN, FAAN: Centers for Disease Control and Prevention, consultant or advisory role
Mark H. Smith: National Coalition for Cancer Research, consultant or advisory role

Contents

Foreword

Advocacy: A Force Multiplier in the Cancer Fight

I have been involved in the cancer fight for more than four decades and have been fortunate during that time to see the tide begin to change—and continue to do so—as we battle this disease. During the first part of my career, we were running *into* the woods, seeking to find out more about a disease that was then a dark and shrouded mystery. But for many years now, we have been running *out* of the woods, toward the light of greater understanding and ability to fight, and beat, cancer.

What changed in the past four decades that enabled this progress? Many things. But one of the most critical—indeed, the most essential to our progress—has been the recognition that public policy plays an essential role in our nationwide efforts to prevent, detect, and treat cancer. Advocacy in support of public policies that help people prevent and fight cancer is a force multiplier that dramatically enhances the value of scientific discovery. Indeed, only by enacting meaningful cancer policy will we bring this disease under control.

In the pages that follow, you will see firsthand the power of public policy at work in the fight against cancer, whether it is the impact of 40-plus years of the U.S. government's war on cancer, the collective lessons we've learned through successful tobacco control efforts, or the major advances made possible through laws such as the Patient Protection and Affordable Care Act. I believe that as you read these insights, the existing opportunity for even greater impact in the cancer fight will be clear.

Cancer mortality rates have been declining in this country for more than two decades, leading to a 20% overall decrease in the cancer death rate, or more than 1.3 million cancer deaths averted (Siegel, Ma, Zou, & Jemal, 2014). That is incredible progress. Yet we can, and we must, do more.

I have long believed that we can at last *finish* the fight against cancer if we can do three things: promote prevention into standard practice nationwide, redouble and balance our nation's cancer research portfolio, and ensure access to quality, affordable health care for everyone. Those are not easy tasks.

But undergirding all three is the absolutely critical need for strong and sustained advocacy in support of effective policies at all levels of government that emphasize disease prevention, fund scientific discovery, and improve access to cancer care.

Effective advocacy is the skillful application of lobbying at all levels of government, policy development and evaluation, grassroots engagement and mobilization, and communications aimed at the media and, by extension, the general public. When the American Cancer Society concluded more than a decade ago that public policy was essential to winning the cancer fight, we created a nonprofit, nonpartisan advocacy organization with expertise in each of these areas. The American Cancer Society Cancer Action Network combines a deep reservoir of experience in lobbying, policy, and media advocacy with a nationwide army of grassroots advocates representing every congressional district in the country. These volunteers—patients with cancer, survivors, and the loved ones of people with cancer—have made it their mission to urge elected officials to make the disease a national priority.

Prevention: Public policy must ensure that we can not only treat cancer but also prevent the disease in the first place. An oft-quoted poem by Joseph Malins highlights the merits of building a fence on a cliff to protect passersby, rather than sending an ambulance to treat those who fall from the precipice. The poem has long been a favorite of mine. An excerpt reads,

"It's a marvel to me
That people give far more attention
To repairing results than to stopping the cause,
When they'd much better aim at prevention.
Let us stop at its source all this mischief."

This is a truth we at the American Cancer Society know all too well. Chronic diseases such as cancer kill more than 1.7 million Americans each year—7 of every 10 deaths in the United States (Partnership to Fight Chronic Disease, n.d.). Cancer alone kills more than 1,600 Americans every day (American Cancer Society, 2014). But half of these deaths could be avoided by taking steps to prevent the disease from occurring in the first place. Good public policy, from laws that mandate insurance coverage of preventive cancer screenings to those that protect people from the harms of secondhand smoke, is a proven way to help create a system that focuses on stopping the cause rather than repairing results.

Research: Scientific discovery always has been, and will always remain, an essential component of the cancer fight. The federal government is by far the largest funder of cancer research in the world. We will accelerate discovery only by redoubling and balancing our national medical research efforts. Historic advances, such as the mapping of the human genome, promise to speed progress against cancer and numerous other diseases. But we can only leverage such advances if we fuel the engine of discovery by fully funding the National Institutes of Health and the National Cancer Institute. We must also complement basic scientific research with funding for translational research and applied behavioral research, which carry medical advances from laboratories to doctors' offices and maximize their use among patients.

Access: The United States has some of the best, if not *the* best, medical care in the world. And yet the promise of high-quality medical care will continue to fall short if we cannot ensure that everyone has access to the latest and best prevention, early detection, and treatment methods that save lives. No one deserves to get cancer, but everyone deserves the right to fight it. The Affordable Care Act dramatically improves access to care by ensuring patients are no longer denied coverage or charged sky-high premiums because they have a preexisting condition such as cancer. We must similarly improve the delivery of care to patients by funding research into the most effective ways to administer care and supporting community health centers that best understand the needs and norms of local populations.

In more than a century fighting cancer, the American Cancer Society has learned the incredible power of advocacy to produce strong public policy and improve public health. From our early years, when we created an unprecedented volunteer force through our Women's Field Army, to the 1960s when we began to aggressively support tobacco control, to the 1970s when we advocated for the National Cancer Act, and so on, our advocacy efforts over the past century have directly led to more lives saved today from cancer. I have no doubt this work will continue to bear fruit in the future.

As you read the chapters in *Cancer and Health Policy: Advancements and Opportunities*, I am confident you will recognize the many opportunities ahead to leverage public policy to make exponential advances in the fight against cancer. One day soon, the combination of public policy and scientific discovery will enable us to finish this fight once and for all. May God, and our good work together, speed that day.

John R. Seffrin, PhD
Chief Executive Officer
American Cancer Society
American Cancer Society Cancer Action Network

References

American Cancer Society. (2014). *Cancer facts and figures 2014*. Retrieved from http://www .cancer.org/research/cancerfactsstatistics/cancerfactsfigures2014/index

Partnership to Fight Chronic Disease. (n.d.). The growing crisis of chronic disease in the United States. Retrieved from http://www.fightchronicdisease.org/sites/fightchronicdisease .org/files/docs/GrowingCrisisofChronicDiseaseintheUSfactsheet_81009.pdf

Patient Protection and Affordable Care Act, Pub. L. No. 111-148, 124 Stat. 119 (2010).

Siegel, R., Ma, J., Zou, Z., & Jemal, A. (2014). Cancer statistics, 2014. *CA: A Cancer Journal for Clinicians, 64*, 9–29. doi:10.3322/caac.21208

Preface

Cancer will remain a major health concern worldwide well into the 21st century. Notably, in 2014, the American Cancer Society estimates that 1,665,540 new cancer cases will be diagnosed in the United States alone. By 2030, the United States is expected to experience a 45% increase in the number of new cancer cases, in part due to an aging population (American Society of Clinical Oncology, 2014). Cancer remains the second most common cause of death in the United States, exceeded only by heart disease. Projections indicate that approximately 585,720 Americans are expected to die from cancer in 2014. This equates to about 1,600 people each day (American Cancer Society, 2014).

The good news is that, as a result of scientific discoveries, more and more people are living longer with a cancer diagnosis. Approximately 13.7 million Americans were living with a history of cancer in 2012. Today, 1 in 23 people are cancer survivors (Sawyers et al., 2013). The five-year survival rate for all cancers diagnosed between 2003 and 2009 was 68%, compared to the 49% five-year survival rate for cancers diagnosed between 1975 and 1977 (American Cancer Society, 2014). While improvements have occurred in the cancer outcomes for some segments of the U.S. population, much work still is needed to eliminate the ongoing unequal burden of cancer, particularly among individuals with lower socioeconomic status.

The recognition of cancer as an ongoing public health concern underscores the need for sound cancer policies that will ultimately improve the cancer profile of our nation and countries across the globe. This text, *Cancer and Health Policy: Advancements and Opportunities*, is designed to highlight the role and impact of health policy and legislation on cancer care, cancer outcomes, and the future of cancer control in the United States. The book extends the discussion in existing oncology textbooks and resources by providing an in-depth overview and discussion of accomplishments in the policy arena, while illuminating opportunities to advance the cancer policy agenda. The book is designed specifically to

1. Elucidate critical milestones in the history of cancer policy.

2. Examine current and emerging topics of relevance to advancing cancer policy.
3. Articulate future directions for shaping cancer policy through research and leadership.

Content

This text consists of 18 chapters that are divided into three sections, followed by an epilogue addressing future directions for cancer policy.

Section I, **Foundations for Shaping Cancer Policy**, highlights the evolution of health policy, cancer policy, and the contributions of key organizations and advisory boards in shaping a national cancer policy agenda.

Section II, **Selected Topics in Cancer Policy**, highlights some of the advancements in the cancer policy arena while identifying implications for shaping the future of cancer policy. The authors address topics such as the policy implications for biospecimen collection, cancer activism, cancer pain management, health reform, cancer survivorship, and the elimination of cancer disparities through legislative action.

Section III, **Current Issues in Cancer Policy**, focuses on advancing cancer policy through research and leadership. Current and emerging legislative issues influencing the future of oncology practice are noted.

The epilogue, **Looking Toward the Future**, provides provocative final thoughts on advancing cancer policy.

Audience

Written by experts in health policy from multiple disciplines, *Cancer and Health Policy: Advancements and Opportunities* is suitable for a number of audiences within the diversity of oncology disciplines, including nursing, medicine, all other healthcare providers, graduate students in oncology, cancer policy makers, and a diverse cadre of stakeholders with an interest in and a commitment to achieving cancer control through advocacy and political activism.

References

American Cancer Society. (2014). *Cancer facts and figures 2014.* Retrieved from http://www.cancer.org/research/cancerfactsstatistics/cancerfactsfigures2014/index

American Society of Clinical Oncology. (2014). The state of cancer care in America, 2014: A report by the American Society of Clinical Oncology. *Journal of Oncology Practice, 10,* 119–142. doi:10.1200/JOP.2014.001386

Sawyers, C.L., Abate-Shen, C., Anderson, K.C., Barker, A., Baselga, J., Berger, N.A., ... Weiner, G.J. (2013). AACR cancer progress report 2013. *Clinical Cancer Research, 19*(Suppl. 20), S1–S88. doi:10.1158/1078-0432.CCR-13-2107

Acknowledgments

The editors want to acknowledge the entire Oncology Nursing Society Publications Department, whose support and wisdom guided the production of this book from start to finish. We also wish to acknowledge the work of Barbara Bittner, whose knowledge of the *Publication Manual of the American Psychological Association* and thoughtful edits contributed greatly to the completion of this project. We thank the Robert Wood Johnson Foundation Health Policy Fellows Program for the excellent training and congressional experiences that contributed to our inspiration to conceive and edit this book. And, to the many contributing authors, thank you for your time and talents in making this book a reality. You all give meaning to the phrase "together everyone accomplishes more." Thank you, TEAM!

Foundations for Shaping Cancer Policy

CHAPTER 1

Introduction to Health Policy

Nancy Ridenour, PhD, APRN, BC, FAAN, and Deborah E. Trautman, PhD, RN

Introduction

Health professionals are consistently rated highly by the public for ethical and professional standards (Swift, 2013). They are in a unique position to advocate for improving health outcomes for patients and the nation. Increasing access to care and improving quality outcomes for patients while decreasing the costs of care requires that healthcare providers become more adept at health policy and advocacy. This chapter provides an overview of the policy process and the basics of healthcare reform. The policy process described by Kingdon (2010) serves as a theoretical backdrop supporting policy analysis. Current policy issues related to oncology provide exemplars illustrating how to become more involved in the policy and advocacy process. Examples relevant to oncology are provided, including resources for developing oncology policy advocacy and evidence-based tools.

Jurisdiction and Oversight

It is important to understand the jurisdictional committees for healthcare issues at the federal level. Most health-related legislation will either originate in these committees or be referred to one or more of them for review.

U.S. House of Representatives

U.S. House of Representatives Committee on Ways and Means: This committee has jurisdiction over taxes. Any health-related legislation that is funded through federal general revenues and taxes will be overseen by Ways and

Means. The committee has jurisdiction over most of the programs authorized by the Social Security Act. The Social Security Act of 1935 has been amended several times; Medicare was introduced in 1965 (Social Security Administration, n.d.). Title II of the Social Security Act covers Old-Age, Survivors, and Disability Insurance. Title XVIII covers Medicare Parts A and B. It also covers tax credit and deduction provisions of the Internal Revenue Code dealing with health insurance premiums and healthcare costs.

U.S. House of Representatives Energy and Commerce Committee: The health-related jurisdiction of this committee includes the selected programs authorized under the Social Security Act: Medicaid, Medicare Part B, child health, long-term care, and peer review. It also includes programs authorized by the Public Health Service Act: hospital construction, biomedical research, allied health and nurse training, medical devices, mental health research, alcoholism, drug abuse, maternal and child health, health maintenance organizations, and environmental protection.

U.S. House of Representatives Education and the Workforce Committee: This committee has influence over workers' health and safety and pension benefits, including health benefits and the Employee Retirement Income Security Act (ERISA).

U.S. Senate

U.S. Senate Committee on Health, Education, Labor, and Pensions (HELP): This committee has jurisdiction over the country's healthcare programs, schools, employment, and retirement programs. All programs authorized under the Public Health Service Act are in the jurisdiction of the Senate HELP Committee. The committee has three subcommittees: Children and Families, Employment and Workplace Safety, and Primary Health and Aging. All three subcommittees may oversee aspects of health-related legislation.

Rule 25 of the Standing Rules of the Senate states the HELP Committee's jurisdiction to include referral of all proposed legislation, messages, petitions, memorials, and other matters related to

• Measures relating to education, labor, health, and public welfare
• Aging
• Agricultural colleges
• Arts and humanities
• Biomedical research and development
• Child labor
• Convict labor and the entry of goods made by convicts into interstate commerce
• Domestic activities of the American National Red Cross
• Equal employment opportunity
• Gallaudet University, Howard University, and St. Elizabeths Hospital

- Individuals with disabilities
- Labor standards and labor statistics
- Mediation and arbitration of labor disputes
- Occupational safety and health, including the welfare of miners
- Private pension plans
- Public health
- Railway labor and retirement
- Regulation of foreign laborers
- Student loans
- Wages and hours of labor.

U.S. Senate Committee on Finance: This committee covers health programs under the Social Security Act and health programs financed by a specific tax or trust fund. These programs may be housed in the Department of Health and Human Services (DHHS), Department of Labor (DOL), or Social Security Administration (SSA). In addition, the Senate Finance Committee oversees numerous advisory committees, boards, and commissions, including the Prospective Payment Assessment Commission and the Physician Payment Review Commission.

Department of Health and Human Services

DHHS includes the Centers for Medicare and Medicaid Services (CMS). CMS is responsible for Medicare Parts A and B; the Medicare Drug Benefit (Part D); Medicare Advantage (Part C); Medicaid; and the State Children's Health Insurance Program. DHHS also oversees the Administration for Children and Families (with the HELP Committee). Programs include Temporary Assistance for Needy Families; Child Welfare Services; Child Support and Paternity; the JOBS Program; Foster Care and Adoption Assistance; Maternal and Child Health; the Title XX Social Services Block Grant Program; the Child Care and Development Block Grant; the Independent Living Program; and Promoting Safe and Stable Families. DHHS also administers title XI of the Social Security Act, which includes demonstration authority, peer review of the utilization and quality of healthcare services, and administrative simplification.

Department of Labor

DOL oversees the health coverage tax credit, ERISA group health plans, the Health Insurance Portability and Accountability Act, and the Consolidated Omnibus Budget Reconciliation Act. With the HELP Committee, it oversees Consumer Protections, the Pension Benefit Guaranty Corporation, and the Pension and Welfare Benefits Administration. It also guarantees payment of nonforfeitable pension benefits in covered private-sector defined benefit pension plans and title IV of ERISA.

Social Security Administration

SSA is responsible for the Old-Age, Survivors, and Disability Insurance Program.

Additional Committees

Other committees may have oversight over portions of health care. For example, the Senate Homeland Security and Governmental Affairs Committee and the House Homeland Security Committee have jurisdiction over the Department of Homeland Security, including emergency preparedness. The Senate Judiciary Committee and the House Committee on the Judiciary cover medical malpractice and product liability.

Kingdon's Three Stream Model

Health-related legislation and regulation involves a complex process. What key factors separate successful policy initiatives from those policy proposals that never make it to law or regulation? How do policy topics come to officials' attention? How are the alternatives from which they choose generated? How is the governmental agenda set? Why does an idea's time come when it does?

Kingdon (2010) provided a model to assist in navigating the policy arena. He proposed that three streams must align for a policy alternative to make it to the agenda. This dynamic process opens a policy window of opportunity, allowing advocates to gain attention to or push their projects. This policy window may open predictably, as in the case of the renewal of Title VIII of the Public Health Service Act, which provides funding for nursing education. This funding bill is introduced every year and advocates work to ensure that the funding continues. In other cases, the window of opportunity is not nearly so predictable. A natural disaster, for example, may lead to a special opportunity to increase funding in a specified area. Health policy advocates need to be alert to the convergence of the three streams and take advantage of the opportunities as they arise. These three streams come together at critical times.

- **Problem stream:** Specific events signify a problem. These events can be a crisis, disaster, or personal experience. This focus occurs when those with power and authority to act believe that the problem is genuine and/or that addressing the issue will further their political careers. This stream focuses on the intricacies of directing the policy makers to specific problems in the midst of the many facing them and their constituents.

- **Policy stream:** Potential solutions, alternatives, ideas, and proposals are discussed, revised, and reintroduced. These ideas float in government looking for a problem to attach to or an event that increases the likelihood of adoption. Researchers, policy analysts, congressional staffers, advocacy groups, and agency representatives continuously generate these ideas, attempting to convince others of their merit.
- **Political stream:** In this context, *political* refers to value streams and distribution of benefits and costs. The political stream occurs when those with the power and authority to act believe that the timing is right. This stream is composed of such things as changes in administration, election results, public sentiment or mood, congressional partisanship or ideology, and advocacy and consensus-building campaigns.

The policy window is a particular time when solutions are joined to problems in a favorable political context. Astute policy advocates must recognize the timing of the policy agenda and pull the three streams together to push the issue to a decision.

Basics of Healthcare Reform

Health Reform

Issues of access, quality, and cost are driving a national agenda for reform in the United States. The simultaneous pursuit of improving the experience of care, improving the health of populations, and reducing per capita costs of health care is gaining momentum across the country (Berwick, Nolan, & Whittington, 2008). Reform initiatives are evident in the federal, state, and local government and private sector.

Why reform, and why now? Concerns about healthcare spending, quality, and access have existed for decades. Prior to the passage of the Patient Protection and Affordable Care Act (ACA) in 2010, presidents had tried but failed to move national health reform forward (Blumenthal & Morone, 2010). In 1993, when President Clinton proposed health reform, there was no consensus that the U.S. healthcare system was a problem and some believed the United States had the best healthcare system in the world (Johnson & Broder, 1997). More recently, as the country faces the challenges of an aging population, mounting debt and deficits, and increasing evidence that more spending does not equate to better health outcomes, consensus has emerged that there is a problem.

While there is consensus that the U.S. healthcare system has problems, disagreement exists as to the preferred policies to address the problems. The passage and enactment of the ACA illustrates this disagreement. Since the passage of the ACA and its enactment into law, the nation remains divided. Political party affiliation matters. Democrats (72%) are more likely to have a favorable opinion of the law, whereas among Republicans, only 12%

view the law favorably (Kaiser Family Foundation, 2013c). In addition to a divided opinion, many Americans are unaware of what is actually in the law (Kaiser Family Foundation, 2013c).

Following is an overview of the characteristics of the current healthcare environment and a review of the major provisions in the ACA.

Characteristics of the U.S. Healthcare System

Health Spending

Total health spending in the United States in 2012 averaged $8,915 per person and $2.8 trillion for the nation (CMS, 2012). Government accounts for the most spending, followed by private health insurance, and lastly out-of-pocket spending (see Figure 1-1). The rise in the growth of health spending has slowed in the last three years (Executive Office of the President of the United States, 2013), but there is concern that future spending will rebound as the economy recovers. Growth in spending has occurred across all payers (Medicare, Medicaid, private insurers, and individual out-of-pocket expenses). A goal of health reform is to slow the rate of growth.

Figure 1-1. Care Coverage and Personal Healthcare Expenditures in the United States, 2011

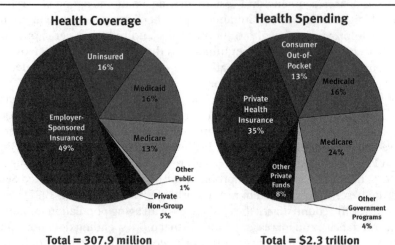

NOTE: Health spending total does not include administrative spending.
SOURCE: Health insurance coverage: KCMU/Urban Institute analysis of 2011 data from 2012 ASEC Supplement to the CPS.
Health expenditures: KFF calculations using 2011 NHE data from CMS, Office of the Actuary

Note. From "Health Care Coverage and Personal Health Care Expenditures in the U.S., 2011," by Kaiser Family Foundation, 2013. Retrieved from http://kff.org/health-costs/slide/health-care-coverage-and -personal-health-care-expenditures-in-the-u-s-2011. Copyright 2013 by Kaiser Family Foundation. Reprinted with permission.

Health Insurance Coverage

The majority of Americans have health insurance coverage; for many (49%), this coverage is provided by their employer (Kaiser Family Foundation, 2013b). Employer-sponsored insurance is the leading source of health insurance, followed by Medicaid (16%), Medicare (13%), and private non-group insurance (5%).

Medicare

Medicare provides coverage to Americans age 65 or older and nonelderly individuals with permanent disabilities. As the U.S. population ages, the number of Americans eligible for Medicare increases. Medicare enrollment in 2013 covered 52 million Americans (see Figure 1-2) (Kaiser Family Foundation, 2013d).

Sustaining Medicare for the future is a key issue in health reform. Medicare eligibility, beneficiary cost sharing, beneficiary premiums, Medicare payments to providers, Medicare delivery system payments, and benefit redesign are among some of the policy issues being considered.

Medicaid

Medicaid covers low-income individuals and families. Medicaid is also the primary source of coverage for nursing home and community-based

Figure 1-2. Medicare Enrollment, 1966–2013

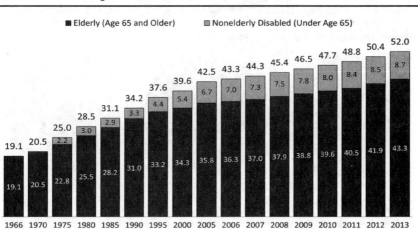

■ Elderly (Age 65 and Older)   ▨ Nonelderly Disabled (Under Age 65)

NOTES: Numbers may not sum to total due to rounding. People with disabilities under age 65 were not eligible for Medicare prior to 1972.
SOURCE: Centers for Medicare & Medicaid Services, Medicare Enrollment: Hospital Insurance and/or Supplemental Medical Insurance Programs for Total, Fee-for-Service and Managed Care Enrollees as of July 1, 2011: Selected Calendar Years 1966-2011; 2012-2013, HHS Budget in Brief, FY2014.

services. Income eligibility for Medicaid varies across the country and is based on the federal poverty level (FPL). In 2013, the FPL was $11,490 for an individual and $19,530 for a family of three (CMS, 2013). Most states cover children at 100% of the FPL or higher, but income eligibility for adults varies, and coverage is either not provided or is limited to the poorest of the poor (income of $3,124 or less). Medicaid covers more than 62 million Americans (CMS, 2014). Reform proposals for Medicaid range from plans for Medicaid expansion to a complete overhaul of the system.

Uninsured Individuals

Almost 50 million Americans (16%) are uninsured. The majority of the uninsured are working Americans, low-wage earners, and age 34 or younger (see Figure 1-3) (Kaiser Family Foundation, 2013a). A goal of reform is to increase the number of Americans with health insurance coverage.

Coverage Matters

Increasing evidence demonstrates that coverage matters. While having an insurance card does not guarantee access to quality medical care, those without coverage are less likely to seek medical care, are more likely to encounter barriers when trying to access care, and have a greater mortality than the insured (Institute of Medicine [IOM], 2011; Sommers, Baicker, & Epstein, 2012).

Figure 1-3. Characteristics of the Nonelderly Uninsured Population, 2011

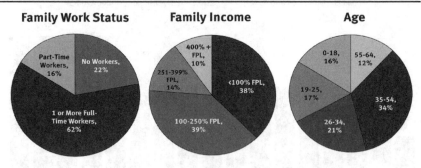

Family Work Status   Family Income   Age

Total = 47.9 Million Uninsured

NOTE: The federal poverty level was $22,350 for a family of four in 2011. Data may not total 100% due to rounding.
SOURCE: KCMU/Urban Institute analysis of 2012 ASEC Supplement to the CPS.

FPL—federal poverty level

Note. From "Characteristics of the Nonelderly Uninsured Population," by Kaiser Family Foundation, 2013. Retrieved from http://kff.org/uninsured/slide/characteristics-of-the-nonelderly-uninsured-population-2011. Copyright 2013 by Kaiser Family Foundation. Reprinted with permission.

What Ails the U.S. Healthcare System?

The U.S. healthcare system has been characterized as expensive, ineffective, and unjust. High cost, fragmentation, variation, disparities, workforce shortages, and an aging and sicker population pose challenges to the delivery of health care and the health of the population. The United States is not alone in facing rising healthcare expenditures. International comparisons of health spending reveal that most industrialized countries are experiencing an increase in healthcare spending (see Figure 1-4). What distinguishes the United States is that it spends more than most other industrialized countries but does not have better outcomes. In recent comparisons, the United States leads all other industrialized nations in adult obesity, is the fourth highest in infant mortality, and is in the bottom third for life expectancy (Organisation for Economic Co-operation and Development, 2014a, 2014b).

The Affordable Care Act

The ACA was signed into law in March 2010. While one policy alone cannot fix all that ails the U.S. healthcare system, supporters contend

Figure 1-4. International Comparison of Spending on Health, 1980–2009

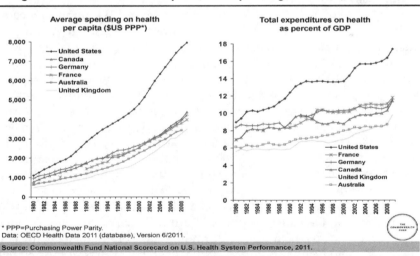

* PPP=Purchasing Power Parity.
Data: OECD Health Data 2011 (database), Version 6/2011.

Source: Commonwealth Fund National Scorecard on U.S. Health System Performance, 2011.

GDP—gross domestic product

Note. From "International Comparison of Spending on Health 1980 to 2009," by Commonwealth Fund, 2014. Retrieved from http://www.commonwealthfund.org/interactives-and-data/chart-cart/report/why-not-the-best-results-from-the-national-scorecard-on-us-health-system-performance-2011/i/international-comparison-of-spending-on-health-1980-to-2009. Copyright 2014 by Commonwealth Fund. Reprinted with permission.

that the implementation of the ACA will increase the number of insured Americans, facilitate the movement toward better care, and contribute to constraining the rising cost of health care. Opponents of the ACA worry that the implementation will exacerbate existing problems, cost more than the country can afford, and unnecessarily expand the role of government. Whether a supporter or opponent, most agree that the ACA is a landmark health reform. As with other major policy, the ACA will be revised and evolve over time. Notably, the ACA and its implementation are complex, and the merits of the law will be debated for quite some time.

Major Provisions in the Affordable Care Act

Major provisions in the ACA can be organized into four key areas (McDonough, 2011; U.S. DHHS, n.d.).

- Health insurance expansion to reduce the numbered of uninsured individuals and improve the affordability of coverage
- Insurance market reforms to provide consumer protections and coverage for preexisting conditions
- Delivery system changes to improve the quality of care and lower the cost of care
- Prevention provisions to improve wellness and prevent disease

Health Insurance Expansion

The ACA requires most U.S. citizens to have health insurance, creates exchanges to help individuals and families purchase insurance, and provides premium and cost-sharing benefits to individuals and families with incomes below 400% of the FPL ($45,960 for an individual or $94,200 for a family of four in 2013). The ACA increases the number of Americans with health insurance coverage through the expansion of public programs (Medicaid) and changes in health insurance. It also provides an opportunity for states to increase Medicaid eligibility to 138% of the FPL ($15,856 for an individual or $32,499 for a family of four in 2013). Beginning in 2014, the federal government will provide states 100% assistance in the cost of the Medicaid expansion for three years. After three years, the federal support drops to 90%. As of December 2014, 27 state governors supported Medicaid expansion (Advisory Board Company, 2014). The ACA also requires all individuals who can afford to purchase health insurance to obtain coverage or pay a fine. Beginning in 2014, the penalty for failure to purchase health insurance will start at $95 per person ($47.50 per child younger than 18) a year or up to 1% of income and will rise each year, reaching $695 per person or 2.5% of taxable income in 2016 and later years. Medicaid expansion and changes in insurance are projected to expand coverage to 30 million of the 50 million uninsured (Congressional Budget Office, 2012).

Insurance Reforms

In addition to the mandate to purchase insurance, key insurance reforms set forth in the law include

- Prohibiting denial of coverage due to a preexisting condition
- Prohibiting lifetime limits
- Prohibiting dropping people when sick
- Requiring extension of coverage for a child on a parent's health insurance until the child's 26th birthday to all existing insurance plans
- Creating benefit tiers and specifying a minimum benefit package
- Limiting insurance rate variations to age and tobacco use
- Providing free coverage of prevention services
- Requiring insurers to spend 80 or 85 cents of premium dollars collected on clinical services.

Delivery System Changes

Delivery system changes in the law are designed to promote coordinated, quality, low-cost care. Key delivery system changes include funding for comparative effectiveness research, grants to states to develop programs to address medical malpractice issues and alternatives to tort litigations, support for patient-centered medical homes and accountable care organizations, investments in health information technology, and the establishment of new payment reforms, such as value-based purchasing, bundled payments, and reduced payments for preventable readmissions and hospital-acquired conditions. The ACA establishes a new center for innovation, the Center for Medicare and Medicaid Innovation, and supports a new research institute, the Patient-Centered Outcomes Research Institute, to promote patient engagement. Title V of the ACA includes key sections to promote innovations in the health workforce, increase the supply of the health workforce, enhance education and training, support the existing workforce, strengthen primary care, and improve access to healthcare services. The law supports the creation and expansion of community health centers, nurse-managed health centers, and nurse home visitations and establishes a National Health Care Workforce Commission (McDonough, 2011; U.S. DHHS, 2013).

Prevention

The ACA expands efforts to promote prevention and includes a number of prevention provisions. The provisions aim to promote wellness and reduce the occurrence of chronic disease. Prevention is addressed at three levels (McDonough, 2011), which are

- Preventing disease from occurring
- Treating illness before it becomes symptomatic through screening
- Reducing disability and restoring function.

Some key prevention measures are coverage for an annual wellness visit, no co-payments or deductibles for certain preventive services, and free access to all preventive services rated A or B by the U.S. Preventive Services Task Force for Medicare patients. The ACA creates incentives for healthier behaviors, such as requiring large restaurant chains to provide menu labeling to disclose calorie counts, and supports employers' ability to vary premium payments of workers with unhealthy behaviors.

Current Health Policy Issues

Identifying Policy Issues

Several avenues exist for identifying policy issues related to oncology. Professional societies, nonprofits, nongovernmental agencies, and agencies within the government address issues related to cancer and the care of patients with a diagnosis of cancer. The following are a few of these sources.

- The **American Cancer Society Cancer Action Network** (www.acscan.org/campaigns) is involved in several federal and state initiatives in prevention, early detection, access to care, quality of life, and research funding.
- The **American Society of Clinical Oncology** (www.cancer.net/advocacy -and-policy/public-policy-advocacy) has outlined advocacy positions in areas of access to care, clinical trials, drug shortages, funding for cancer research, palliative care, and quality care.
- The **National Cancer Policy Forum** (www.iom.edu/Activities/Disease/NCPF.aspx), sponsored by IOM, is designed to identify high-priority issues in the national effort to combat cancer and examine these issues through convening experts with mutual interest to promote discussion and develop opportunities for action. A sampling of topics includes
  - Convening 2013 National Cancer Policy Summit
  - Implementing a national cancer clinical trials system for the 21st century
  - Delivering affordable cancer care in the 21st century
  - Reducing tobacco-related cancer incidence and mortality.
- The **Oncology Nursing Society (ONS)** (www.ons.org/advocacy-policy) is active in advocating for issues related to oncology. The ONS *Health Policy Agenda for the 113th Congress* (ONS, 2014) includes three major policy initiatives:
  - Promote and improve cancer symptom management and palliative care.
  - Advance and ensure access to quality cancer prevention and care.
  - Bolster the nation's nursing workforce to safeguard public health.

Health Affairs is the leading journal of health policy, reaching a broad audience that includes leaders in government, health advocacy, health research, and provision of health care. The journal focuses on timely topics related to cost, quality, and access to care. In April 2012, it published an issue titled *Issues in Cancer Care: Value, Quality and Costs* (see www.healthaffairs .org/Media/toc/2012_04_toc.pdf).

Triple Aim Initiative

Discussions related to health reform and the ACA center on the triad of quality, cost, and access. Several provisions in the ACA address improving access to care, improving quality outcomes of health care, and reducing, or at least not increasing, cost of care. These ideas of balancing cost, quality, and access are related to the Triple Aim Initiative of the Institute for Healthcare Improvement (IHI). IHI proposes that redesign in healthcare delivery models must include three dimensions developed simultaneously (IHI, n.d.):

• Improving the patient experience of care (including quality and satisfaction)
• Improving the health of populations
• Reducing the per capita cost of health care.

The three dimensions outlined in the Triple Aim are interconnected. If a health system, for example, focuses only on cost reduction, the patient experience or quality may suffer. The introduction of improving the health of populations requires individual healthcare providers and health systems to intervene across social determinants of health, not just individually focused interventions. Population health includes factors such as literacy, health behaviors, environment, housing, transportation, and education. Mortality and morbidity outcomes are analyzed at a specified population level. By taking the population approach in addition to the individual approach, issues of health equity emerge. For example, why do Black women have higher morbidity rates from breast cancer than White women? Why do Navajos living in uranium mining areas have higher incidences of lung cancer? By expanding policy makers' and providers' understanding to include population-level considerations, we can begin to address health disparities and achieve health equity.

The Triple Aim Initiative has influenced health policy at the highest levels. CMS has adopted the Triple Aim approach in the newly created Center for Medicare and Medicaid Innovation (the Innovation Center). This center supports the development and testing of "new models of care and payment that provide better health and better health care at lower costs" (CMS, n.d.).

Several innovation projects are currently underway with Innovation Center funding. For example, studies focused on smoking cessation include programs in California (Medicaid Incentives for Prevention of Chronic Diseases: Increasing Quitting Among Medi-Cal Smokers), Connecticut (Incentives to Quit Smoking for Connecticut Medicaid Program [iQUIT]), and Wisconsin (Striving to Quit), among others (CMS, 2011).

The *Future of Nursing* Report

Policy work includes analyzing reports and developing recommendations to further the work of the initial report. IOM published *The Future of Nursing: Leading Change, Advancing Health* in 2011. This report included the following four key messages (IOM, 2011).
• Nurses should practice to the full extent of their education and training.
• Nurses should achieve higher levels of education and training through an improved education system that promotes seamless academic progression.
• Nurses should be full partners, with physicians and other health professionals, in redesigning health care in the United States.
• Effective workforce planning and policy making require better data collection and an improved information infrastructure.

These key messages provide the framework for the following eight major recommendations (IOM, 2011).
• Remove scope-of-practice barriers.
• Expand opportunities for nurses to lead and diffuse collaborative improvement efforts.
• Implement nurse residency programs.
• Increase the proportion of nurses with a bachelor's of science in nursing degree to 80% by 2020.
• Double the number of nurses with a doctorate by 2020.
• Ensure that nurses engage in lifelong learning.
• Prepare and enable nurses to lead change to advance health.
• Build an infrastructure to collect and analyze healthcare workforce data.

ONS has developed a detailed action plan in response to the IOM report and is actively working with the Action Coalitions, groups of nurse and non-nurse stakeholders from different sectors at the local, state, and regional levels that determine best practices and research needs, to implement the recommendations (ONS, 2014).

Evidence-Based Practice

The ACA (§ 4301) outlines funding for research and describes the need to examine evidence-based practices related to Healthy People 2020. The use of evidence to support practice has gained credence and is promoted in the ACA. *Evidence* is defined as "the practice of health care in which the practitioner systematically finds, appraises, and uses the most current and valid research findings as the basis for clinical decisions" ("Evidence," 2009).

The Cancer Control P.L.A.N.E.T. (Plan, Link, Act, Network with Evidence-based Tools) portal provides evidence-based tools for comprehensive cancer control programs. Topics covered include individual- and population-based approaches to physical activity, tobacco control, diet and nutrition, sun safety, screening, and informed decision making (National Cancer Institute, Division of Cancer Control and Population Sciences, n.d.). In addition, ONS has developed reference materials and resources for evidence-based practice (ONS, n.d.). Policy analysis, use of evidence to change practice, and advocacy are all skills vital to the policy process. It is also important to develop political competence.

Political Competence: What Is It, and Why Do Health Professionals Need It?

Political competence is an important and necessary skill for healthcare professionals. While perhaps not a term that first comes to mind when thinking about the nursing profession, its importance cannot be overstated. As early as the 18th century, Florence Nightingale recognized the value of political competency and advised nurses accordingly. Two quotes from Florence Nightingale, the first from a letter to a friend in 1844 and the second from her writings on India in 1896, illustrate her belief in the profession's responsibility to take action and bring about change:

> You ask me why I do not write something. . . . I think one's feelings waste themselves in words; they ought all to be distilled into actions, and into actions which bring results. (as cited in Cook, 1913a, pp. 93–94)

> So I never lose an opportunity of urging a practical beginning, however small, for it is wonderful how often in such matters the mustard-seed germinates and roots itself. (as cited in Cook, 1913b, p. 406)

Many of the same skills that enable a nurse to be an effective patient advocate are applicable to advocacy at an organizational and governmental level. The following sections review three key lessons to consider about political competence and guide healthcare providers in developing an effective advocacy role.

First Lesson: Not All Politics Are Negative

What is political competence? Samuel Bacharach (as cited in Harvard Management Update, 2008) defined it in far more positive terms than some managers might:

> It's the ability to understand what you can and cannot control, when to take action, who is going to resist your agenda, and whom you need on your side. It's about knowing how to map the

political terrain and get others on your side, as well as lead coalitions. Examine the vocabulary that's part and parcel of our business mindset—words like uncertainty, risk, change, action, and execution. At every level, businesses need people who are willing to take action and who know how to create change—people who feel secure enough to take risks in an uncertain environment. (para. 2)

Bacharach's statements have meaning and applicability to healthcare professionals. Possessing political competence is critical to advocate for and influence institutional, professional, and governmental policy. In the IOM report *The Future of Nursing*, it is recognized that "nurses should be full partners, with physicians and other health professionals, in redesigning health care in the United States" (IOM, 2011, p. 221).

Redesigning health care is complex and provides numerous opportunities for influence. The process of influencing can occur in many ways. Common to any effort to influence is the ability to develop a clear and compelling message.

Second Lesson: Words Matter

Effective communication requires active listening and the ability to craft and deliver a persuasive message. Figure 1-5 illustrates steps to consider when communicating with policy makers. First, it is important to have a clear, specific message: What is the problem, and how should it be addressed? Second, the audience should be identified: What does the audience know about the issue? Generally, coupling nursing's content expertise with personal stories and data will provide a great start to the dialogue. Third, set the stage: Why is this matter of importance? Fourth, stay on track, and do not ramble. Be concise and logical. Include brief, evidence-based points to clarify the issue. Fifth, identify three key points for the audience to remember about the issue. Sixth, repeat these points in the message. Finally, conclude on a positive note (see Figure 1-5).

Third Lesson: Advocate for the Public and the Profession

Nurses are well positioned to advocate for a wide range of health reform initiatives. Continuing to advocate for the profession is important, but should not be the limit of nursing's advocacy efforts. Key policy areas where nursing has and should continue to influence the direction of reform include patient-centered care and engagement, interdisciplinary practice and education, and innovative approaches to care coordination. Engaging nurses in policy discussions and demonstrating the profession's commitment to achieving the Triple Aim will facilitate reform efforts and help lead the way toward a healthier nation.

Figure 1-5. Communications With Policy Makers

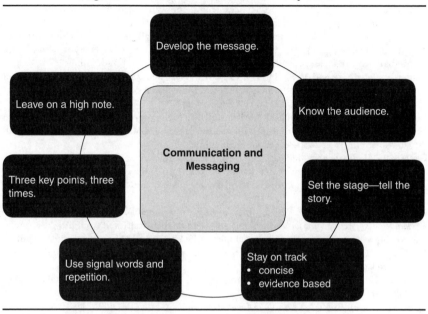

Note. Figure courtesy of Deborah E. Trautman, 2013. Used with permission.

Conclusion

Several influences are converging to provide an opportune time for healthcare providers to improve health care. The policy streams are coming together to support legislative and regulatory change. *The Future of Nursing* report and its recommendations foster nursing taking an active role in healthcare improvement. The IHI Triple Aim approach has gained wide backing, and future research will continue to provide evidence to validate current practices or provide new information to promote practice changes.

References

Advisory Board Company. (2014, December 17). Where the states stand on Medicaid expansion: 27 states, D.C. expanding Medicaid. Retrieved from http://www.advisory.com/daily-briefing/resources/primers/medicaidmap

Berwick, D.M., Nolan, T.W., & Whittington, J. (2008). The Triple Aim: Care, health, and cost. *Health Affairs, 27,* 759–769. doi:10.1377/hlthaff.27.3.759

Blumenthal, D., & Morone, J.A. (2010). *The heart of power: Health and politics in the Oval Office.* Los Angeles, CA: University of California Press.

Centers for Medicare and Medicaid Services. (n.d.). Innovation center: Share your ideas. Retrieved from http://innovation.cms.gov/Share-Your-Ideas/index.html

Centers for Medicare and Medicaid Services. (2011). Medicaid incentives for prevention of chronic diseases grants [Fact sheets]. Retrieved from http://www.cms.gov/Newsroom/ MediaReleaseDatabase/Fact-sheets/2011-Fact-sheets-items/2011-09-13.html

Centers for Medicare and Medicaid Services. (2012). *National health expenditures 2012.* Retrieved from http://www.cms.gov/Research-Statistics-Data-and-Systems/Statistics-Trends-and-Reports/ NationalHealthExpendData/Downloads/highlights.pdf

Centers for Medicare and Medicaid Services. (2013). 2013 poverty guidelines. Retrieved from http://www.cms.gov/Outreach-and-Education/Training/CMSNationalTrainingProgram/ Downloads/2013-Federal-Poverty-Guidelines.pdf

Centers for Medicare and Medicaid Services. (2014). Medicaid Statistical Information System (MSIS) state summary datamarts. Retrieved from http://www.cms.gov/Research-Statistics -Data-and-Systems/Computer-Data-and-Systems/MedicaidDataSourcesGenInfo/MSIS -Mart-Home.html

Congressional Budget Office. (2012, July). *Estimates for the insurance coverage provisions of the Affordable Care Act updated for the recent Supreme Court decision.* Retrieved from http://www.cbo .gov/sites/default/files/cbofiles/attachments/43472-07-24-2012-CoverageEstimates.pdf

Cook, E. (1913a). *The life of Florence Nightingale* (Vol. I, 1820–1861). London, England: Macmillan and Co.

Cook, E. (1913b). *The life of Florence Nightingale* (Vol. II, 1862–1910). London, England: Macmillan and Co.

Evidence. (2009). In *Mosby's medical dictionary* (8th ed.). St. Louis, MO: Elsevier Mosby.

Executive Office of the President of the United States. (2013, November). *Trends in health care cost growth and the role of the Affordable Care Act.* Retrieved from http://www .whitehouse.gov/sites/default/files/docs/healthcostreport_final_noembargo_v2.pdf

Harvard Management Update. (2008, February 27). Sharpen your political competence. *Harvard Business Review Blog Network.* Retrieved from http://blogs.hbr.org/2008/02/sharpen-your -political-compete-1

Institute for Healthcare Improvement. (n.d.). The IHI Triple Aim. Retrieved from http://www .ihi.org/engage/initiatives/TripleAim/Pages/default.aspx

Institute of Medicine. (2011). *Future of nursing: Leading change, advancing health.* Retrieved from http://books.nap.edu/openbook.php?record_id=12956

Johnson, H., & Broder, D.S. (1997). *The system: The American way of politics at the breaking point, with a new foreword and afterword.* Boston, MA: Little, Brown & Co.

Kaiser Family Foundation. (2013a). Characteristics of the nonelderly uninsured population, 2011. Retrieved from http://kff.org/uninsured/slide/characteristics-of-the-nonelderly- uninsured-population-2011

Kaiser Family Foundation. (2013b). Health care coverage and personal health care expenditures in the U.S., 2011. Retrieved from http://kff.org/health-costs/slide/health-care-coverage -and-personal-health-care-expenditures-in-the-u-s-2011

Kaiser Family Foundation. (2013c). Kaiser health tracking poll: March 2013. http:// kaiserfamilyfoundation.files.wordpress.com/2013/03/8425-t1.pdf

Kaiser Family Foundation. (2013d). Medicare enrollment, 1966–2013. Retrieved from http:// kff.org/medicare/slide/medicare-enrollment-1966-2013

Kingdon, J. (2010). *Agendas, alternatives, and public policies* (Updated 2nd ed.). Upper Saddle River, NJ: Pearson Longman.

McDonough, J.E. (2011). *Inside national health reform.* Los Angeles, CA: University of California Press.

National Cancer Institute, Division of Cancer Control and Population Sciences. (n.d.). Cancer Control P.L.A.N.E.T. Retrieved from http://cancercontrolplanet.cancer.gov

Oncology Nursing Society. (n.d.). ONS PEP—Putting evidence into practice. Retrieved from https://www.ons.org/practice-resources/pep
Oncology Nursing Society. (2014, January). *Health policy agenda, 113th Congress, 2nd session.* Pittsburgh, PA: Author.
Organisation for Economic Co-operation and Development. (2014a). OECD Health Statistics 2014: How does the United States compare? Retrieved from http://www.oecd.org/unitedstates/briefing-note-united-states-2014.pdf
Organisation for Economic Co-operation and Development. (2014b, June 30). OECD Health Statistics 2014 online database. Retrieved from http://www.oecd.org/els/health-systems/health-data.htm
Patient Protection and Affordable Care Act, Pub. L. No. 111-148, 124 Stat. 119 (2010).
Social Security Administration. (n.d.). Legislative history. Retrieved from http://www.ssa.gov/history/law.html
Sommers, B.D., Baicker, K., & Epstein, A.M. (2012). Mortality and access to care among adults after state Medicaid expansions. *New England Journal of Medicine, 367,* 1025–1034. doi:10.1056/NEJMsa1202099
Swift, A. (2013). Honesty and ethics rating of clergy slides to new low. Retrieved from http://www.gallup.com/poll/166298/honesty-ethics-rating-clergy-slides-new-low.aspx
U.S. Department of Health and Human Services. (n.d.). Key features of the Affordable Care Act. Retrieved from http://www.hhs.gov/healthcare/facts/timeline/index.html
U.S. Department of Health and Human Services. (2013). Creating jobs by addressing primary care workforce needs. Retrieved from http://www.hhs.gov/healthcare/facts/factsheets/2013/06/jobs06212012.html

CHAPTER 2

Public Policy, Public Health, and Health Policy

Sally S. Cohen, PhD, RN, FAAN, and Karen McKeown, MSN, RN

Introduction

The world of public policy is fascinating, complex, and essential for all those interested in any facet of health policy. To work effectively within health policy arenas, policy stakeholders, including individuals and organizations, must understand certain tenets and structures of public policy. Effectively analyzing and changing health policies also requires knowledge of certain key public health principles and issues.

This chapter (a) provides an overview of the policy process, including a brief summary of two policy frameworks, (b) discusses major issues in public health and health policy, and (c) offers suggestions for getting involved in health policy.

Overview of the Policy Process

Policy competency requires knowledge of certain core principles. This section will define policy and explain core public policy structures, discuss the policy process, and summarize two major policy models. Discussion will focus on the national level of government, with reference to states and localities as needed.

Defining Policy and Policy Structures

Definitions of public policy abound. One policy scholar defined it as "authoritative decisions made in the legislative, executive, or judicial branches of government that are intended to direct or influence the actions, behaviors, or decisions of others" (Longest, 2006, p. 7). Health policy comprises the subset of these decisions dealing with health.

Although this definition of health policy focuses on government policies, many health policies are created in the private sector (although these too may be influenced by government policy). For example, a grocery store might choose to display low-fat milk more prominently than whole or chocolate milk; a convenience store might decide to add a large fresh produce section; or a health insurance plan might offer incentives for enrollees to participate in physical activities. All of these represent nongovernmental policy decisions to promote health and healthy lifestyles.

Furthermore, each level of government—local, state, and federal—develops health policies. The outcomes (laws, regulations, or court decisions) are often the result of collaboration, negotiation, and bargaining among individuals at different levels of government. For example, each state makes policy decisions for its Medicaid program, but significant changes require approval of the federal government. As another example, the Centers for Disease Control and Prevention (CDC) works collaboratively through funding grants with state and local governments to address public health issues. Although CDC sets program guidelines, each grant recipient implements programs and policy that make sense in the local environment. Thus, organizations in the private sector and all levels of government are involved with health policies. Moreover, health policies must be examined within the context of socioeconomic conditions, political environments, and different ideologic and philosophical perspectives.

Politics are an important component of any policy analysis. Harold Lasswell's classic definition of politics has endured for nearly a century. According to Lasswell, politics is "the process by which society determines who gets what, when they get it, and how they get it" (Lasswell, 1958, as cited in Birkland, 2011, p. 42). Building on Lasswell's definition, it is important for those engaged in health policy to be mindful of the politics of issues in order to understand power dynamics and bargaining outcomes, regardless of the setting or clinical focus.

Stages of the Policy Process

Typically, when we discuss the policy process, we envision it as a linear sequence of stages. But as most people who work in national health and other policy domains know, it is actually a cyclical process (Longest, 2006) with modification and feedback loops throughout. The classic stages of the policy process are agenda setting, policy formation, policy implementation, and policy evaluation. Sometimes, agenda setting is considered part of policy formation, and implementation and evaluation often are linked together. Consider how key players in each stage described in the following text also influence other stages of the process through informal or formal mechanisms, thereby demonstrating the cyclical nature of the policy process.

Agenda setting: Problems and issues can rise to the attention of policy makers in a number of ways. The news media may report on a new problem, or a constituent may raise a novel concern. Alternatively, emerging scientific research or successful local or pilot programs may suggest potential solutions to long-standing problems.

Important to note is that a clinical problem does not usually translate to a policy problem for lawmakers. Therefore, knowing how to define a problem or frame policy for policy audiences is the first key step to the policy process.

If an issue is particularly compelling, or if it resonates with a legislator's personal priorities, legislators and their staff may take the initiative to introduce legislation. Other times, interested stakeholders, often led by professional or special interest associations, provide the driving force to craft legislation. In these cases, the individuals or groups seeking to spur the creation of a new bill must first do their homework to learn as much as possible about both the issues and the legislators. The most compelling arguments often comprise scientific evidence, demographic data, and personal stories or anecdotes. Communication should focus on only one problem or issue at a time to prevent distracting lawmakers and constituents from the priority at hand.

Given the bargaining nature of politics, it is always best to have a backup or contingency solution in case one's first choice is not politically feasible. It is wise to indicate whether there is support for a given proposal among other interest groups, the lawmaker's constituents, and other legislators and executive branch officials. And, it is also wise to acknowledge what one's opponents or critics of the solution might say and to suggest possible responses.

Policy formation: Once a legislator (or group of legislators) has decided to introduce a bill, the next goal is to gain adequate support from other lawmakers to pass the bill and from the president to sign it. Savvy advocates know how to work with the media by providing compelling facts and narratives. Individual constituents can communicate with their elected officials to describe anticipated effects of the proposed legislation and to express support for or opposition to the bill; special interest groups will do likewise.

Constituents have more leverage than advocates who are not from that lawmaker's district. One can advocate for a position to legislators by telephone calls or emails, as face-to-face interactions with lawmakers or their staff may be most effective but may not be feasible. Working with the legislator's district offices, one can attempt to either schedule a time to meet when the legislator is in the home office or arrange an appointment in Washington, DC, with staff, and the legislator if she or he is available. Advocates should focus on talking with the staff, who generally carry tremendous influence with lawmakers. A very important rule of thumb is to establish ongoing communications with staff and legislators. It is not sufficient to comment only once when advocating for legislative action. Rather, one should be a regular source of knowledge and expertise.

Policy implementation: After members of Congress pass a bill and the president signs it into law, it goes to the relevant executive branch agency for implementation through rule making. However, less than 10% of all proposed bills become law. The 113th Congress (2013–2014) has been one of the least productive in terms of number of bills enacted (125 as of September 10, 2014). But assessing congressional productivity is difficult because of the many different measures that one can use, such as number of pages or words per law or the ratio of introduced to enacted bills (Tauberer, 2014). Rules are established to guide implementation of the law at state or local levels, or in delivery systems where Medicare, Medicaid, and other federal beneficiaries, such as veterans, receive care. Rule making usually provides details or specifics of a law that the lawmakers, perhaps intentionally, omitted in the policy formation stage. It can be difficult for executive and legislative branch officials, interest group representatives, and others to agree on the intent of the law. That is one reason why rule making can be so politically challenging, yet important.

Usually, healthcare bills are referred to an agency in the Department of Health and Human Services (DHHS), but some go to other agencies, such as the Department of Veterans Affairs, Department of Defense, or Department of Agriculture.

The rulemaking process differs significantly from the legislative process. First, it occurs within the executive branch, often with legislative oversight. Second, it tends to be a more closed process than lawmaking because access to the executive branch is not as easy as to the legislative branch, where elected officials are eager to work with members of their district and organizations with expertise in a designated area.

Nevertheless, an important—and often overlooked—means of influencing health policy is to comment on proposed rules. This pertains to both those who supported the enacted law and those who opposed the legislation. Most often, there are sections of the law that legislators, organizations, or individuals oppose. Comments to the executive branch regarding proposed rules usually address specific sections of the law in an attempt to mitigate what interested parties consider the law's adverse effects or to revise a proposed rule.

It is important to watch for proposed rules relevant to one's area of interest. One way to do this is by being a member of or supporting a professional organization or other group that is following the rulemaking process. Its government affairs staff will likely send members notices that explain rules, the organization's position, and how to respond or communicate with executive branch officials.

Policy evaluation: Once a policy is implemented at the federal, state, or local level (or a combination of them), executive branch officials often seek evaluation information to determine the policy's effectiveness and the extent to which it has reached the intended populations. Executive branch officials may also want to know about any unintended outcomes, such as undue enrollment burdens on target populations, and whether federal funds were used efficiently. Did bureaucratic obstacles make implementation an unwieldy and unnecessarily difficult process?

Interagency coordination is also an area for evaluation. How well did federal and state administrators from different agencies responsible for implementation work together? What systems might be needed to enhance such coordination for the good of improving population outcomes? With this type of evidence, lawmakers, interest group representatives, and individual citizens can advocate for changes in laws or rules or the introduction of new bills, thereby demonstrating the cyclical nature of the policy process.

Policy Frameworks

Policy frameworks are useful for enhancing understanding of and planning how to attain policy change. The summaries of the two frameworks described here, multiple streams and punctuated equilibrium, are not meant to be complete descriptions. Readers are referred to the original works (Baumgartner & Jones, 2009; Kingdon, 2010; Sabatier, 2007) for more detailed explanations.

Kingdon's Framework

John W. Kingdon (2010) developed one of the most well-known policy frameworks, focusing on agenda setting, or how issues catch the attention of lawmakers. His model is based on decades of research on federal agenda setting for several issues, including health care. Kingdon posited that three "streams" are needed for issues to land on the national agenda. According to Kingdon, each stream is independent of the others. The three streams pertain to a different aspect of agenda setting: problems, policies, and politics. At critical and often unpredictable junctures, a "window of opportunity" opens when two or more streams overlap. This open window, which is short-lived, enables lawmakers to push an issue onto the legislative agenda.

Problem stream: Kingdon distinguished between *conditions*, which people may know about and discuss, and *problems*, which catch the attention of lawmakers and then prompt them to act. The successful transformation of a condition to a policy problem is a main characteristic and process of the problem stream.

Kingdon also specified that interest groups are mainly responsible for pushing an issue onto the national agenda. They do this by forming coalitions with each other and with legislators who might be interested in introducing a bill, developing succinct ways of conveying evidence to legislators, and bringing to congressional hearings and meetings with legislators individuals who can tell compelling stories that might convince legislators to support a bill. Interest groups also can develop model legislation for congressional staff to use in drafting an official bill.

Policy stream: The policy stream consists of a mix of ideas that are "generated by specialists in policy communities (networks that include bureaucrats, congressional staff members, academics, and researchers in think tanks)" (Zahariadas, 2007, p. 72). Although many ideas float within the policy stream, only a few will endure. Those that are technically and politically feasible have the most likelihood of success.

Individuals and organizations in the policy stream are continually developing ideas and policy solutions for different conditions or problems. That way, when a problem lands on the government agenda, members of the policy stream are ready to offer a policy solution.

Politics stream: The politics stream has three major components: national mood, interest group campaigns, and legislative or executive branch turnover. Changes in national mood, usually detected by public opinion polls, can create changes in the problem stream. An example is the ideologic shifts of the 1980s when the national mood became increasingly conservative. This meant that policy solutions that were left of center were unlikely to be feasible. National mood changes also can be the result of sudden or dramatic shifts in the economy or economic indicators, such as increases in inflation or unemployment rates, which can lower people's trust in government and national policies.

Major public campaigns on behalf of interest groups or coalitions can generate changes in the political stream. An example is Mothers Against Drunk Driving (known as MADD), whose members drew attention to the dangers of driving while under the influence of alcohol and set into action a new type of awareness among the public at large and especially among teens.

Last, changes in the party in control of the White House or Congress, swings in ideology, and turnover in the presidency or an influx of a new cohort in Congress can prompt changes in the politics stream. These partisan or political shifts can be sudden or occur gradually over years. Nonetheless, they can contribute to action on the national government agenda.

Policy entrepreneurs: For a problem to land on the government agenda, two or more streams need to couple, and a policy entrepreneur, or broker, needs to make use of a window of opportunity to push the problem through to the agenda. Policy entrepreneurs have keen policy and political bargaining skills, persevering until their issue lands on the agenda.

It often takes more than one attempt for an issue to land on the government agenda. In the process, actors in each stream—problem, policy, and politics—can strategize how to work the coupling of the streams to their advantage. For example, actors in the policy stream might interact in the political stream by campaigning for the election of a president or legislator who supports their policy goals.

A major limitation of Kingdon's framework is the assumption that the streams are independent. To the contrary, the policy and political actors often interact with each other in more than one stream. Moreover, sometimes Kingdon's model blurs the line between agenda setting and policy formation. Nonetheless, it is a well-known and useful model for health policy analysts and activists—including clinicians, researchers, and academicians— seeking to get their proposed problem solutions on the government agenda.

Punctuated-Equilibrium Framework

Another useful public policy model is the punctuated-equilibrium theory, which Bryan Jones and Frank Baumgartner developed (Baumgartner & Jones, 2009). This theory offers a way of understanding how and why policy change occurs. It claims that political processes are characterized by periods of rapid change followed by periods of "stability and incrementalism" (True, Jones, & Baumgartner, 2007, p. 155).

Baumgartner and Jones were interested in what caused these waves of policy change and the subsequent periods of relative stasis, characterized by issues and actors settling into a state of equilibrium. They claimed that periods of equilibrium are also reinforced by American political institutions, such as Congress, that "were conservatively designed to resist many efforts at change and thus to make mobilizations necessary if established interests are to be overcome" (True et al., 2007, p. 157).

Interest groups are important in the punctuated-equilibrium framework. They are necessary for mobilization of individual actors and organizations, changes in issue definition, agenda setting, and subsequent policy change. In analyzing the rise and fall of issues on the agenda, Baumgartner and Jones (2009) identified positive and negative feedback effects. Policy feedback effects occur when several events coalesce to enhance the visibility and rise of an issue on a government agenda; they resemble Kingdon's policy windows. Negative feedback effects function as brakes on rapid policy change.

The value of the punctuated-equilibrium theory for those interested in health policy is that it offers ways of conceptualizing policy structures, players, and events. It also provides ways of strategizing how to prompt policy change. Specifically, if a policy issue is in a lull or state of relative equilibrium, then one might plan how to work with interest groups and members of Congress to revise a problem definition, widen an issue network, and accelerate policy change.

Major Issues in Public Health and Health Policy

Health policy is complex and dynamic—constantly changing. Clinicians and policy makers can analyze health policy through many different and overlapping perspectives. For example, those engaged in policies for children and youth aim to ensure that all children get screening for chronic or acute conditions that can impair their development. Those working with older adults know that events and patterns of childhood affect adult lifestyles and health. From another perspective, studying access to care necessarily involves understanding the financing of care. Similarly, quality of care entails understanding patient safety, health literacy, relationships between patients and clinicians, and more recently, electronic health records.

Policy stakeholders bring different perspectives to health policy. The politics of health policy making reflect the interactions, alliances, and negotiations among individuals and groups in a particular health policy arena. Understanding the politics of a particular health policy can enhance one's appreciation of why certain policy outcomes (e.g., laws, regulations, and court decisions) prevail over others.

Different ways of categorizing health policy abound, and none is better than another. The following section will discuss public health, access, financing, and quality. We chose these topics because they span most areas of health policy and encompass diverse populations, delivery settings, and clinical specialty areas.

Public Health

Public health encompasses many aspects of public and health policy, not just issues assigned to public health agencies. The Institute of Medicine (IOM) defined the mission of public health as "fulfilling society's interest in assuring conditions in which people can be healthy" (IOM Committee for the Study of the Future of Public Health, 1988, p. 7). The work required to carry out this mission is broad and includes forming and implementing policies aimed at preventing infection and illness, ensuring access to safe food and water, developing healthcare delivery infrastructures, improving healthcare systems, and preparing for threats to health (Turnock, 2012).

In 1999, CDC released a list of the 10 greatest achievements of public health in the 20th century. Among them were vaccination and control of infectious diseases, motor vehicle and workplace safety, and recognition of tobacco as a health hazard. As a result of these and other initiatives, public health has been credited with 25 of the 30-year increase in Americans' life expectancy during the 20th century (CDC, 1999).

A major impetus for many public health policies is the Healthy People plan. In 1979, Surgeon General Julius B. Richmond released *Healthy People: The Surgeon General's Report on Health Promotion and Disease Prevention*, which identified specific population health goals that the nation was to achieve by the end of the next decade. In 1980, U.S. DHHS (2014) operationalized this under *Healthy People 1990: Promoting Health/Preventing Disease: Objectives for the Nation*. Each decade since then, DHHS has revised *Healthy People* in response to changes in society's health needs and priorities and progress in attaining previous Healthy People goals. In 2010, DHHS released the most current version, *Healthy People 2020: Objectives for Improving Health.* Many states and localities develop similar plans specific to their jurisdiction.

One of the most important indicators of population health is infant mortality. It is "associated with a variety of factors such as maternal health, quality and access to medical care, socioeconomic conditions, and public health practices" (MacDorman & Mathews, 2008, p. 1). In 1900, the United States had an infant mortality rate of 100 per 1,000 live births, meaning that 10% of infants died before their first birthday. By 2000, the rate had improved and dropped to 7 deaths for every 1,000 live births. Yet, closer analysis reveals disparities among infant mortality rates for different populations. The largest infant mortality disparities were between non-Hispanic Black populations and other groups. Non-Hispanic Black infants are two to three times more likely to die by one year of age than White infants. Maternal child health specialists and practitioners have a dual goal: to reduce the national infant mortality rate and eliminate the disparities so that babies of all racial and ethnic groups have the opportunity to thrive (Health Resources and Services Administration [HRSA], 2012).

In the aftermath of the terrorist attacks of September 11, 2001, and the subsequent anthrax threats, "bioterrorism preparedness and emergency response [rose] to the top of the national agenda" (Turnock, 2012, p. 424). Since 2001, enhanced federal funding has strengthened the infrastructure for public health preparedness for any health crisis, whether a disease outbreak, natural disaster, or act of terrorism. Under this all-hazards strategy, public health officials assess risk and plan to prevent or mitigate disaster.

Access to Coverage and Care

Access to care is a complex issue with no single definition (Medicare Payment Advisory Commission, 2003). IOM has defined access to care as "the timely use of personal health services to achieve the best possible health outcomes" (Millman, 1993, p. 4). Access to care includes both availability of services and their actual use. Although coverage is an important component of access, the two are not the same. One can have coverage but lack access to appropriate care due to rurality, lack of culturally congruent care, or other structural barriers. Similarly, one can lack coverage and still access care through safety net providers.

Some covered individuals report that they delay or forgo care because of cost concerns (Kaiser Commission on Medicaid and the Uninsured, 2012). Also, providers may opt not to work with specific payers (Borchgrevink, Snyder, & Gehshan, 2008). Provider shortages can also create access problems. By increasing the number of people who may have access to health insurance, the Patient Protection and Affordable Care Act (ACA) in 2010 increased the need for primary care clinicians. In response, many states have increased the funding for physician, nurse practitioner, and physician assistant training, but lack of available providers in rural and certain inner-city areas are likely to represent ongoing access policy challenges.

The United States has historically had a combination of private and public coverage policies. In 2011 (prior to implementation of the ACA), almost 50% of Americans had employer-provided insurance coverage, and an additional 5% purchased health insurance through the individual market (Kaiser Family Foundation, n.d.). Virtually all of the older adults in America have coverage through Medicare (Kaiser Commission on Medicaid and the Uninsured, 2012). Most Medicare beneficiaries also have privately purchased supplemental coverage (Medicare Payment Advisory Commission, 2013).

In 2011, 16% of Americans had Medicaid coverage (Kaiser Family Foundation, n.d.). Under the Medicaid programs, states are required to cover specific categories of people (pregnant women, infants and children, seniors, and individuals with disabilities) who meet certain income guidelines (Centers for Medicare and Medicaid Services [CMS], n.d.-c). States have the option to expand eligibility to people not meeting traditional coverage requirements. Such expansions are subject to federal review and approval. Additionally, the Children's Health Insurance Program (CHIP) provides coverage to children whose families cannot afford insurance, even though their annual incomes exceed Medicaid eligibility cutoff levels (CMS, n.d.-a).

In 2011, approximately 16% of Americans (30 million people) lacked coverage (Kaiser Family Foundation, n.d.). The primary goal of the ACA, and one metric by which its success will be measured, is to reduce the number of uninsured individuals. In addition to the planned expansion of Medicaid, as of January 2014, government subsidies based on income are available to help eligible individuals purchase their own health insurance through state, federal, or state or federal exchanges (Kaiser Family Foundation, 2013).

The ACA extended Medicaid coverage to all individuals with incomes up to 138% of the federal poverty level (Kaiser Family Foundation, 2014b). In July 2012, the Supreme Court ruled that the federal government could not require states to change the eligibility for their Medicaid program, giving states the option not to participate in the Medicaid expansions under the ACA (see Figure 2-1). As of August 2014, 28 states, including the District of Columbia, had implemented Medicaid expansions, 2 states were still holding debates, and 21 states had decided not to expand at this time (Kaiser Family Foundation, 2014a).

The safety net for the uninsured varies by location. Scattered throughout every state are federally qualified health centers (FQHCs), which receive federal grants from public health funds and "qualify for enhanced reimbursement from Medicare and Medicaid, as well as other benefits" (HRSA,

---

Figure 2-1. Federalism

The Tenth Amendment in the U.S. Bill of Rights provides that "the powers not delegated to the United States by the Constitution, nor prohibited by it to the States, are reserved to the States respectively, or to the people" (U.S. Const. amend. X). This is the clearest legal formulation of federalism, "a system of government in which sovereignty is constitutionally divided between a central governing authority and constituent political units (e.g., states), and in which the power to govern is shared between the national and state governments" (Teitelbaum & Wilensky, 2013, p. 267).

Over the years, the Supreme Court has defined the separation of powers described as "federalism" with varying degrees of strictness. As a result of looser definitions, the boundaries may become blurred, and some government programs better fit the description of "cooperative federalism . . . in which state agencies take primary responsibility for the enforcement of federal laws" (Krotoszynski, 2012, p. 1602).

The Roberts Court has returned to a stricter definition of federalism (Krotoszynski, 2012), and one example of this is the decision regarding the ACA. The sections of the ACA dealing with Medicaid provided that if states did not expand their Medicaid programs as prescribed by the act, they would lose not only the new federal dollars, but all federal funding for their existing Medicaid programs. The majority decision of the Supreme Court described this approach as "a gun to the head" of the states (*National Federation of Independent Business v. Sebelius*, 2012, p. 51). The Court ruled that it was unconstitutional for the ACA to require state participation in the expansion:

> As for the Medicaid expansion, that portion of the Affordable Care Act violates the Constitution by threatening existing Medicaid funding. Congress has no authority to order the States to regulate according to its instructions. Congress may offer the States grants and require the States to comply with accompanying conditions, but the States must have a genuine choice whether to accept the offer. (*National Federation of Independent Business v. Sebelius*, 2012, p. 58)

ACA—Patient Protection and Affordable Care Act

n.d.-b). In exchange, among other requirements, "FQHCs must serve an underserved area or population, offer a sliding fee scale, [and] provide comprehensive services" (HRSA, n.d.-b).

The Emergency Medical Treatment and Labor Act of 1986 provides "public access to emergency services regardless of ability to pay" (CMS, 2012a). Hospitals that participate in Medicare are required to provide examination upon request and treatment and stabilization of any emergency medical condition, including active labor (CMS, 2012a).

Historically, states have been the primary insurance regulators. This has meant that insurance regulation could vary from one state to another. One area of wide state variation has been mandated coverage of specific services, meaning that a specific condition or treatment that is required to be covered by insurance in one state may not be covered in another. Although the precise effects of the ACA are not yet known, it is likely to reduce variation in mandated coverage across state lines because the ACA, itself, mandates uniform coverage of "essential benefits" (National Conference of State Legislatures, 2014).

Financing of Care

In 1970, the average healthcare spending per person was $356 per year, and healthcare spending represented 7.2% of the total economy. Over the next 40 years, healthcare spending steadily grew faster than the economy. By 2010, yearly spending averaged $8,402 per person, and healthcare spending represented 17.9% of the total economy (Kaiser Family Foundation, 2012). In addition to improving coverage, many health policy analysts and public policy makers see controlling healthcare costs as a high priority (see Figure 2-2).

Controlling the cost of care for their clients is an especially high-priority focus for both public and private healthcare payers. Many models exist by which payers attempt to accomplish this goal; each strategy can have far-reaching and unintended effects. For example, a payer can set a lower reimbursement for a given service. The risk of this approach is that providers may determine that the fee is too low, and opt not to serve that population. Alternatively, a payer can attempt to reduce utilization, either by improving members' health or by sharing costs with members, which can lead to members forgoing needed care. Or, a payer may partner with providers to increase the quality and efficiency of care and then share the savings with the providers.

Given that more than half of Americans have some form of private insurance coverage, private insurance companies and employers who purchase insurance for their employees are powerful health policy decision makers. Working together, these groups have been able to test innovative ways to achieve

---

Figure 2-2. Choosing Wisely

There is broad consensus that projected healthcare costs will consume too much of the national income and that healthcare dollars are often spent on unnecessary care. Nevertheless, many Americans are uncomfortable with the idea of government involvement in "appropriate care" discussions, fearing that intervention could lead to rationing. They often express this unease by asserting that such discussions should take place only between clinicians and patients.

Traditionally, clinicians have not considered the larger context of healthcare delivery and policy. In 2009, physician Howard Brody challenged his colleagues to identify commonly ordered tests and treatments that are both expensive and lack evidence to support them. He asked each medical specialty society to develop a "top five" list for their specialty and to work with providers to reduce the use of these procedures (Brody, 2009). Now called the Choosing Wisely initiative and led by the American Board of Internal Medicine Foundation, more than 30 medical specialty organizations have taken on this challenge (American Board of Internal Medicine Foundation, n.d.).

---

lower healthcare costs for their members. Many employers have implemented employee wellness plans, partly in an effort to reduce their healthcare costs and keep their employees healthy, thereby reducing absenteeism and enhancing worker productivity. Some insurance plans offer financial or other incentives to members who engage in health-promoting activities, such as healthful eating, physical activity, or health screenings. Some plans and employers offer consumer-driven plans, in which high deductibles coupled with health savings accounts are designed to decrease utilization by making patients aware of cost and engaging them in decisions about their care.

Because government expenditures (primarily through Medicare and Medicaid) represent approximately half (American Hospital Association, 2013) of all healthcare expenditures in the United States, payment systems and structures represent a significant means by which federal and state governments direct health policy.

Medicare is the largest single payer for hospital care, paying a larger proportion of hospital costs than all private insurance combined (American Hospital Association, 2013). Because of this, Medicare policies have long wielded great influence in hospital care and beyond. Medicare payment policies can affect how health care is delivered to all patients, partly because private payers often follow Medicare's lead and partly because hospital systems and processes developed for Medicare patients may affect all patients. A notable example of the latter occurred with Medicare's transition in the 1980s from paying billed charges, or fee-for-service, to using a prospective payment system using diagnosis-related groups, or DRGs. This new system, which paid hospitals based on patient diagnoses rather than services rendered, removed some incentives for providing unnecessary treatments and tests and created new incentives to reduce the length of hospital stay. This massive change caused hospitals to reconfigure how they provided care to all patients (Kahn et al., 1990).

Quality of Care

The recent emphasis on improving healthcare quality began with the release in 1999 of IOM's seminal report *To Err Is Human* (Kohn, Corrigan, & Donaldson, 2000), which estimated that as many as 98,000 Americans died in hospitals each year as a result of medical error. This publication, together with IOM's report *Crossing the Quality Chasm* (IOM Committee on Quality of Health Care in America, 2001), profoundly affected the world of health policy by highlighting the vital importance of quality (Gardner, Wakefield, & Gardner, 2007).

Improving healthcare quality depends on close collaboration between government and the private sector. Government plays a key role in holding healthcare providers to minimum standards. Both the federal and state governments develop regulations to govern healthcare organizations and clinicians and exert direct oversight and inspection to ensure compliance with all relevant requirements.

Private organizations have also played a role in quality assurance. In 1951, a group of professional associations, including the American College of Surgeons, American College of Physicians, American Hospital Association, and American Medical Association, formed what is today known as The Joint Commission (TJC). Originally, TJC only offered accreditation to those hospitals that voluntarily met its standards. In 1965, however, when Congress created the Medicare and Medicaid programs, it also stipulated that hospitals holding accreditation from TJC would not require additional review and would be deemed to have met program standards (TJC, 2013b). Today, although hospitals can choose to undergo routine surveys by state agencies or be accredited by any of several organizations, most hold TJC accreditation (TJC, 2013a).

Many professional organizations set standards for quality care provided by various types of practitioners (e.g., American Dental Association, American Medical Association, American Nurses Association) and specialties (e.g., American Society of Clinical Oncology, Oncology Nursing Society, American Pain Society, Hospice and Palliative Nurses Association). These organizations have used various approaches to achieve quality care, including publishing research related to the field or specialty, offering continuing education opportunities for members, and often offering certification in specialty practice.

In 1999, as the quality imperative took hold, Congress and President Clinton quickly took action. One result was the creation of the Agency for Healthcare Research and Quality (AHRQ) (Gardner et al., 2007) within DHHS. The mission of this agency is "to produce evidence to make health care safer, higher quality, more accessible, equitable, and affordable, and to work within the U.S. Department of Health and Human Services and with other partners to make sure that the evidence is understood and used" (AHRQ, n.d., "Mission and Budget" section).

Many private organizations also focus primarily or solely on improving healthcare quality. These include the National Committee for Quality Assurance (n.d.), which monitors the quality of care delivered by health insurance plans; the National Quality Forum (n.d.), which focuses on quality in care delivery at the bedside; and the Leapfrog Group (n.d.), a consortium of employers who purchase employee health plans.

Leveraging Payment Structures to Achieve Quality Goals

Payment policy decisions can affect more than cost. At times, these decisions can have unintended consequences (see Figure 2-3), but in recent

---

Figure 2-3. Hospice

In 1967, Dame Cicely Saunders founded the first modern hospice in England. Florence Wald, dean of Yale University School of Nursing from 1959 to 1965, so admired Saunders's work with the dying that she left her position as dean to work with and learn from Saunders in London. Wald then returned to Connecticut and in 1974 was instrumental in founding Connecticut Hospice, the first modern hospice in the United States. The mission of the first hospices was to provide specialized, holistic care, with a focus on symptom control, to the terminally ill (Biewen, n.d.; National Hospice and Palliative Care Organization, n.d.; Yale School of Nursing, 2009).

In 1982, Congress enacted legislation to provide a Medicare hospice benefit (National Hospice and Palliative Care Organization, n.d.). Today, approximately 44% of all people who die are receiving hospice services at the time of their death. Yet because a large majority of hospice patients are Medicare beneficiaries, the parameters of the Medicare hospice benefit have largely defined hospice care, limiting it to patients who are willing to forgo any curative treatment and whose physicians certify that their life expectancy is six months or less. These two requirements have contributed to the problem of terminally ill patients entering hospice care at the very end of their lives, when there is little opportunity for them or their family members to benefit from hospice services. Most receive hospice services for less than a month, and more than a third receive them for only a week or less (National Hospice and Palliative Care Organization, 2012).

---

years, groups representing other areas of policy—such as quality and public health—have viewed Medicare and Medicaid (and, to a lesser extent, private insurance) payment policy as a way to effect changes in healthcare practice and delivery more quickly than might be possible through education of providers alone (see Figure 2-4).

Because quality and financing issues necessarily overlap, the quality movement has joined forces with public and private purchasers of health care to improve the quality of care through pay-for-performance. Under this approach, purchasers determine priority quality metrics for a given provider type (e.g., hospital, clinician, or homecare agency) and adjust payments based on how well the provider meets the quality standard. Several pay-for-performance models exist. In one, the payer withholds a small percentage of payment throughout the year and, at the end of the year, disburses the withheld funds based on performance. This means that high-performing providers receive more than they would have otherwise, while low performers receive less (Cromwell, Trisolini, Pope, Mitchell, & Greenwald, 2011).

Adoption of health information technology (HIT) is another example. Although organizations such as IOM and the Leapfrog Group were advocating adoption of HIT, especially computerized physician order entry (Thompson et al., 2007), and President George W. Bush took steps to advance HIT through his Health Information Technology Plan (U.S. DHHS, Office of the Assistant Secretary for Planning and Evaluation, 2004), progress in the early

---

Figure 2-4. Early Elective Deliveries

In 1979, the American College of Obstetricians and Gynecologists began to warn against electively (without medical need) delivering babies before 39 weeks of gestation, either by induction or Cesarean section. Physicians and patients may choose to deliver early for a variety of reasons, including convenience or relief of the discomfort associated with the late stages of pregnancy. Yet, early elective deliveries bring increased risk of complications for both mother and infant, and infant complications can require stays in neonatal intensive care. Moreover, evidence suggests that even when they do well at birth, infants born before 39 weeks are more likely to struggle academically (Centers for Medicare and Medicaid Services [CMS], 2012b; Galewitz, 2013). Nevertheless, changing societal norms and medical practice is not easy; despite the evidence and recommendations, early elective deliveries have been "stubbornly persistent" (Galewitz, 2013, para. 1).

A growing number of organizations have been working to bring attention to the problem and identify solutions. This group includes professional associations such as the Association of Women's Health, Obstetric and Neonatal Nurses (AWHONN), quality organizations such as the Leapfrog Group, and advocacy groups led by the March of Dimes (CMS, 2012b). In September 2011, David Lakey, commissioner of the Texas Department of State Health Services and president of the Association of State and Territorial Health Officials (ASTHO), challenged states to reduce prematurity in the United States by 8% by 2014; one component of the challenge was to reduce early elective deliveries (ASTHO, n.d.). On May 1, 2013, the American Academy of Family Physicians, American Academy of Pediatrics, American College of Nurse Midwives, American College of Obstetricians and Gynecologists, American Hospital Association, AWHONN, and March of Dimes sent a letter to hospital executives outlining actions that hospitals can take to reduce early elective deliveries (American Academy of Family Physicians et al., 2013).

In addition to working with hospitals, clinicians, and the public, advocates identified state Medicaid programs as essential partners in reducing elective deliveries. Nationwide, Medicaid pays for about 45% of all births (CMS, 2012b), making Medicaid payment policy an important lever for groups attempting to improve care for mothers and infants. Options available to state Medicaid programs include performance monitoring and public reporting; regulatory/contracting approaches; education, outreach, and training; and payment/purchasing approaches (CMS, 2012b). As an example of the latter, in Texas, "Medicaid will deny payment for claims [for] non-medically necessary early elective deliveries, but allow retrospective reviews for reconsideration" (CMS, 2012b, Appendix C). Together, these initiatives seem to be yielding results. In 2012, early elective deliveries represented 11.2% of births, down from 17% in 2010. The goal set by the Leapfrog Group is to get this below 5% (Galewitz, 2013).

2000s was slow. The HIT movement gained momentum and prominence when the American Recovery and Reinvestment Act of 2009 made billions of dollars available for hospitals and clinicians to implement and use electronic health records (EHRs) and systems (Hersh, 2009).

Medicare has offered incentive payments, for a limited time, for providers to transition to EHRs. Those who do not make the transition by 2015 will face penalties in the form of reduced Medicare payments (HRSA, n.d.-a). Proponents anticipate that with time, the increasing use of HIT will result in improved quality and reduced cost of health care (CMS, n.d.-b).

Getting Involved in Health Policy

Equipped with knowledge of the policy process, insights into two major policy frameworks, and familiarity with major principles in public health and health policy, readers are now ready to consider how they might get involved with health policy. Many options are available to pursue: Some involve individual strategies, and others entail working with organizations to advance an issue on the policy agenda.

Individual Action

One of the most important and easiest ways to engage in health policy is to be well versed in current issues relevant to one's area of interest. Reading a daily national newspaper is a first step in that regard. National newspapers (such as the *New York Times, Washington Post,* and *Wall Street Journal*) provide feature stories and editorials on economic, political, and social issues that provide the context for national health policy. They offer analyses of Congress, the presidency, and national economic indicators such as unemployment, inflation, and changes in the consumer price index.

Another individual strategy is to read and follow websites for organizations that continually update their online resources and provide useful data. It is usually best to follow websites for nonpartisan organizations so that the information is as balanced as possible. One of the most frequently used organizational websites for obtaining national and state health policy data is the Kaiser Family Foundation (www.kff.org). The foundation's website contains tutorials; interactive maps for comparisons among states; summaries and fact sheets on Medicare, Medicaid, CHIP, and other health programs; and updates on ACA implementation. Other entities that offer innovative ideas and in-depth analyses on health research and policy are the Robert Wood Johnson Foundation (www.rwjf.org) and the Commonwealth Fund (www.commonwealthfund.org).

Collective Action

Interest groups and organizations representing healthcare professionals, providers (e.g., hospitals, home health, or federally qualified health centers), payers, insurers, and specific populations are very important. They provide a collective voice for many health policy stakeholders and can speak with the force of numbers behind them.

Professional organizations and associations can provide opportunities for networking and meeting health policy leaders and may also offer continuing education in health policy. Typically these groups keep members informed about policy related to their field or specialty and may assist members in becoming active in policy efforts.

It is a good idea to be active with and visible in organizations. Participating in the development of policy positions, briefing papers, and other health policy materials can establish one's reputation as a leader or expert in a given area and may lead to opportunities for nomination to boards or government entities.

Conclusion

This chapter covered many issues, ranging from the stages of the policy process and policy frameworks to core principles of public health and health policy. No single component or issue discussed is sufficient for unraveling the complexities of public policy or ensuring successful advocacy. Moreover, much of the content presented is a summary of more detailed reports, monographs, or other publications.

One takeaway message is that to advance health, advocates need to have bold action plans. One can always look up facts and figures, but there is also a need for ideas, models, and frameworks to give structure and perspective to raw data. Although it is easy to become absorbed in the details of public health and health reform policies when forming strategies for getting involved, it is important to balance the quest for data and evidence with the human side. After all, the ultimate goal of getting involved in health policy and politics is to improve the health and well-being of people and populations.

References

Agency for Healthcare Research and Quality. (n.d.). About us. Retrieved from http://www.ahrq.gov/about/index.html

American Academy of Family Physicians, American Academy of Pediatrics, American College of Nurse Midwives, American College of Obstetricians and Gynecologists, American Hospital Association, Association of Women's Health, Obstetric and Neonatal Nurses, & March of Dimes. (2013, May 1). Joint statement: Strong start in America's hospitals. Retrieved from https://www.magnetmail.net/actions/email_web_version.cfm?recipient_id=829470608&message_id=2607586&user_id=AHA_MR&group_id=0&jobid=13926148

American Board of Internal Medicine Foundation. (n.d.). Choosing wisely: Lists. Retrieved from http://www.choosingwisely.org/doctor-patient-lists

American Hospital Association. (2013). Chapter 4: Trends in hospital financing. In *Chartbook: Trends affecting hospitals and health systems*. Retrieved from http://www.aha.org/research/reports/tw/chartbook/ch4.shtml

American Recovery and Reinvestment Act of 2009, Pub. L. No. 111-5, 123 Stat. 115.

Association of State and Territorial Health Officials. (n.d.). ASTHO healthy babies initiative. Retrieved from http://www.astho.org/healthybabies/?terms=healthy+babies

Baumgartner, F.R., & Jones, B.D. (2009). *Agendas and instability in American politics* (2nd ed.). Chicago, IL: University of Chicago Press.

Biewen, J. (n.d.). The hospice experiment: A revolution in dying: Florence Wald. American Radio-Works. Retrieved from http://americanradioworks.publicradio.org/features/hospice/a4.html

Birkland, T.A. (2011). *An introduction to the policy process: Theories, concepts, and models of public policy making* (3rd ed.). Armonk, NY: M.E. Sharpe.

Borchgrevink, A., Snyder, A., & Gehshan, S. (2008, March). The effects of Medicaid reimbursement rates on access to dental care. Retrieved from http://www.nashp.org/sites/default/files/CHCF_dental_rates.pdf

Brody, H. (2009). Medicine's ethical responsibility for health care reform—The top five list. *New England Journal of Medicine, 362,* 283–285. doi:10.1056/NEJMp0911423

Centers for Disease Control and Prevention. (1999, April 2). Ten great public health achievements—United States, 1900–1999. *Morbidity and Mortality Weekly Report, 48,* 241–243. Retrieved from http://www.cdc.gov/mmwr/preview/mmwrhtml/00056796.htm

Centers for Medicare and Medicaid Services. (n.d.-a). Children's Health Insurance Program (CHIP). Retrieved from http://www.medicaid.gov/Medicaid-CHIP-Program-Information/By-Topics/Childrens-Health-Insurance-Program-CHIP/Childrens-Health-Insurance-Program-CHIP.html

Centers for Medicare and Medicaid Services. (n.d.-b). CMS eHealth roadmap. Retrieved from www.cms.gov/eHealth/downloads/eHealth-Roadmap.pdf

Centers for Medicare and Medicaid Services. (n.d.-c). Eligibility. Retrieved from http://www.medicaid.gov/Medicaid-CHIP-Program-Information/By-Topics/Eligibility/Eligibility.html

Centers for Medicare and Medicaid Services. (2012a). Emergency Medical Treatment and Labor Act (EMTALA). Retrieved from http://www.cms.gov/Regulations-and-Guidance/Legislation/EMTALA/index.html?redirect=/emtala

Centers for Medicare and Medicaid Services. (2012b). Reducing early elective deliveries in Medicaid and CHIP. Retrieved from http://www.medicaid.gov/Medicaid-CHIP-Program-Information/By-Topics/Quality-of-Care/Downloads/EED-Brief.pdf

Cromwell, J., Trisolini, M.G., Pope, G.C., Mitchell, J.B., & Greenwald, L.M. (Eds.). (2011). *Pay for performance in health care: Methods and approaches.* Retrieved from http://www.rti.org/pubs/rtipress/mitchell/bk-0002-1103-ch02.pdf

Galewitz, P. (2013, February 21). Hospitals clamp down on dangerous early elective deliveries. Retrieved from http://www.kaiserhealthnews.org/stories/2013/february/21/early-elective-deliveries-leapfrog-group.aspx

Gardner, D.B., Wakefield, M.K., & Gardner, B.G. (2007). Contemporary issues in government. In D.J. Mason, J.K. Leavitt, & M.W. Chaffee (Eds.), *Policy and politics in nursing and health care* (pp. 622–646). St. Louis, MO: Elsevier Saunders.

Health Resources and Services Administration. (n.d.-a). Health information technology. Retrieved from http://www.hrsa.gov/ruralhealth/resources/healthit

Health Resources and Services Administration. (n.d.-b). What are federally qualified health centers (FQHCs)? Retrieved from http://www.hrsa.gov/healthit/toolbox/RuralHealthITtoolbox/Introduction/qualified.html

Health Resources and Services Administration. (2012). Region IV and VI Infant Mortality Summit 2012. Retrieved from http://mchb.hrsa.gov/infantmortalitysummit2012.html

Hersh, W. (2009). A stimulus to define informatics and health information technology. *BMC Medical Informatics and Decision Making, 9,* 24. Retrieved from http://www.biomedcentral.com/1472-6947/9/24

Institute of Medicine Committee for the Study of the Future of Public Health. (1988). *The future of public health.* Retrieved from http://www.nap.edu/catalog.php?record_id=1091

Institute of Medicine Committee on Quality of Health Care in America. (2001). *Crossing the quality chasm: A new health system for the 21st century.* Retrieved from http://www.nap.edu/catalog.php?record_id=10027

Joint Commission. (2013a). Facts about hospital accreditation. Retrieved from http://www.jointcommission.org/facts_about_hospital_accreditation

Joint Commission. (2013b). The Joint Commission history. Retrieved from http://www.jointcommission.org/assets/1/6/Joint_Commission_History.pdf

Kahn, K.L., Draper, D., Keeler, E.B., Rogers, W.H., Rubenstein, L.V., Kosecoff, J., ... Brook, R.H. (1990, October). *A summary of the effects of DRG-based prospective payment system on quality of care for hospitalized Medicare patients.* Retrieved from http://www.rand.org/content/dam/rand/pubs/notes/2007/N3132.pdf

Kaiser Commission on Medicaid and the Uninsured. (2012, October). *The uninsured: A primer: Key facts about Americans without health insurance.* Retrieved from http://kaiserfamilyfoundation.files.wordpress.com/2013/01/7451-08.pdf

Kaiser Family Foundation. (n.d.). Health insurance coverage of the total population. Retrieved from http://kff.org/other/state-indicator/total-population

Kaiser Family Foundation. (2012, May). *Health care costs: A primer: Key information on health care costs and their impact.* Retrieved from http://kaiserfamilyfoundation.files.wordpress.com/2013/01/7670-03.pdf

Kaiser Family Foundation. (2013, April 25). Summary of the Affordable Care Act. Retrieved from http://kff.org/health-reform/fact-sheet/summary-of-the-affordable-care-act

Kaiser Family Foundation. (2014a, August 28). Current status of state Medicaid expansion decisions. Retrieved from http://kff.org/health-reform/slide/current-status-of-the-medicaid-expansion-decision

Kaiser Family Foundation. (2014b, April 7). How will the uninsured fare under the Affordable Care Act? Retrieved from http://kff.org/health-reform/fact-sheet/how-will-the-uninsured-fare-under-the-affordable-care-act

Kingdon, J.W. (2010). *Agendas, alternatives, and public policies* (Updated 2nd ed.). Upper Saddle River, NJ: Pearson Longman.

Kohn, L.T., Corrigan, J.M., & Donaldson, M.S. (Eds.). (2000). *To err is human: Building a safer health system.* Retrieved from http://www.nap.edu/catalog.php?record_id=9728

Krotoszynski, R.J., Jr. (2012). Cooperative federalism, the new formalism, and the separation of powers revisited: Free enterprise fund and the problem of presidential oversight of state-government officers enforcing federal law. *Duke Law Journal, 61,* 1599–1669. Retrieved from http://scholarship.law.duke.edu/dlj/vol61/iss8/1

Lasswell, H.K. (1958). *Politics: Who gets what, when, how.* New York, NY: Meridian Books.

Leapfrog Group. (n.d.). About Leapfrog. Retrieved from http://www.leapfroggroup.org/about_leapfrog

Longest, B.B. (2006). *Health policymaking in the United States* (4th ed.). Chicago, IL: Health Administration Press.

MacDorman, M.F., & Mathews, T.J. (2008, October). *NCHS Data Brief, No. 9. Recent trends in infant mortality in the United States.* Retrieved from http://www.cdc.gov/nchs/data/databriefs/db09.htm

Medicare Payment Advisory Commission. (2003). *Report to the Congress: Medicare payment policy.* Retrieved from http://www.medpac.gov/publications%5Ccongressional_reports%5CMar03_Ch3.pdf

Medicare Payment Advisory Commission. (2013, June). *A data book: Health care spending and the Medicare program.* Retrieved from http://www.medpac.gov/documents/Jun13DataBookEntireReport.pdf

Millman, M.L. (Ed.). (1993). Access to health care in America. Retrieved from http://www.nap.edu/catalog.php?record_id=2009

National Committee for Quality Assurance. (n.d.). About NCQA. Retrieved from http://www.ncqa.org/AboutNCQA.aspx

National Conference of State Legislatures. (2014, June). State health insurance mandates and the ACA essential benefits provisions. Retrieved from http://www.ncsl.org/issues-research/health/state-ins-mandates-and-aca-essential-benefits.aspx

National Federation of Independent Business v. Sebelius, 132 S. Ct. 2566 (2012). Retrieved from http://www.supremecourt.gov/opinions/11pdf/11-393c3a2.pdf

National Hospice and Palliative Care Organization. (n.d.). History of hospice care. Retrieved from http://www.nhpco.org/history-hospice-care

National Hospice and Palliative Care Organization. (2012). NHPCO facts and figures: Hospice care in America. Retrieved from http://www.nhpco.org/sites/default/files/public/Statistics _Research/2012_Facts_Figures.pdf

National Quality Forum. (n.d.). Who we are. Retrieved from http://www.qualityforum.org/who_we_are.aspx

Richmond, J.B. (1979). *Healthy people: The Surgeon General's report on health promotion and disease prevention.* Retrieved from http://profiles.nlm.nih.gov/ps/retrieve/ResourceMetadata/NNBBGK/p-segmented/true

Sabatier, P.A. (Ed.). (2007). *Theories of the policy process* (2nd ed.). Boulder, CO: Westview Press.

Tauberer, J. (2014, July 8). Congressional productivity, 3/4ths into the 113th Congress [Web log post]. Retrieved from https://www.govtrack.us/blog/2014/07/08/congressional -productivity-34ths-into-the-113th-congress

Teitelbaum, J.B., & Wilensky, S.E. (2013). *Essentials of health policy and law* (2nd ed.). Burlington, MA: Jones & Bartlett Learning.

Thompson, P., Caramanica, L., Cohen, E., Hychalk, V., Ponte, P.R., Schmidt, K., & Sherman, R. (2007). Contemporary issues in the health care workplace. In D.J. Mason, J.K. Leavitt, & M.W. Chaffee (Eds.), *Policy and politics in nursing and health care* (5th ed., pp. 449–474). St. Louis, MO: Elsevier Saunders.

True, J.L., Jones, B.D., & Baumgartner, F.R. (2007). Punctuated-equilibrium theory: Explaining stability and change in public policymaking. In P.A. Sabatier (Ed.), *Theories of the policy process* (2nd ed., pp. 155–187). Boulder, CO: Westview Press.

Turnock, B.J. (2012). *Public health: What it is and how it works* (5th ed.). Burlington, MA: Jones & Bartlett Learning.

U.S. Const. amend. X.

U.S. Department of Health and Human Services. (2010). HHS announces the nation's new health promotion and disease prevention agenda. Retrieved from http://www .healthypeople.gov/2020/about/DefaultPressRelease.pdf

U.S. Department of Health and Human Services. (2014). History and development of Healthy People. Retrieved from http://www.healthypeople.gov/2020/about/history.aspx

U.S. Department of Health and Human Services, Office of the Assistant Secretary for Planning and Evaluation. (2004, April 26). The President's health information technology plan. Retrieved from http://www.aspe.hhs.gov/sp/nhii/news/presidentshealthitplan4-26-2004.pdf

Yale School of Nursing. (2009, December 1). YSN researchers reflect on Florence Wald's impact. Retrieved from http://nursing.yale.edu/ysn-researchers-reflect-florence-walds-impact-0

Zahariadas, N. (2007). The multiple streams framework: Structure, limitations, prospects. In P.A. Sabatier (Ed.), *Theories of the policy process* (2nd ed., pp. 65–92). Boulder, CO: Westview Press.

CHAPTER 3

A Brief History of Major Federal Cancer Policy— 1970s to Present

Ilisa Halpern Paul, MPP, and Mark H. Smith

Authors' note: Although hundreds of health and cancer legislative proposals are introduced in the U.S. Congress every year, very few—if any—see action and result in a new policy or program. As such, this chapter seeks to provide an overview of the major federal cancer policies enacted into law during the past four decades and offer insight into how those policies garnered support. Given that this is only a chapter, we, as authors, are inherently unable to provide a comprehensive history of all federal cancer policy and associated advocacy efforts. Any omissions of particular policies are not meant to intentionally leave out any specific cancer site or organization, but are merely because of our limitations in chapter length.

Introduction

Ask someone involved in oncology and health policy about when cancer issues first "got on the map," and you are likely to get one of three answers: (a) Mary Lasker in the 1950s and 1960s, (b) the 1971 National Cancer Act, or (c) the breast cancer movement in the 1990s. The correct answer is (d) all of the above. Indeed, U.S. cancer policy has a long history going back to the post–World War II era; however, few people realize that major federal cancer policy actually dates back to 1937, when the first National Cancer Act created the National Cancer Institute (NCI) (NCI Office of Government and Congressional Relations, n.d.-a).

The National Institutes of Health (NIH) traces its roots to 1887 with the creation of a one-room laboratory within the Marine Hospital Service. Established in 1789 to provide for the medical care of merchant seamen, the Marine Hospital Service was the predecessor agency to the U.S. Public Health Service (NIH Office of History, n.d.). In 1891, the Hygienic Laboratory, as it came to be called, was moved to Washington, DC. In 1901, the laboratory was belatedly recognized in law when Congress authorized $35,000 for construction of a new building in which the laboratory could investigate "infectious and contagious diseases and matters pertaining to the public health" (NIH Office of History, n.d., "The Move to Washington"). The following year, it was renamed the Public Health and Marine Hospital Service, moving it toward its status as the chief U.S. public health agency. The act also launched a formal program of research by designating the pathologic and bacteriologic work as the Division of Pathology and Bacteriology and creating three new components that represented the most fruitful research areas at that time: the Divisions of Chemistry, Pharmacology, and Zoology (NIH Office of History, n.d.). In 1930, legislation (Public Law [P.L.] 71-251) sponsored by Senator Joseph Ransdell (D-LA) changed the name of the Hygienic Laboratory to the National Institute (singular) of Health and authorized the establishment of fellowships for research into basic biologic and medical problems. The name was changed to plural, National Institutes of Health, in 1948 by the National Heart Act (NIH Office of History, n.d.).

The passage of the National Cancer Act of 1937 (P.L. 75-244) marked the "first time Congress appropriated funds to fight a non-transferable epidemic disease" (NCI Office of Government and Congressional Relations, n.d.-a, para. 1). NCI was to serve as the principal federal agency responsible for addressing the myriad challenges associated with diagnosing and treating cancer. In 1944, Congress made NCI an operating division of NIH. Hence, the inception of NCI created the foundation upon which much subsequent federal cancer policy would be based, as the search for the causes of—and better treatments, diagnostic tools, and screening tests for—cancer has proved to be a multigenerational quest. Although NCI dates to before World War II, the most influential oncology policy developments have occurred in the past 40 years and generally fall into one of three categories: research, risk reduction and prevention efforts, and access to care.

The First Modern Cancer Lobbyist

The majority of cancer policy and advocacy in the post–World War II era generally is attributed directly or indirectly to the efforts of Mary Lasker (1900–1994), a Radcliffe College graduate with a degree in art history. Lasker came to biomedical research advocacy, like most, through a personal experience with a life-threatening disease: her housekeeper had been diagnosed with cancer at a time when the disease was not mentioned in society (National Library of Medicine, n.d.). Determined to bring public attention and funding to cancer, Lasker sought to create a national infrastructure for cancer research, and she focused her efforts on convincing Congress to boost its investment in the then-National Institute of Health (not yet plural) (National Library of Medicine, n.d.). In doing so, she became the cancer community's first major lobbyist.

> Lasker acted as a catalyst for the growth of the world's largest and most successful biomedical research enterprise, with the National Institutes of Health (NIH) as its centerpiece. . . . She developed a compelling political rationale for federal sponsorship of medical research, [and] built a powerful lobby that won large research appropriations [for NIH]. (National Library of Medicine, 2007)

Lasker also pushed for programmatic and agency changes to facilitate cancer research. Her legacy includes the role of laypeople in NIH scientific advisory panels and the National Cancer Act of 1971 (National Library of Medicine, n.d.). Today, the prestigious Lasker Awards Program of the Lasker Foundation recognizes the contributions of scientists, physicians, and public servants who have made major advances in the understanding, diagnosis, treatment, cure, or prevention of human disease.

National Cancer Act of 1971

Known best for being the official launch of the "War on Cancer," the enactment of the second National Cancer Act in December 1971 was the culmination of numerous forces at play—the decades-long advocacy of Mary Lasker and her allies, key Congressional champions pushing for a "conquest of cancer," a State of the Union call to action directed at Congress by President Nixon, and scientific and clinical developments illustrating that some cancers could be defeated through the use of chemotherapy (National Library of Medicine, n.d.; Nixon, 1971a). In the late 1960s, Lasker and her Citizens Committee for the Conquest of Cancer took out ads in major newspapers urging "Mr. Nixon: You can cure cancer" (National Library of Medicine, n.d.).

In response to growing public and policymaker interest in greater federal response to the scourge of cancer, in April 1970, the Senate enacted, by unanimous consent, a resolution (S. Res. 376) in which the Senate Committee on Labor and Public Welfare (now the Senate Committee on Health, Education, Labor, and Pensions) authorized $250,000 to "study cancer research activities, calling for a report on the present status of scientific research conducted by governmental and nongovernmental agencies to ascertain the causes and develop means for the treatment, cure, and elimination of cancer" (NCI Office of Government and Congressional Relations, n.d.-b, "Legislative Background to the Conquest of Cancer Act"). To conduct the study, the committee convened a National Panel of Consultants on the Conquest of Cancer composed of 26 members, half scientists and half laypeople (NCI Office of Government and Congressional Relations, n.d.-b). The panel first met on June 29, 1970, and was directed to submit its findings in a report to the Senate by December 15, 1970. Shortly after this first meeting, a concurrent resolution (H. Con. Res. 675) expressing the unanimous sense of the Congress that the "conquest of cancer is a national crusade" passed both the House and Senate (National Cancer Crusade, 1970).

Senator Ralph W. Yarborough (D-TX) led the panel, which in November 1970 delivered its report, *A National Program for the Conquest of Cancer*, to the Senate Committee on Labor and Public Welfare (NCI Office of Government and Congressional Relations, n.d.-b). The report contained numerous recommendations, including calling for "the development of a comprehensive national program for the conquest of cancer" requiring "major ingredients that are not present today: effective administration with clearly defined authority and responsibility, a comprehensive national plan, and necessary financial resources" (NCI Office of Government and Congressional Relations, n.d.-b, "Legislative Background to the Conquest of Cancer Act"). Specifically, the Panel urged that "an independent agency—a National Cancer Authority—be established, which would absorb all functions of the National Cancer Institute, and be separate from the National Institutes of Health" (Rettig, 1978, p. 2). The panel also recommended "that funds for cancer research be increased at an annual rate of $100 million to $150 million until the budget reached a level of $800 million to $1 billion per year" (Rettig, 1978, p. 2). Following the panel's report, in the waning days of the 91st Congress, Senator Yarborough introduced S. 4564, the Conquest of Cancer Act, to implement the Panel's recommendations (NCI Office of Government and Congressional Relations, n.d.-b). Similar legislation (S. 34) was introduced at the beginning of the 92nd Congress. Building on this effort, during his 1971 State of the Union address, President Nixon called upon members of the U.S. House of Representatives and U.S. Senate to provide an additional $100 million for "an intensive campaign to find a cure for cancer" (Nixon, 1971a). The president went on to state,

> The time has come in America when the same kind of concentrated effort that split the atom and took man to the moon should be turned toward conquering this dread disease. Let us make a total national commitment to achieve this goal. (Nixon, 1971a)

Over the course of the 92nd Congress, members of Congress, the NCI director, the White House, and cancer advocates engaged in a heated debate over whether NCI should receive earmarked funding and whether a separate cancer research agency should be created (National Library of Medicine, n.d.). On May 11, 1971, Senators Peter Dominick (R-CO) and Robert Griffin (R-MI), on behalf of the Nixon Administration, introduced S. 1828, an "Act to Conquer Cancer" (NCI Office of Government and Congressional Relations, n.d.-b). The bill was reviewed and revised by the Senate Committee on Labor and Public Welfare and reported out the legislation in late June 1971 (NCI Office of Government and Congressional Relations, n.d.-b). The bill passed the Senate in July; the House subsequently held hearings in the fall and voted on its version of the measure in November (Rettig, 1978). Because the House and Senate versions differed, a conference committee of members of the House and Senate was convened to create a single uniform measure (Rettig, 1978). After months of debate and numerous meetings of the committees of jurisdiction, both the House and Senate passed the final compromise legislation on December 8, 1971, and sent it to President Nixon for his signature.

The president, upon signing the National Cancer Act into law (P.L. 92-218) on December 23, 1971, stated,

> As a result of signing this bill, the Congress is totally committed to provide the funds that are necessary, whatever is necessary, for the conquest of cancer. . . . For those who have cancer and who are looking for success in this field, they at least can have the assurance that everything that can be done by government, everything that can be done by voluntary agencies in this great, powerful, rich country, now will be done and that will give some hope, and we hope those hopes will not be disappointed. (Nixon, 1971b)

According to the written statement issued by the president upon signing the bill into law, the genesis of the National Cancer Act was his State of the Union message in January 1971 in which he called upon the Congress "to launch an unprecedented attack against cancer" (Nixon, 1971c). The National Cancer Act created the three-member President's Cancer Panel to oversee the newly expanded National Cancer Program, authorized an additional $100 million in research funding, provided authority for the president to name the head of the NCI, granted the NCI director the ability to submit the budget directly to the President, bypassing (to become known in the vernacular as the *NCI Bypass Budget*) the usual channels of the budget bureaucracy of the then-Department of Health, Education, and Welfare (now Health and Human Services) (Nixon, 1971c). Nixon spoke of these components as putting in "place the full weight of the Presidency behind the national cancer program" and allowing the president to "take personal command of the Federal effort to conquer cancer so that its activities need not be stymied by the familiar dangers of bureaucracy and red tape" (Nixon, 1971c).

Following the passage of the 1971 National Cancer Act, Congress appropriated $337.5 million in fiscal year 1972 to NCI. Funding was designated to three major categories—$142.8 million for grants, $178.7 million for direct operations (including intramural collaborative studies), and $16 million for construction. By 1974, appropriations to NCI had increased to $551.1 million, an increase of 63% from fiscal year 1972. Funding for NCI increased steadily, topping $1 billion for the first time in fiscal year 1984; $2 billion in fiscal year 1994; $3 billion in fiscal year 1999; $4 billion in fiscal year 2002; and $5 billion in fiscal year 2010. However, because of federal budgetary constraints, annual appropriations for NCI have been relatively flat since fiscal year 2004 (NCI Office of Budget and Finance, 2012).

It is important to note that each year since enactment of the 1971 National Cancer Act, NCI has been required to prepare a plan and corresponding budget, which is submitted directly to the President for consideration in determining the Congressional budget request (NCI Office of Budget and Finance, 2013). As noted previously, the report is better known as the *bypass budget*, named so because it bypasses the traditional NIH Institute or Center process. This bypass budget and plan (also known as the Professional Judgment Budget) together describe the resources the agency needs in order to undertake activities for "building on research successes, supporting the cancer research workforce with the technologies and resources it needs, and ensuring that research discoveries are applied to improve human health" (NCI Office of Budget and Finance, 2013, para. 1). Each year, the budget and plan are made available to the public, which gives researchers, policy makers, and advocates significant insight into the operations and vision of the agency. Virtually no other federal agency has the authority to bring its budget request and plan for the coming fiscal year into the public domain. This transparency can serve the agency well for those who approve of the plans and requests, but it also can put the agency under greater scrutiny if advocates or policy makers disagree with what is presented. Traditionally, a number of advocacy organizations, including the National Coalition for Cancer Research, use the official agency request contained in the bypass budget as the baseline for determining their own NCI federal funding requests to submit to Congress during the annual appropriations process.

Tobacco Control Policy

It is generally acknowledged that the Surgeon General's landmark report of 1964 was a watershed moment in federal public health policy by linking smoking to adverse health consequences. The report placed the dangers of smoking squarely in the public, but another two decades passed before a lesser-known but equally compelling and important study by the National Research Council was released. The report, titled *The Airliner Cabin Environ-*

ment: Air Quality and Safety (National Research Council Committee on Airliner Cabin Air Quality, 1986), found that "a flight attendant working full-time is receiving an integrated exposure . . . approximately equal to that associated with living with a 1.0-pack/d smoker" (p. 146) and recommended "a ban on smoking on all domestic commercial flights" (p. 151). According to Americans for Nonsmokers' Rights (2005), following the release of the report, a grassroots advocacy campaign to ban smoking on airplanes was launched. U.S. Secretary of Transportation Elizabeth Dole, serving in the cabinet of President Reagan, did not accept the National Research Council's recommendation and stated that the issue is "best left to the marketplace" ("Study Expected to Urge Smoking Ban," 1986). However, the ban enjoyed broad support from the public health community, and its passage was supported by organizations such as Americans for Nonsmokers' Rights, the American Cancer Society, the American Lung Association, the American Public Health Association, the American Medical Association, and the American Heart Association (Holm & Davis, 2004). Other supporters included then-U.S. Surgeon General C. Everett Koop, who commissioned a clinical study of flight attendants' exposure to passive smoke (Cimons, 1987). In January 1987, Koop went on record as saying, "It's my suspicion that a young lady who works in the smoking end of a plane in the galley is probably 'smoking' three or four cigarettes a flight . . . just by inhaling the passive smoke" (as cited in Cimons, 1987). His statements, coupled with the study he requested, were considered essential factors in securing support within the Congress (Cimons, 1987).

Then-U.S. Representative Richard Durbin (D-IL) was elected to the House of Representatives in 1982 and to the U.S. Senate in 1996, reelected in 2002 and 2008, and served as the Senate Majority Whip/Assistant Majority Leader through 2014. Durbin, motivated by his father's death from lung cancer, had been an anti-tobacco advocate for years. However, a personal experience in 1986 prompted him to take action to ban smoking on airplanes. When he was unable to get a seat in the nonsmoking section of a plane, he appealed to the gate agent, "Can't you do anything about it?" The gate agent looked at his ticket and said, "No, I can't, but you can, Congressman" (Scherer, 1989). So, in July 1987, Representative Durbin offered an amendment to the Federal Aviation Act of 1958 to ban smoking on domestic flights of two hours or less duration for a period of two years (Americans for Nonsmokers' Rights, 2005). The first ban was attached to a federal funding bill for the U.S. Department of Transportation; there was a great deal of procedural maneuvering. (For more information about how the initial and subsequent bans were secured, see Holm and Davis, 2004, available online at www.ncbi.nlm.nih.gov/pmc/articles/PMC1766149/pdf/v013p00i30.pdf.)

In the Senate, the provision was championed and passed as a result of the advocacy of U.S. Senator Frank Lautenberg (D-NJ), also a long-standing antismoking advocate (Pagan, 2009). Despite significant opposition from the tobacco lobby, in 1988 President Reagan signed the airline smoking ban into law and the provision became effective on April 23, 1988 (Americans for Nonsmokers' Rights, 2005). In October 1988, in an open letter, Durbin attributed the smoke-free policy's success to "strong grassroots support" and stated that "hard work on the local level is what led to an unprecedented public health victory in Congress" (Americans for Nonsmokers' Rights, 2005).

Building on this initial success and the growing popularity of the ban among the nonsmoking and smoking public, members of Congress, again under the leadership of Congressman Durbin in the House of Representatives and with the support of the medical and public health advocacy communities, took action in 1989 by passing H.R. 160, which made the ban permanent on flights of two hours or less; therefore, no subsequent reauthorization was required (Americans for Nonsmokers' Rights, 2005). Following the House action, on the Senate side, again with Senator Lautenberg as the lead champion, an amendment passed that banned smoking on all domestic airline flights of six hours or less (Pagan, 2009). The amendment, again facing vigorous opposition from the tobacco lobby, was filibustered, and the Senate invoked a parliamentary procedure known as *cloture* to end floor debate and move to a final vote (Pagan, 2009). Despite these challenges, the amendment passed, and in November 1989, President George H.W. Bush signed legislation into law, making all domestic flights of six hours or less smoke-free (the provision subsequently became effective in February 1990) (Americans for Nonsmokers' Rights, 2005). Following these federal legislative actions, numerous airlines—both domestic and international— voluntarily adopted smoke-free policies for all domestic and trans-Atlantic flights (Americans for Nonsmokers' Rights, 2005). The final chapter in federal smoke-free airline policy occurred in 2000, when President Clinton enacted the Wendell H. Ford Aviation Investment and Reform Act for the 21st Century (2000), which contained a provision to make all flights between the United States and foreign destinations 100% smoke-free (Americans for Nonsmokers' Rights, 2005).

Although federal policy made the skies a safer place to fly, advocates had been pushing for other ways to reduce the adverse public health impact of tobacco. In May 1994, Mississippi Attorney General Michael Moore filed a suit against the tobacco industry to recover $940 billion the state claimed its Medicaid program had paid to provide health care to treat citizens who had used tobacco products. This was the first of many such state suits alleging that the damaging health complications of tobacco use had created a large systemic increase in states' Medicaid health spending. Toward the end of 1994, attorneys general for Minnesota, West Virginia, and Florida followed with similar legal action against the tobacco industry. In 1996, the Liggett Group reached a settlement with 67 private firms and five states suing the industry. In 1997, Philip Morris Chief Executive Officer Geoffrey Bible, RJR Nabisco Chief Executive Officer Steven Goldstone, and their attorneys met with the attorneys general of the more than 20 states that had filed suit by that time to discuss national settlement terms. One of the largest individual settlements with a state was for $3.4 billion with Mississippi in 1997. The Texas attorney general also filed suit, bringing the total to more than 40 states (Frontline, 1998b).

In the midst of growing legal action by the states on behalf of their respective Medicaid programs, the Clinton administration and Congress were preparing legislation to address the public health issues caused by tobacco products. In 1998, Senator John McCain (R-AZ), then chair of the Senate Commerce Committee, with the support and involvement of the public health community introduced comprehensive tobacco-control legislation with a wide range of provisions, new regulations, and programs to reduce the scourge of tobacco use on American society. The bill, the National Tobacco Policy and Youth Smoking Reduction Act (1998), included broad regulation of the tobacco industry, including specific restrictions on tobacco product advertising targeted at youth; requirements for new tobacco product warnings, labels, and packaging; an increase in the federal tobacco excise tax (due to long-standing evidence that as the price of tobacco increases, purchase and consumption decrease); and efforts to reduce tobacco smuggling. The bill also established a National Smoking Cessation Program, a Tobacco-Free Education Board, and a National Tobacco-Free Public Education Program—initiatives targeted at discouraging people from starting tobacco use and encouraging current users to quit (Congressional Research Service, 1998). During a 1998 PBS *Frontline* interview, Senator McCain asserted the importance of public health advocacy involvement in the drafting of the legislation: "These advocacy groups, the American Lung Association, the National Cancer Society, all of these other organizations. . . . They're there at the table. They're in constant consultation with us. They've testified at the hearings. They will be, to some degree anyway, the arbiters or the referees as to whether this is good for America or not" (Frontline, 1998a). Illustrating his point, during a Senate Commerce Committee hearing on the proposed tobacco bill, the American Cancer Society referred to young people using cigarettes as a "pediatric epidemic" and urged support for the legislative proposal as the remedy for this public health problem (Staff of Senate Committee on Commerce, Science, and Transportation, 1998).

While many of the provisions of the McCain tobacco-control legislation enjoyed support, the questions of whether to provide the tobacco industry with liability protection and whether to increase the federal tobacco excise tax would prove to be two of the major sticking points. The legislation was brought before the full Senate for consideration over the course of a month and an estimated 80 hours of floor time; the bill was debated, amended, and ultimately defeated by procedural votes. Typically, for most legislation, 60 votes are needed to move proposals forward for a final vote. The vote was 57–42 to limit the floor debate and to proceed toward final consideration of the measure. With three votes shy of the threshold necessary to vote on S. 1415, in July 1998, the public health community's hopes of comprehensive tobacco legislation died along with the measure (Cancer Network, 1998).

With the federal legislative arena no longer an option for action, the states' attorneys general moved forward to craft a Master Settlement Agreement (MSA) with the tobacco industry. In November 1998, attorneys general from 46 states, five U.S. territories, and the District of Columbia joined together as parties to an agreement with the nation's largest tobacco companies (Brown & Williamson Tobacco Corporation, R.J. Reynolds Tobacco Company, Lorillard Inc., and Philip Morris) regarding

the advertising, marketing and promotion of tobacco products. In addition to requiring the tobacco industry to pay the settling states approximately $10 billion annually for the indefinite future, the MSA also set standards for, and imposed restrictions on, the sale and marketing of cigarettes by participating cigarette manufacturers. (Public Health Law Center, n.d.)

Another public health component of the MSA is Legacy (originally called American Legacy Foundation), a nonprofit organization based in Washington, DC, charged with undertaking tobacco-control research and public health education and advertising programs. According to the official history of the organization, "the states requested that a portion of the money they received from the tobacco industry be used to establish and fund an organization primarily dedicated to studying and providing public education about the impact of tobacco in order to reduce its use and associated death and disease" (Legacy, n.d.). Since 1999, the organization has undertaken numerous initiatives to reduce the adverse societal impact of tobacco, including launching the award-winning Truth® youth smoking prevention campaign. Legacy's efforts have been effective in reducing tobacco use among children, youth, and young adults (Legacy, n.d.).

While the MSA helped advance tobacco-control efforts, the public health community remained steadfast in its commitment to seek federal legislation to secure U.S. Food and Drug Administration (FDA) regulation of tobacco. This tenacity and focus culminated on June 22, 2009, when President Obama signed the Family Smoking Prevention and Tobacco Control Act (U.S. FDA, 2014b). The law, advocated by organizations such as the Oncology Nursing Society, the American Cancer Society, the American Public Health Association, and the National Association of County and City Health Officials, granted broad and specific authority to FDA "to regulate the manufacture, distribution, and marketing of tobacco products to protect public health" (U.S. FDA, 2014b), finally enacting many of the types of regulatory restrictions and requirements that the Mc-Cain legislation included a decade earlier. Advocacy efforts were not limited to groups in favor of the legislation. In fact, some entities opposed the legislation on the basis that it was a presumptive attack on the First Amendment. Following the bill's enactment, the Association of National Advertisers filed an amicus or "friend of the court" brief in the Western District of Kentucky, joining six major tobacco companies in challenging the constitutionality of the act. The American Association of Advertising Agencies and the American Advertising Federation also joined the brief (Association of National Advertisers, 2009). Ultimately, the advocates for the Tobacco Control Act and the government prevailed when the Sixth Circuit Court of Appeals ruled that "the 2009 Family Smoking Prevention and Tobacco Control Act (Pub. L. No. 111-31, 123 Stat. 1776 [2009]) does not violate the companies' First Amendment right against compelled speech" in a similar case (Lefkowitz, 2012). The FDA's Center for Tobacco Products oversees implementation of the act. FDA's responsibilities include "setting performance standards, reviewing premarket applications for new and modified risk tobacco products, requiring new warning labels, and establishing and enforcing advertising and promotion restrictions" (U.S. FDA, 2014a).

With federal regulatory authority over tobacco products finally achieved and helping to reduce tobacco use, public health advocates continue to seek other effective ways to prevent tobacco use, particularly among children and youth. Tobacco excise taxes at both the state and federal levels continue to be a favorite mechanism of the public health community to reduce tobacco consumption, decrease healthcare costs associated with tobacco use, and increase revenue for tobacco-control efforts. The World Health Organization (n.d.) has cited tobacco price increases, including consumption taxes, as "the most potent and cost-effective option for governments everywhere" in reducing tobacco use. On April 1, 2009, according to the Centers for Disease Control and Prevention's (CDC's) *Morbidity and Mortality Weekly Report*, "the largest federal cigarette excise tax increase in history went into effect, bringing the combined federal and average state excise tax for cigarettes to $2.21 per pack" (CDC, 2009, para. 1). Furthermore, a 10% increase in the real price of cigarette packs can reduce total consumption by almost 4% (CDC, 2009) and youth consumption by about 7% (Campaign for Tobacco-Free Kids, n.d.). As such, the public health and tobacco-control communities consider these taxes to be an important component to preventing and reducing tobacco use and, in turn, decreasing the adverse public health effects associated with tobacco. While the current federal political environment is not favorable to an increase in the federal tobacco tax, public health advocates continue to seek tobacco tax increases at the state level (Campaign for Tobacco-Free Kids, n.d.). Chapter 18 provides additional discussion of policy related to tobacco cessation and control.

Medicare Coverage of Cancer-Related Care

The Medicare program, created in 1965, traditionally has provided coverage for treatment of healthcare problems, and for the most part Congress has maintained a general statutory ban on reimbursement for most services associated with prevention or early detection of disease. Changes to the Medicare program have been made through numerous legislative approaches, including stand-alone legislation; provisions as part of a broader package affecting the underlying Social Security Amendments of 1965, which created the Medicare program (Social Security Administration, n.d.); and as part of an otherwise seemingly arcane Congressional procedure known as *budget reconciliation* (Krutz, 2001). Budget reconciliation has been used consistently over the past three decades to enact changes to the Medicare program with respect to cancer care. To that end, Glen Krutz, author of *Hitching a Ride: Omnibus Legislating in the U.S. Congress*, found that "every single budget reconciliation bill enacted from 1980 to 1994 contained healthcare policy provisions. Almost all reconciliation bills contained what many health policy experts would likely consider significant changes" (p. 108). Budget reconciliation is the process by which Congress—through policy-authorizing committees such as the Senate Finance Committee and the House Ways and Means Committee (the two committees that have jurisdiction and authority to create tax policy)—creates a legislative measure that meets (or "reconciles") the tax and spending targets outlined in a Congressional budget resolution, which has been approved by both chambers. Individual committees create their respective legislative measures, and they are woven together into a single proposal known as an *omnibus bill*. Because a budget reconciliation bill contains legislative language to modify taxes and change spending levels for federal programs, these measures serve as a natural vehicle for other program alterations (known sometimes as "policy riders," as they hitch a ride on another bill).

In 1983, a Congress controlled in both houses by the Democrats worked with President Reagan to enact the Social Security Amendments of 1983 (University of Texas, Ronald Reagan Presidential Library and Museum, 1983). Among myriad other policy changes, the legislation created a new mechanism for Medicare reimbursement for inpatient care, known as the inpatient prospective payment system (IPPS) (Office of Inspector General, Office of Evaluation and Inspections, 2001). Importantly, the legislation included language that initially exempted four cancer centers from the new payment system, under which hospitals are paid a fixed amount for each patient based on the patient's particular condition, categorized as a specific diagnosis-related group, or DRG (Alliance of Dedicated Cancer Centers, 2011; Centers for Medicare and Medicaid Services [CMS], 2012, 2014). This change was in response to policymaker and cancer advocate concerns that moving from a cost-based payment system to a prospective payment system would leave certain cancer centers without the resources they needed to maintain their efforts in cancer research (Alliance of Dedicated Cancer Centers, 2011). An additional four cancer centers subsequently were excluded from the Medicare IPPS based on the initial implementing 1984 legislation (CMS, 2012). Three more cancer hospitals were excluded from the payment system in 1989, 1997, and 1999—with the 1989 and 1997 changes achieved through budget reconciliation and the 1999 change included in the Miscellaneous Appropriations Act of 2001, through which Congress "enacted on a permanent basis, a 'hold harmless' floor on the Centers' payments under the new outpatient prospective payment system (OPPS)" (Alliance of Dedicated Cancer Centers, 2011; Consolidated Appropriations Act of 2001).

The Omnibus Budget Reconciliation Act of 1989 contained numerous provisions pertaining to cancer policy, including new coverage of Pap smears for some female Medicare beneficiaries to be screened for cervical cancer, effective July 1, 1990 (CMS, 2009; Omnibus Budget Reconciliation Act of 1989). This addition of Pap smear coverage to the Medicare program marked an important turning point for Medicare payment policy, moving the program more into the prevention and early detection sphere. Further, the Omnibus Budget Reconciliation Act of 1989 also contained an exemption for certain "hospitals involved extensively in cancer treatment or cancer research from the prospective payment system" and created a "formula for establishing the target amount to be used in determining the amounts of payments to be made to such hospitals" (Congressional Research Service, 1989, Title VI). This precedent laid the foundation for future cancer advocacy efforts during consideration of the Omnibus Budget Reconciliation Act of 1993 and the Balanced Budget Act of 1997, which established coverage for pelvic examinations and increased frequency of Pap smears for high-risk women.

In the Omnibus Budget Reconciliation Act of 1993, under a section titled "Oral Cancer Drugs," Congress provided Medicare coverage to self-administered chemotherapeutic oral anticancer therapies that have the same active ingredient as drugs previously available and covered by Medicare in injectable or IV forms. In addition, the act included statutory language to clarify and provide uniform Medicare coverage for off-label uses of anticancer therapies. Although FDA has the authority to determine whether a drug is safe and effective, the agency generally cannot limit the conditions for which the drug is prescribed and used in the practice of medicine. *Off-label* use of a prescription drug or device refers to the ability of licensed healthcare providers to prescribe or use the drug for indications, conditions, patients, dosages, or routes of administration not yet evaluated and approved by FDA (American Cancer Society, 2013; U.S. FDA, 2011). In 1993, relatively few anticancer therapies were available. However, emerging science showed that certain anticancer drugs were effective in managing forms of cancer beyond those included in the FDA-approved labeling. Members of Congress learned that Medicare coverage for off-label uses was being inconsistently applied by contractors, who, absent a national coverage determination, decide whether services are reasonable and necessary and therefore covered under Medicare (American Cancer Society, 2013; CMS Medicare Payment Advisory Commission, 2003). The Omnibus Budget Reconciliation Act of 1993 provision made it clear that Medicare would cover FDA-approved drugs

> used appropriately in an anticancer chemotherapeutic regimen for a medically accepted indication, regardless of whether the drug has been approved by the FDA specifically for such use, as long as such use is supported either by clinical evidence in peer reviewed medical literature or by one or more of three specified major medical compendia. (Congressional Research Service, 1993, Subpart E: Other Provisions)

In 1997, Congress worked with President Clinton to craft a balanced budget deal. One area that enjoyed some bipartisan support was the expansion of Medicare coverage for certain cancer-related benefits and services. The Balanced Budget Act of 1997 contained a section titled "Prevention Initiatives," which outlined new Medicare coverage and payment policies for annual screening mammography for women older than age 39, triennial screening Pap smear and pelvic examinations for all women (annually for women with cervical or vaginal cancer or at high risk for developing such a cancer), annual prostate cancer screening tests for men older than age 50, and annual colorectal cancer screening tests for people older than age 50 (O'Sullivan et al., 1997). For years, the American Cancer Society, working alongside other national organizations such as the American Gastroenterological Association, the Crohn's and Colitis Foundation of America, and the United Ostomy Association, pushed Congress to expand Medicare coverage for colorectal and other cancer screening-related services and successfully secured coverage with the waiver of any deductible (National Task Force on CME Provider/Industry Collaboration, n.d.). The Balanced Budget Act of 1997 also included expanded coverage of certain oral cancer drugs, including antinausea drugs used as part of cancer treatment (Bagley & McVearry, 1998; Balanced Budget Act of 1997; O'Sullivan et al., 1997).

The majority of the Medicare cancer-related provisions that were contained in the final Balanced Budget Act of 1997 had been introduced as stand-alone, bipartisan legislation in previous years and past sessions of Congress. For example, Senator John Chafee (R-RI) introduced the Cancer Screening and Prevention Act of 1995 (S. 1178) to provide Medicare coverage of "prevention and early detection of colorectal cancer services" (Cancer Screening and Prevention Act of 1995, p. S12275). The senator introduced the bill on behalf of himself and a bipartisan group of five senators: Connie Mack (R-FL), Strom Thurmond (R-SC), Claiborne Pell (D-RI), Dale Bumpers (D-AR), and Joseph Lieberman (D-CT). That same year, then-Representative (now U.S. Senator) Ben Cardin (D-MD) introduced the Medicare Preventive Benefits Improvement Act of 1995 (H.R. 2777), which would have amended Medicare by adding new preventive benefits including but not limited to mammography, screening Pap smears, colorectal cancer screening, and prostate cancer screening, in addition to a number of noncancer-related services (Introduction of the Medicare Preventive Benefits Improvement Act, 1995). The Cardin bill garnered a group of 36 cosponsors, including a number of Republicans, such as then-Representative (now Senator) Tom Coburn (R-OK). Building on this previous bicameral and bipartisan Congressional interest, President Clinton, in his February 1997 State of the Union speech, informed Congress that his Medicare plan (as provided for in his budget for the coming fiscal year) would "fully pay for annual mammograms" ("State of the Union Address by the President of the United States," 1997). As such, the president set the stage for Medicare coverage for breast cancer screening, along with other cancer early detection services, to be included in the Balanced Budget Act of 1997, which would be crafted later in the year. The previous bipartisan support and interest in expanding Medicare coverage of cancer screening, coupled with leadership from the president, paved the way for the inclusion of such benefits in the final Balanced Budget Act of 1997.

Department of Defense Congressionally Directed Medical Research Programs

Seeing the success of those involved in the HIV/AIDS movement, in the late 1980s, women affected by breast cancer began their own grassroots advocacy effort to garner greater federal attention to and funding of breast cancer research (Bardin, 2012; Hughes, 2013; Riter, 2014). Following societal changes in the 1970s, when it became acceptable to discuss breast cancer in public, the late 1980s and 1990s saw a shift toward women demanding greater investment in their health and well-being, with a particular focus on breast cancer (Riter, 2014). Key players in the movement included Fran Visco, first president of the National Breast Cancer Coalition; Rose Kushner, author of the book *Why Me? What Every Woman Should Know About Breast Cancer to Save Her Life*; and the model Matuschka, who in 1993 showed her mastectomy scar on the cover of the *New York Times Magazine*, bringing the disfigurement of breast cancer into the public's view and consciousness (Kolata, 1990; Riter, 2014). A 1997 Institute of Medicine report credited the National Breast Cancer Coalition for the successful creation of the first major breast cancer funding earmark, stating, "A massive grassroots and lobbying effort, coordinated by the National Breast Cancer Coalition, resulted in a $210 million appropriation for a peer-reviewed breast cancer research program in the 1993 Department of Defense budget" (Institute of Medicine, 1997, p. v). The National Breast Cancer Coalition, founded in 1991 by a group of breast cancer survivors, shares the credit on its website with Congressional champions Senators Tom Harkin (D-IA) and Alfonse D'Amato (R-NY) (National Breast Cancer Coalition, 2013b). This grassroots effort also led to the creation of the Department of Defense Congressionally Directed Medical Research Programs in 1992 (CDMRP) (U.S. Department of Defense CDMRP, 2013a). The federal fiscal year 1993 appropriation was an almost 10-fold increase in breast cancer program funds, and as part of the funding, Congress required the Department of Defense to conduct external peer review for the funded projects (Institute of Medicine, 1997). This initial funding, coupled with subsequent federal appropriations, has been used to "support peer-reviewed scientific research focusing on the causes, prevention, detection, treatment, and outcome of breast cancer" (Institute of Medicine, 1997, p. 18).

Subsequently, Congress expanded the CDMRP to include additional cancer sites, including chronic myeloid leukemia (CML), lung cancer, ovarian cancer, and prostate cancer. In 1997, with a group of prostate cancer advocates under the leadership of Senator Ted Stevens (R-AK), Congress provided $45 million to support the first prostate cancer–specific funding at the Department of Defense (U.S. Department of Defense CDMRP, 2010). That same year, due to the steadfast advocacy of Representative Rosa DeLauro (D-CT) and ovarian cancer advocates, Congress provided an initial $7.5 million to create an ovarian cancer research program (Baird, 2010; U.S. Department of Defense CDMRP, 2013b). In federal fiscal year 2002, Representative Jerry Lewis (R-CA), then a senior member of the House Appropriations Committee whose brother died of CML, led the effort to have Congress create the Chronic Myelogenous Leukemia Research Program and worked to secure funding for it from fiscal years 2002 to 2006 (a total of $22.05 million for the effort) (U.S. Department of Defense CDMRP, n.d.). In fiscal year 2009, Congress provided $20 million to the Department of Defense to initiate the Lung Cancer Research Program (U.S. Department of Defense CDMRP, 2012a). That same year, Congress also established the Peer Reviewed Cancer Research Program to support research in cancers that Congress designates as relevant to military service members and their families because of military members' exposure to hazardous environments due to the nature of their service and deployments that place them at risk for developing different types of cancers (U.S. Department of Defense CDMRP, 2012b). In total, since its inception through the current federal fiscal year, the CDMRP has expanded to include other disease states and has received a total of $8.22 billion (U.S. Department of Defense CDMRP, 2014).

Many people understandably wonder why and how cancer research programs were established at the Department of Defense. Together, the Balanced Budget and Emergency Deficit Control Act of 1985, known more popularly as Gramm-Rudman-Hollings (named for the three senators who led the effort), the Balanced Budget and Emergency Deficit Control Reaffirmation Act of 1987, and the Budget Enforcement Act of 1990 created a budgetary environment in the early 1990s in which federal discretionary spending was significantly constrained and any new spending was required to be offset with revenue legislation (Lynch, 2011). Therefore, boosting discretionary research spending at NIH and NCI was exceedingly difficult. Moreover, members of Congress and scientists within the federal government became increasingly reluctant to earmark NIH spending for a particular disease or condition. The Department of Defense has long maintained a strong biomedical and clinical research operation focusing on combat- and service-related healthcare needs, such as wound care, infectious disease, limb loss, paralysis, and post-traumatic stress disorder (U.S. Department of Defense Military Health System, n.d.). With a robust Department of Defense research program as a foundation—coupled with spending caps and firewalls between discretionary and mandatory spending and non-defense and defense spending—members of Congress and advocates recognized an opportunity to boost biomedical research spending in a creative and effective manner. By creating cancer-related research programs at the Department of Defense, Congress earmarked federal funding for specific diseases and expanded the agency's biomedical research portfolio with a focus on site-specific cancers.

Centers for Disease Control and Prevention Breast and Cervical Cancer Programs

CDC maintains a robust cancer prevention and control program with efforts spanning numerous cancer sites, including colorectal cancer, skin cancer, prostate cancer, and ovarian cancer, as well as cancer survivorship. However, many of these initiatives have not been authorized by Congress through specific statutes but rather have been created and maintained through the annual appropriations measures and the broad authority provided to CDC under the Public Health Service Act (CDC, 2014b; Mensah et al., 2004).

As part of the breast cancer advocacy movement of the 1990s, Representative Henry Waxman (D-CA) introduced the Breast and Cervical Cancer Mortality Prevention Act of 1990. The legislation (P.L. 101-354) was enacted to establish CDC's National Breast and Cervical Cancer Early Detection Program (NBCCEDP) (CDC NBCCEDP, 2013). The act stemmed from a series of government findings that certain women, particularly older, low-income women and members of racial and ethnic minority populations, were not receiving breast and cervical cancer screening and therefore were needlessly suffering from advanced-stage cancers. For example, a January 1990 study by the General Accounting Office (now the Government Accountability Office) found that approximately 60% of American women older than 40 had never had a mammogram (U.S. General Accounting Office, 1990). The report also concluded that only approximately 9.2% of women with household incomes of less than $10,000 had a mammogram during the previous year (U.S. General Accounting Office, 1990). Furthermore, the report found wide variations for fees charged for mammograms, ranging from $50 to more than $150, with an average charge of $104 (U.S. General Accounting Office, 1990). At the time, the Pap smear was recognized as the universal screening tool for cervical cancer in asymptomatic women. Yet, according to a 1990 Office of Technology Assessment study, only slightly more than half of older adult women had had a Pap smear within the past three years (U.S. Congress Office of Technology Assessment, 1990).

In addition to providing breast and cervical cancer screening, the grant program included appropriate treatment referrals for women screened, created educational initiatives, improved training of health professionals, and established mechanisms to monitor the quality of screening procedures and surveillance mechanisms (CDC NBCCEDP, 2013). To receive federal grant funding, states were required to provide $1 of matching contributions for every $3 of federal funds (CDC NBCCEDP, 2013). The program provided both a physical examination of the breasts and screening mammography (CDC NBCCEDP, 2013). For cervical cancer screening, both a pelvic examination and a Pap smear were required. Initially, $50 million in funding was authorized for the program in fiscal year 1991, with "such sums as may be necessary" in both fiscal years 1992 and 1993 (Breast and Cervical Cancer Mortality Prevention Act of 1990). The legislation was approved unanimously by the House of Representatives and the Senate and was signed into law by President George H.W. Bush on August 10, 1990.

In 1991, CDC provided funding for implementation of the program in eight states, with four additional states added in 1992 (CDC NBCCEDP, 2014). That same year, CDC provided funding to 18 more states to build capacity to implement the screening programs (CDC NBCCEDP, 2014). In 1993, Congress unanimously passed the Preventive Health Amendments of 1993 (P.L. 103-183) to expand the program to provide direct grant funding to American Indian and Native Alaskan tribes and tribal organizations (Preventive Health Amendments of 1993). The legislation directed that priority be given to states with high rates of breast and cervical cancer incidence and mortality (Preventive Health Amendments of 1993). It also established a coordinating committee that was charged with coordinating the efforts of all agencies of the Public Health Service to achieve the objectives established by the secretary of Health and Human Services for reductions in the mortality rate from breast and cervical cancer in the United States by 2000 (Preventive Health Amendments of 1993). By 1997, NBCCEDP funding was provided to 50 states, the District of Columbia, 5 territories, and 13 tribes or tribal organizations. Case management services were added as an allowable component of programmatic funding in 1998 (Ryerson, Benard, & Major, n.d.; Women's Preventive Health Amendments of 1993). Participation in the program grew steadily (Ryerson et al., n.d.). In its first year (1991–1992), 38,476 women had received an initial or at least one subsequent mammogram. During that same period, 62,842 women received an initial or at least one subsequent Pap smear. In 1995, 145,614 women received mammograms and 175,190 women received Pap smears. In 1977, the first year in which the program was operational in all 50 states, 225,198 women were screened for breast cancer, while 224,525 were screened for cervical cancer. By 2000, the number of women receiving mammograms was 234,887, and 257,376 had received Pap smears (Ryerson et al., n.d.).

The Breast and Cervical Cancer Mortality Prevention Act of 1990 required that states provide appropriate referrals of women screened through the program for medical treatment and follow-up services (CDC NBCCEDP, 2014; Ryerson et al., n.d.). At the time the bill was passed, however, the House Committee on Energy and Commerce and breast cancer advocates expressed concern that those women who required follow-up treatment would go unserved, given that the program, at the time, did not include funding for treatment for those found to have cancer. The committee, in its report to accompany the legislation, stated its intention that "grantees take all appropriate measures to ensure provision of services required by women who have abnormal screening results" (CDC, 1998, p. 217).

In 1996, CDC began a case study to determine how early detection programs in seven participating states (California, Michigan, Minnesota, New Mexico, New York, North Carolina, and Texas) identified resources and obtained diagnostic and treatment services (CDC, 1998). Respondents in these states reported that treatment had been initiated for almost all NBCCEDP clients in whom cancer was diagnosed. However, respondents also expressed concern that the strategies used to obtain these services as short-term solutions were labor intensive and diverted resources away from screening activities. Survey respondents reported that the lack of coverage for diagnostic and treatment services negatively affected recruitment of providers and restricted the number of women screened. Furthermore, respondents believed that, because of changes in the healthcare system, an increasing number of physicians would not have the autonomy to offer free or reduced-fee services to NBCCEDP clients (CDC, 1998).

In response, breast cancer and other advocacy organizations, such as the National Breast Cancer Coalition and the American Cancer Society, began an effort to secure treatment through the federal Medicaid program for women diagnosed with breast or cervical cancer through the NBCCEDP (National Breast Cancer Coalition, 2013a). In March 1999, the Breast and Cervical Cancer Prevention and Treatment Act of 2000 (H.R. 1070/S. 662) was introduced in the House of Representatives by Representative Rick Lazio (R-NY) and Senator John Chafee (R-RI). The legislation garnered strong bipartisan support, with 317 House cosponsors and 76 Senate cosponsors. Although members of Congress expressed concerns about creating disease-specific Medicaid eligibility categories, Congress concluded that the new Medicaid eligibility category was unique because it specifically was linked to an existing federal screening program (Breast and Cervical Cancer Treatment Act, S. Rep. No. 106-323, 2000). In the accompanying report, the Senate Committee on Finance, which has jurisdiction over the Medicaid program, stressed that the Medicaid expansion "shall not be viewed as a precedent for extending Medicaid eligibility body-part by body-part" (Breast and Cervical Cancer Treatment Act, S. Rep. No. 106-323, 2000, section B, para. 3).

After nearly a decade, breast cancer advocates successfully secured enactment of the Breast and Cervical Cancer Prevention and Treatment Act of 2000, which established a new optional categorically needy coverage group under Medicaid (Breast and Cervical Cancer Prevention and Treatment Act of 2000). Eligible individuals included women who were younger than 65, had been screened under the CDC's NBCCEDP, and needed treatment for breast or cervical cancer. The legislation also included an "enhanced match" for states that opted to participate in the treatment program (Breast and Cervical Cancer Prevention and Treatment Act of 2000). Medicaid, a federal-state matching program, has its share of program payments determined by the federal medical assistance percentage, which is based on a formula that considers the state's per capita income compared to the national average. As originally introduced, the legislation would have provided for a 75% federal matching rate for Medicaid services provided. However, because of budgetary constraints, the final legislation used an existing matching rate structure used for the State Children's Health Insurance Program, which averaged a 68% federal to 32% state match rate (compared to the Medicaid average match of 57% federal to 43% state) (Breast and Cervical Cancer Prevention and Treatment Act of 2000).

The House of Representatives approved the legislation on May 9, 2000, by a vote of 421–1; H.R. 1070 and S. 662 were subsequently merged into a new bill, H.R. 4386, introduced by Representative Sue Myrick (R-NC), a breast cancer survivor. On October 4, 2000, the Senate approved the legislation unanimously, and it was signed into law by President Clinton on October 24, 2000 (Breast and Cervical Cancer Prevention and Treatment Act of 2000).

Given the states' role in the Medicaid program, as well as providing funding for public health education and awareness programs, since the inception of the NBCCEDP, numerous cancer advocacy organizations and oncology professional societies have engaged in state-level advocacy efforts to encourage state investment in the program, as well as to provide expanded Medicaid access for women who need access to treatment.

The impact and effectiveness of the NBCCEDP has been significant. Since 1991, NBCCEDP-funded programs have served more than 4.3 million women, provided more than 10.7 million breast and cervical cancer screening examinations, and diagnosed more than 56,662 breast cancers, 3,206 invasive cervical cancers, and 152,470 premalignant cervical lesions, of which 41% were high-grade (CDC NBCCEDP, 2014).

With the advent of the Patient Protection and Affordable Care Act (ACA) in 2010 and expanded access to health insurance coverage through state exchanges and those states opting to expand their Medicaid programs, the future role and scope of the NBCCEDP has been discussed and debated among policy makers in Congress and staff at CDC and the Office of Management and Budget, as well as within the advocacy community. If the promise of the ACA comes to fruition, policy makers and advocates anticipate that many of the women served by the NBCCEDP will have health insurance and therefore should have access to breast and cervical cancer screening and treatment. However, because many states have not adopted the Medicaid expansion and some individuals will opt not to purchase insurance, the nation will continue to have a significant uninsured population. According to a Commonwealth Fund study and results of the National Health Interview Survey, the number of people with health insurance has increased since enactment of the ACA; however, by early 2014, 40.7 million Americans remained uninsured (Collins & Rasmussen, 2014).

Despite the persistent uninsured population, some elected officials believe that the need for the NBCCEDP has diminished and that its purpose of serving uninsured women will become obsolete. These policy makers have proposed reducing NBCCEDP funding and eventually phasing out the program. Yet, cancer community advocates and other members of Congress have asserted that the program and its funding should be maintained because uninsured women still will need breast and cervical cancer screening services, as well as cancer education and awareness information. Congress has allocated NBCCEDP funding in each of the federal fiscal years since the ACA was enacted; yet, as health reform is implemented further, funding for the program may be more difficult to sustain because of the perception among some that demand for the program will decrease. Cancer community advocates are working with elected officials and CDC to ensure the program reflects current and anticipated needs. These discussions include consideration of changes that could be made through program reauthorization. Given the difference of opinion and the changing landscape, the future scope of and funding for the NBCCEDP remains uncertain.

The 340B Drug Discount Program

To assist safety net providers and low-income patients with the increasing cost of prescription drugs, Congress established the 340B drug discount program as part of the Veterans Health Care Act of 1992.

The program requires drug manufacturers to sell their products to certain providers at the lowest price offered to other purchasers. The covered entities originally included federally qualified community health centers, critical access hospitals, sole community hospitals, rural referral centers, and nonprofit hospitals that provide a disproportionate share of care to Medicaid and uninsured patients.

Since the program's inception, the number of participating facilities and patients has grown rapidly. From 2005 to 2011, the number of hospitals in the 340B program grew from 591 to 1,673 (U.S. Government Accountability Office, 2011). Overall, the number of covered entity sites that participate in the program has increased from 8,605 in 2001 to 16,572 in 2011 (U.S. Government Accountability Office, 2011).

The ACA (P.L. 111-148 and P.L. 111-152) expanded the number of 340B-eligible entities, assuming they meet other programmatic requirements, for certain children's hospitals, freestanding cancer centers, critical access hospitals, rural referral centers, and sole community hospitals (Health Care and Education Reconciliation Act of 2010; Patient Protection and Affordable Care Act of 2010).

General agreement exists that the 340B drug discount program has significantly benefited safety net providers and low-income patients. However, because of the program's rapid growth, additional future oversight by the Health Resources and Services Administration (the federal agency that administers the program) and members of Congress is needed to ensure the program is meeting Congress's intent when the program was established in 1992.

Mammography Quality Standards Act of 1992

As part of the broader breast cancer advocacy movement of the 1990s, Congress enacted the Mammography Quality Standards Act (MQSA) of 1992, which subsequently was amended and reauthorized in 1998 and 2004 (American College of Radiology, n.d.). Before the MQSA was enacted, "an uneven and conflicting patchwork of standards for mammography jeopardized the technology and its efficacy. No national quality standards for personnel or equipment existed and the quality of mammograms varied widely" (Susan G. Komen Breast Cancer Foundation, 2004, p. 10). This challenge, coupled with public and provider concerns about patient safety and mammography screening quality and anecdotal stories of women not receiving the results of their mammograms in a timely fashion, led Congress to seek to create national standards to ensure high-quality mammography screening (American College of Radiology, n.d.; U.S. Senate Committee on Labor and Human Resources, Subcommittee on Aging, 1992).

The original version of the bill was introduced on October 1, 1991, by Representative Patricia Schroeder (D-CO) as the Breast Cancer Screening Safety Act of 1991 (H.R. 3462), and it eventually garnered a bipartisan group of 110 cosponsors. A hearing on the measure was held on June 5, 1992. Meanwhile, Senator Barbara Mikulski (D-MD) introduced the landmark Women's Health Equity Act of 1991, which included provisions to require the certification and accreditation of mammography facilities. On October 1, 1991, Senator Brock Adams (D-WA) introduced the MQSA companion measure, S. 1777, to H.R. 3462, and on October 24, 1991, secured a hearing on the measure before the Senate Labor and Human Resources Subcommittee on Aging (Congressional Research Service, 1992).

Subsequently, House Energy and Commerce Committee Chairman John Dingell (D-MI) took up the effort, and on September 15, 1992, introduced a modified version of the bill, now called the MQSA of 1992 (H.R. 5938). The bill was considered, amended, and reported out of the Energy and Commerce Committee by September 22, 1992, and two days later was passed by the House of Representatives by a vote of 390–18. It then went to the Senate for consideration. Meanwhile, on September 16, 1992, the Senate Committee on Labor and Human Resources (now called the Committee on Health, Education, Labor, and Pensions), under the leadership of Senator Edward Kennedy (D-MA), reported out a modified version of S. 1777. The bill, which eventually garnered 63 bipartisan cosponsors, was placed on the Senate calendar.

The versions of the House and Senate bills differed, and instead of convening a formal conference committee through which members of the House and Senate reconcile differences and create a single uniform measure, Representative Dingell and Senator Kennedy and their staff worked informally to create a consensus measure that could pass both chambers. This compromise bill became the MQSA of 1992 (H.R. 6182) and was introduced on October 6, 1992, by Representative Dingell. It passed the full House and Senate on October 6 and 7, respectively. The bill was signed by President George H.W. Bush on October 27, 1992, and became P.L. 102-539. The final bill contained numerous provisions, which, taken together, seek to "ensure that all women have access to quality mammography for the detection of breast cancer in its earliest, most treatable stages" (U.S. FDA, 2012). Specifically, the law requires facilities that perform or interpret mammograms to meet certain requirements for certification and creates standards for the safety and accuracy of mammograms (MQSA [P.L. 102-539], 1992). FDA maintains responsibility for implementing the MQSA and enforcing the accreditation and certification provisions of mammography facilities; final regulations promulgated by FDA established the national quality standards for mammography services (U.S. FDA, 2012).

Congress subsequently amended and reauthorized the MQSA in 1998 (P.L. 105-248) and 2004 (P.L. 108-365); both times, the measures were titled the "Mammography Quality Standards Reauthorization Act." MQSA reauthorization efforts have enjoyed broad bipartisan support and were advocated by numerous national organizations, including the American Cancer Society, Susan G. Komen, the National Alliance of Breast Cancer Organizations, and the American College of Radiology ("Statements on Introduced Bills and Joint Resolutions" [Senator Barbara Mikulski on S. 1879], 2003).

Efforts to Double the National Institutes of Health Budget

Prior to the now well-regarded and successful effort to double the NIH budget, which began in the late 1990s, individual diseases and causes would press Congress to fund their respective priorities—placing members of Congress in the unenviable position of having to "choose among their children." Moreover, many times this disease-specific effort pitted members against one another, put constituents at odds, and placed otherwise friendly communities in competition with one another over scarce resources. In response, in 1997, advocates and key bipartisan members of Congress identified a broad-based effort to bring everyone together around a mutually beneficial goal: doubling the NIH budget by 2003. On May 21, 1997, Senators Connie Mack (R-FL) and Dianne Feinstein (D-CA), joined by 16 bipartisan Senate cosponsors, proposed Amendment 315 to the Budget Resolution that it was the "sense of the Senate that . . . appropriations for the National Institutes of Health should be increased by 100 percent over the next 5 fiscal years" (Mack [and others] Amendment No. 315, 1997, para. (b)(1)). The nonbinding amendment passed by a vote of 98–0 (S. Amdt. 315, 1998). In an unprecedented fashion, this goal brought under one umbrella hundreds of organizations, medical and specialty societies, associations, and companies together with a bipartisan group of elected officials. In 1997, Senator Arlen Specter (then R-PA) spoke to the Ad Hoc Group for Medical Research and committed to providing a 7.5% increase for NIH in the coming federal fiscal year (fiscal year 1998) ("Specter Pledges [Again] to Boost NIH," 1997). At the time, Senators Specter and Tom Harkin (D-IA) served as the senior members of the Labor, Health and Human Services, Education, and Related Agencies Appropriations Subcommittee, which has jurisdiction over NIH funding. Hence, Specter's announcement demonstrated a real commitment to making the objective to double the NIH budget over five years a reality. Over the next five years, the biomedical research advocacy community, which included dozens of national cancer organizations, was steadfast in its efforts to secure the annual appropriations necessary to accomplish this historic effort (see Table 3-1).

Table 3-1. Annual National Institutes of Health (NIH) and National Cancer Institute (NCI) Budget Increases From 1998 to 2003

Fiscal Year	NIH	Annual Increase	NCI	Annual Increase
1998	$13.7 billion	7.33%	$2.5 billion	6.98%
1999	$15.6 billion	14.29%	$2.9 billion	14.84%
2000	$17.8 billion	14.15%	$3.3 billion	13.31%
2001	$20.5 billion	14.67%	$3.8 billion	13.27%
2002	$23.3 billion	13.99%	$4.2 billion	11.37%
2003	$27.2 billion	16.49%	$4.6 billion	9.83%

Note. Based on information from National Institutes of Health Office of Budget, n.d.

Women's Health and Cancer Rights Act

In response to reports from women and breast cancer advocates that breast reconstructive surgery following mastectomy was not being covered by health insurance policies, members of Congress introduced legislation to require that private health insurance plans cover these costs (Women's Health and Cancer Rights Act [H.R. 616, S. 249], 1997). These proposals were both individual legislative proposals, as well as provisions contained in various "patients' bill of rights" that were popular at the time, crafted in response to what was perceived to be the unfair policies and practices of managed care organizations. A comprehensive "patients' bill of rights" did not pass the Congress, as the measure was considered by many Republicans to be too expansive and prescriptive and therefore could not garner enough bipartisan support.

Senator D'Amato initially was spurred to action because of the advocacy appeals of grassroots breast cancer survivors and breast cancer surgeons in New York. Originally introduced by D'Amato as S. 249, the Women's Health and Cancer Rights Act of 1997, the bill garnered the support of a bipartisan group of 26 cosponsors spanning the political spectrum (Women's Health and Cancer Rights Act [S. 249], 1997). Across the Capitol in the House of Representatives, the companion bill, H.R. 616, was introduced by Representative Susan Molinari (R-NY), also prompted to action by her affected constituents, with 146 bipartisan cosponsors (Women's Health and Cancer Rights Act [H.R. 616], 1997). Despite the broad support across the aisle, the House bill did not see committee action. However, the Senate version of the bill had a hearing before the Senate Finance Subcommittee on Health. D'Amato worked with Senator Dianne Feinstein (D-CA) to expand the legislation to include a provision prohibiting "drive-through mastectomies" and successfully attached, as an amendment, the revised broader bill to tobacco-related legislation that was debated on the Senate floor. The underlying tobacco bill failed to garner the requisite 60 votes for cloture, which effectively ends unlimited debate and requires the Senate to proceed to a final vote. Therefore, the D'Amato bill appeared dead. However, as a result of Senator D'Amato's tenacity and support from a broad contingent of House members, the Women's Health and Cancer Rights Act of 1998 was passed as part of a larger legislative package (P.L. 105-277). The enacted legislation required private group health plans to cover "reconstruction of the breast on which the mastectomy was performed," as well as "surgery and reconstruction of the other breast to produce a symmetrical appearance" and "prostheses and physical complications of mastectomy, including lymphedemas" (Women's Health and Cancer Rights Act of 1998, § 713(a)(1)–(3)). As part of the legislative compromise, the measure did not include the requirements related to length of stay in the hospital following mastectomy.

Medicare Coverage of Clinical Trials

On June 7, 2000, President Clinton issued an Executive Memorandum requiring the Medicare program to cover the routine patient care costs associated with participation in clinical trials (White House Office of the Press Secretary, 2000). Prior to his action, the Medicare program did not cover such costs (e.g., blood work) if a beneficiary enrolled in a clinical trial (Pear, 2000). This lack of coverage was considered a significant barrier to older Americans participating in research studies to examine new cancer therapies. The Executive Memorandum was a result of long-standing advocacy efforts by the cancer community; numerous coalitions, such as the Cancer Leadership Council and the National Coalition for Cancer Survivorship; and individual organizations, such as the American Cancer Society. These advocacy efforts were coupled with an Institute of Medicine report "recommending policy changes to encourage the greater use of clinical trials by older Americans" (White House Office of the Press Secretary, 2000).

Prior to the Executive Memorandum, cancer community advocates had been pushing for enactment of the Medicare Cancer Clinical Trial Coverage Act, which was introduced numerous times in the Senate by Senators Jay Rockefeller (D-WV) and Connie Mack (R-FL) and in the House by Representatives Ben Cardin (D-MD) and Nancy Johnson (R-CT) (Federal Coverage for Clinical Trials Act of 1996 [H.R. 3958]; Medicare Cancer Clinical Trial Coverage Act of 1996 [S. 1963]; Medicare Cancer Clinical Trial Coverage Act of 1997 [H.R. 1628, S. 381]; Medicare Cancer Clinical Trial Coverage Act of 1999 [S. 784]). In the press release for the Executive Memorandum, the White House noted that the president's memorandum builds on the legislation sponsored by these senators and representatives (White House Office of the Press Secretary, 2000). Individual cancer advocacy organizations and the major cancer coalitions rejoiced upon hearing the news (Cancer Leadership Council, 2000).

Building upon the success of the Medicare clinical trials coverage, advocates renewed their efforts to expand commercial insurance coverage for clinical trials in the ACA, P.L. 111-148 and P.L. 111-152, signed into law on March 23, 2010 (Health Care and Education Reconciliation Act of 2010; Patient Protection and Affordable Care Act of 2010). Section 2709 of the legislation prohibits, beginning in 2014, private health plans or issuers of health plans in the group and individual market from denying coverage for routine items and services in connection with participation in qualified clinical trials for cancer or other life-threatening conditions. The provision also applies to federal employees who obtain coverage by health plans offered through the Federal Employees Health Benefits Program (Health Care and Education Reconciliation Act of 2010; Patient Protection and Affordable Care Act of 2010). Because more than 25 states had already enacted clinical trial coverage laws for plans under state regulation, the federal program does not preempt state laws that provide coverage that is in addition to the federal law (Health Care and Education Reconciliation Act of 2010; Patient Protection and Affordable Care Act of 2010; Purcell & Staman, 2008). States maintain authority to regulate some health insurance plans, generally those that are not employer-sponsored or self-insured plans. However, some health plans fall outside the jurisdiction of state legislative and regulatory authority because of the Employee Retirement Income Security Act, a federal statute that regulates employer-sponsored health care and other benefits and preempts state laws to, as explained by the U.S. Supreme Court, "avoid a multiplicity of regulation in order to permit the nationally uniform administration of employee benefit plans" (*New York State Conference of Blue Cross & Blue Shield Plans v. Travelers Insurance Co.*, 1995).

Medicare Modernization Act of 2003

Until the Medicare Prescription Drug, Improvement, and Modernization Act of 2003 (P.L. 108-173), also known as the Medicare Modernization Act (MMA), was enacted, Medicare coverage of oral anticancer therapies was extremely limited. With the addition of "Part D"—or prescription drug coverage—Medicare beneficiaries gained coverage and reimbursement for a wide range of prescription therapies, including anticancer, antinausea, and pain management drugs, among others. The MMA also included a number of watershed changes to Medicare reimbursement for outpatient infused chemotherapy, also known as "Part B" drugs. Medicare Part B pays for "certain doctors' services, outpatient care, medical supplies, and preventive services" (American Society of Clinical Oncology [ASCO], 2013, "Introduction," para. 1). A number of factors, including government reports, media coverage, and patient testimonials, contributed to policy makers seeking to enact change to the payment policy for outpatient infused chemotherapy.

Until 2005, physician-based oncology practices were paid a percentage of a drug's average wholesale price (AWP), but because of how the formula and prices were set, Medicare payments were often greater, sometimes much greater, than what practices actually paid for a particular drug (ASCO, 2013). Many policy makers considered this overpayment inappropriate and a waste of taxpayer and Medicare beneficiary dollars (as seniors typically pay a 20% coinsurance on Part B services), despite oncology community explanations that the margins "were used to cover both drug administration and critical patient support services not recognized or compensated adequately by Medicare" (ASCO, 2013, "How MMA Changed Medicare Payment for Chemotherapy Drugs," para. 1). In response to policymaker concern and in an effort to bring reimbursement levels closer to the actual cost of the drugs, the MMA contained provisions that modified the AWP system to an average sales price, or ASP, formula (ASCO, 2013). To address the change in payment and make up for underpayment for certain other outpatient oncology services, the MMA also boosted reimbursement for some chemotherapy administration codes (ASCO, 2013). In the years since enactment of the MMA, physician-based oncology practices have expressed concern regarding diminished resources and the adverse impact on Medicare beneficiary access to care (ASCO, 2013; Medicare Payment Advisory Commission, 2006).

On the positive side of the ledger, in addition to prescription drug coverage, the MMA included other new benefits for those served by the Medicare program. Long advocated by the American Cancer Society and championed by Representative Nancy Johnson (R-CT), a "Welcome to Medicare" physical examination was added to the roster of preventive benefits provided under the program (American Cancer Society Cancer Action Network, 2009). Otherwise known as an initial preventive physical examination (IPPE), the examination is a covered benefit so long as it occurs in the first year of Medicare Part B enrollment (American Cancer Society, 2014). During this time with the patient, in addition to a physical examination that includes an electrocardiogram (ECG), the physician is expected to review medical and social history; risk factors for depression; functional ability and level of safety; and the results of the examination, ECG, and the other components (Card, 2005). In addition, during the IPPE, the physician is supposed to engage in "education, counseling, and referral" regarding any issues raised during the examination, as well as the preventive services covered under Part B, including screening for breast, cervical, prostate, and colorectal cancer (Card, 2005). The ACA built upon the IPPE concept and included a new "Annual Wellness Visit" benefit, which includes the same components as the IPPE and allows for the provision of personalized prevention plan services (CMS Medicare Learning Network, 2011).

Recent Developments

Oncology-related federal policy, programs, and payment continue to evolve and garner significant time and attention within the nation's capital. For example, as a result of changes contained in the ACA, numerous Medicare preventive benefits and services now are covered without out-of-pocket expenses to beneficiaries. As part of this new policy, the Medicare program now covers tobacco cessation counseling for any beneficiary who seeks such assistance. Specifically, Medicare covers "two individual tobacco cessation counseling attempts per year, and each attempt may include as many as four sessions, for a maximum of eight sessions per year" (Mitchell, 2010). Prior to the ACA, Medicare coverage for tobacco cessation was narrower and was available only to individuals who had been diagnosed with an illness or disease related to or complicated by tobacco use or who showed symptoms of such a disease (CMS, n.d.; Mitchell, 2010).

Under the ACA, screening colonoscopies are a covered benefit, and patients may not be charged a co-payment or coinsurance. However, there was uncertainty regarding coverage for removal of polyps found during the screening colonoscopy. On February 20, 2013, the administration issued a clarification stating,

> Based on clinical practice and comments received from the American College of Gastroenterology, American Gastroenterological Association, American Society of Gastrointestinal Endoscopy, and the Society for Gastroenterology Nurses and Associates, polyp removal is an integral part of a colonoscopy. Accordingly, the plan or issuer may not impose cost-sharing with respect to a polyp removal during a colonoscopy performed as a screening procedure. (U.S. Department of Labor, 2013, Answer to Question 5)

The ACA also included a section titled "The Education and Awareness Requires Learning Young (EARLY) Act," sponsored by Representative Debbie Wasserman Schultz (D-FL) (Schultz, 2014). The EARLY Act "authorizes CDC to develop initiatives to increase knowledge of breast health and breast cancer among women, particularly among those under the age of 40 and those at heightened risk for developing the disease" (CDC, 2014a, para. 1).

Most recently, in December 2012 in the waning days of the 112th Congress, the Recalcitrant Cancer Research Act passed both chambers of the Congress. President Obama signed it into law in January 2013 as part of the National Defense Authorization Act for Fiscal Year 2013 (P.L. 112-239,

§ 1083). The bipartisan bill originally focused solely on pancreatic cancer but was broadened to include other cancer sites to address policymaker concerns about "earmarking" for one single disease (Viebeck, 2012). The legislation was attached to the National Defense Authorization Act and "calls for the scientific frameworks, or strategic plans, for pancreatic and lung cancers to be created under the direction of the NCI Director by July 2014 and to be updated within five years" (Pancreatic Cancer Action Network, 2013, "The New Statute Will Provide Strategic Direction," para. 1).

Tying It All Together

What Motivates Congress to Act?

One of the most effective means to enact change in public policy is for like-minded organizations and individuals to coalesce around a broad objective. Perhaps no public policy initiative best exemplifies this approach than the initiative to double the budget of NIH over a five-year period. Achieving this goal required the active commitment and participation of dozens of diverse organizations representing biomedical researchers, patient advocates, academia, healthcare professionals, the life sciences industry, and many others. These entities committed the time, resources, and dedication to advance a single, unified message to Congress: "double the NIH budget over five years." Doing so required some organizations to temporarily set aside advocacy for other policy priorities specific to their constituencies. Many of them had never worked together. Indeed, in some cases, these organizations had engaged in efforts that were divergent in nature. Some also had to accept the reality that research funding on their specific disease or condition might not double along with the NIH budget, as Congress traditionally defers to the NIH peer-review system for allocating appropriated funds. Yet, over the five-year period, these organizations engaged in an effective advocacy and communications strategy to ensure that all involved were speaking with one voice and with the same message. It is widely accepted that this unprecedented coalition of organizations and individuals was perhaps the single most significant factor in achieving the objective.

The old adage "politics makes strange bedfellows" could not have been truer in the NIH doubling effort. A strong bipartisan Congressional coalition of Republicans, Democrats, and Independents; liberals, moderates, and conservatives; and budget "hawks" and budget progressives all coalesced around the unified message of doubling the NIH budget. It brought together lawmakers who, in the past, had engaged in opposing, and sometimes fractious, confrontations over other policy issues. However, members of Congress actively engaged in a coordinated manner to persuade their colleagues in helping to secure the necessary annual appropriations, an approximately 15% increase to the NIH budget every year for five years, to achieve success.

Another example of what motivates Congress to act is to address issues of urgent national importance. For example, in recent years the United States has experienced severe shortages of drugs to treat many diseases, including cancer. The media were reporting on a near-daily basis the impact that drug shortages were having on patients and medical research. Members of Congress were hearing from constituents, including patients with life-threatening conditions, who were unable to obtain a drug they were prescribed. Medical practices and hospital pharmacies were being placed in the unconscionable position of having to decide which patients would receive their limited supply of sometimes lifesaving drugs that were in shortage. Researchers were reporting that clinical trials of innovative new therapeutics were being delayed or halted because of shortages. Clinical trial protocols were being altered to limit the number of patients participating in a particular study involving a drug frequently in shortage. These voices—those of constituents, trusted medical professionals, respected researchers, and other key stakeholders—created an echo chamber, a chorus calling for congressional action to address the adverse impact of drug shortages. This spurred Congress to quickly enact bipartisan legislation that would require manufacturers to report actual or potential drug shortages to FDA in a timelier basis (Food and Drug Administration Safety and Innovation Act, 2012). It also provided FDA with additional authorizations to avert or mitigate drug shortages (Food and Drug Administration Safety and Innovation Act, 2012). As a result, the number and duration of drug shortages have declined.

Members of Congress also respond to administration policies that they find objectionable. For example, on June 20, 2007, President George W. Bush issued Executive Order No. 13435 (2008), "Expanding Approved Stem Cell Lines in Ethically Responsible Ways," which addressed the allocation of federal funding for research on stem cells obtained from human embryos. Specifically, the executive order permitted federal funding for human embryonic stem research, but only on lines that are "derived without creating a human embryo for research purposes or destroying, discarding, or subjecting to harm a human embryo or fetus" (Executive Order No. 13435, 2008, section 1(a)). The ban had the effect of limiting government funding for research on embryonic stem cells to stem cell lines already in existence. Furthermore, federal dollars could not be used to start any new embryonic stem cell lines or to conduct research on any newly derived cell lines (Executive Order No. 13435, 2008). The executive order, which did not require congressional approval, sparked a strong outcry from researchers and patient organizations alike. It pitted those who believed embryonic stem cell research destroyed human life (human embryos) against those who believed that this area of scientific exploration could yield important new methods of treatment, such as regenerating damaged muscle tissue in patients with heart disease. Many religious organizations, such as the United States Conference of Catholic Bishops, argued forcefully that it was an improper, and perhaps illegal, use of federal dollars to destroy human embryos for any purpose (*Human Embryo Research Is Illegal*, 2001). However, organizations such as the Juvenile Diabetes Research Foundation waged a grassroots national effort to reverse the Bush policy on the grounds that such research had the potential for curing diseases such as diabetes, heart disease, and Parkinson disease. Scientific organizations, such as the Federation of American Societies for Experimental Biology, objected to the precedent of banning any particular form of research and expressed concern that such policies could drive scientists away from the United States. The ethical, legal, and social implications of embryonic stem cell research became a major public policy issue. For many members of Congress, the issue presented a personal dilemma that caused them to reevaluate the very meaning of when they believe life begins. As with the effort to double the funding for NIH, the issue of federal funding of embryonic stem cell research brought together a diverse group of members of Congress, including Senator Orrin Hatch (R-UT) and Representative Diana DeGette (D-CO), to overturn the ban established by President Bush. Following numerous failed attempts to overturn the policy through legislation, President Obama issued Executive Order No. 13505 on March 9, 2009, "Removing Barriers to Responsible Scientific Research Involving Human Stem Cells," which revoked the 2001 executive order issued by President Bush.

Lastly, nothing is more compelling, in many ways, than being directly affected by an issue or policy to motivate a policy maker to support a particular policy, program, or proposal. This is illustrated in Senator Durbin's loss of his father to lung cancer, which inspired him to enact the airline smoking ban; Senators Mack and Feinstein and Representative Lewis having family members diagnosed with cancer; and Representative Schultz being a breast cancer survivor. Personal experience with the disease is often what prompts policy makers, or their staff, to take action in the oncology policy sphere.

Budget Sequestration

Unsustainable federal budget deficits, a near-catastrophic downturn in the American economy, turmoil within the financial industry, and congressional gridlock, along with other factors, created the "perfect storm" that led Congress to pass the Budget Control Act (BCA) of 2011. Signed into law (P.L. 112-25) on August 2, 2011, the legislation required $917 billion in spending cuts over a 10-year period ("Statement from Cochairs of the Joint Select Committee on Deficit Reduction," 2011). The BCA also established the Joint Select Committee on Deficit Reduction, known as the "supercommittee," which was required to produce legislation by late November 2011 that would decrease the annual budget deficit by $1.2 trillion over 10 years (Bipartisan Policy Center, n.d.).

If Congress failed to produce a deficit reduction bill with at least $1.2 trillion in cuts, then it would trigger across-the-board cuts, known as *sequestration* (Bipartisan Policy Center, n.d.). These cuts would apply to mandatory and discretionary spending from 2013 to 2021; the cuts would be split evenly (by dollar amounts, not by percentages) between the defense and nondefense categories (Bipartisan Policy Center, n.d.). There would be some exemptions: Social Security, Medicaid, civil and military employee pay, veterans' benefits, and Medicare provider payments would be limited to a 2% reduction (Bipartisan Policy Center, n.d.). The intent of the sequester was to secure the commitment of both sides to future negotiations by means of an enforcement mechanism that would be unpalatable to Republicans and Democrats alike.

On November 21, 2011, the Joint Select Committee on Deficit Reduction concluded its work, issuing a statement that began, "After months of hard work and intense deliberations, we have come to the conclusion today that it will not be possible to make any bipartisan agreement available to the public before the committee's deadline" ("Statement from Cochairs of the Joint Select Committee on Deficit Reduction," 2011). The committee was formally terminated on January 31, 2012.

The failure of the "supercommittee" to reach a $1.2 trillion deficit reduction agreement triggered the automatic sequestration cuts provided for in the BCA (Bipartisan Policy Center, n.d.). While the sequestration cuts were set to begin on January 1, 2013, the cuts were postponed two months by the American Taxpayer Relief Act of 2012 (P.L. 112-240) until March 1, 2013, when the BCA went into effect (Bipartisan Policy Center, n.d.). As a result, NIH was forced to implement cuts of approximately $1.5 billion, or 5.5%, of its $30.8 billion fiscal year 2012 budget. The NCI budget was cut by approximately $288 million, or 5.7%, of its $5 billion budget when compared to fiscal year 2013. The first-year impact of the budget sequestration cuts was dramatic. In fiscal year 2013 alone, approximately 700 (8.5%) fewer research project grants were funded compared to fiscal year 2012. About 750 fewer patients (7.5%) were admitted to the NIH Clinical Center. Most scientific areas will be reduced by about 5% because the sequester is being applied broadly at the NIH institute and center level. NIH-funded noncompeting research project grants will be reduced, on average, by approximately 4.7% (NIH Office of Budget, n.d.). The cuts have, among other actions, forced cancer centers to curtail vital research, close laboratories, reduce the number of postdoctoral fellowships, and put the careers of young scientists at risk (NIH, 2013). Furthermore, while no published data currently exist, there is strong concern that cuts due to sequestration have impacted cancer clinical trials by delaying the start of new trials, limiting the number of participants in clinical trials, or curtailing the completion of ongoing clinical trials.

While strong bipartisan support for increased funding for NIH remains, the budgetary constraints under which Congress operates also persist. Without intervening action to craft a long-term legislative solution to meet the requirements of the BCA, automatic annual budget sequestration provisions remain in place through 2021 (Bipartisan Policy Center, n.d.). Congress also has the option to replace across-the-board sequestration cuts with targeted programmatic reductions to meet deficit targets, but doing so will require significant concessions from all parties involved.

Within the biomedical research advocacy community, there is a unified, sustained commitment to work with all members of Congress to help find the thus-far elusive middle ground. However, unlike in past efforts, the challenges are not merely numbers. There is an intensely combative political environment unlike any time before. For many lawmakers, including those who have been the strongest congressional champions, the current debate is focused not only on budgetary issues, but also on the larger fundamental question of the right balance of the role, scope, and function of the federal government. For advocates, this is a difficult, if not impossible, factor to overcome as members must decide, in their opinion and those of their constituents, what that right balance should be.

Future Cancer Advocacy

Future federal cancer advocacy and policy efforts will likely be dictated extensively by outside economic factors, which will determine the amount of federal resources available for cancer-related initiatives. Spiraling debt, unconstrained growth in entitlement program spending, instability in the financial sector, and an increasingly fractious political climate are just some of the challenging elements that cancer advocates face.

Even with bipartisan support, fiscal constraints will make it especially difficult to enact new and expanded programs for cancer research, education, prevention, awareness, detection, and treatment. These and other factors have added a new dimension to advocacy strategy. To address this new economic environment, advocacy organizations also highlight the significant impact that cancer research, for example, has on federal, state, and local job creation, economic growth, and its positive contribution to international trade. Using data from respected health economists, it is hoped that lawmakers not only will view cancer research as good for the health and well-being of its citizens, but that they also will recognize and appreciate its residual positive impact on the American economy. This dual-benefit strategy will likely be employed for the foreseeable future. Collaboration, data development, and unity of messaging among health policy advocacy communities will be essential as nondefense discretionary federal dollars continue to dwindle in the future.

Irrespective of the federal budgetary environment, some key factors will continue to play a role in the shape, scope, and success of federal oncology policy: constituent advocacy, health professional expertise and recommendations, and policy makers' personal experiences with cancer.

Conclusion

The impact that patients, oncology healthcare providers, researchers, and the public have should not be underestimated. As seen during the deficit reduction era of the 1990s, oncology policy still enjoyed attention, and positive changes and funding increases were achieved. As American cultural anthropologist Margaret Mead was famous for saying, "Never doubt that a small group of committed people can change the world. Indeed, it is the only thing that ever has" (Sommers, 1984, p. 158). From Mary Lasker to today's advocates, the American cancer advocacy movement exemplifies this vision.

We wish to acknowledge the research conducted by Samantha Mendell and Amy Walker and express our gratitude and recognize the extensive work by Jenna Dickinson on the references and citations contained in the chapter; we thank them all for their contributions to this important work.

References

Alliance of Dedicated Cancer Centers. (2011). About the Alliance of Dedicated Cancer Centers. Retrieved from http://www.aodcc.org/AboutADCC.aspx

American Cancer Society. (2013). Off-label drug use: What is off-label drug use? Retrieved from http://www.cancer.org/treatment/treatmentsandsideeffects/treatmenttypes/chemotherapy/off-label-drug-use

American Cancer Society. (2014). Medicare coverage for cancer prevention and early detection. Retrieved from http://www.cancer.org/healthy/findcancerearly/cancerscreening guidelines/medicare-coverage-for-cancer-prevention-and-early-detection

American Cancer Society Cancer Action Network. (2009). Winning the fight against cancer: Understanding the Medicare program. Retrieved from http://action.acscan.org/site/DocServer/medicare.pdf?docID=8162

American College of Radiology. (n.d.). Mammography Quality Standards Act. Retrieved from http://www.acr.org/advocacy/legislative-issues/mqsa

American Society of Clinical Oncology. (2013, February 22). ASCO in action brief: Physician administered drugs—The evolution of buy and bill. Retrieved from http://www.asco.org/advocacy/asco-action-brief-physician-administered-drugs-%E2%80%94-evolution-buy-bill

American Taxpayer Relief Act of 2012, Pub. L. No. 112-240, 126 Stat. 2313 (2013).

Americans for Nonsmokers' Rights. (2005). Smokefree transportation chronology. Retrieved from http://no-smoke.org/document.php?id=334

Association of National Advertisers. (2009). ANA argues that Tobacco Control Act violates First Amendment. Retrieved from http://www.ana.net/content/show/id/570

Bagley, G.P., & McVearry, K. (1998). Medicare coverage for oncology services. *Cancer, 82,* 1991–1994.

Baird, C. (2010, September 29). The Ovarian Cancer National Alliance gives Hope Award to Congresswoman Rosa DeLauro. Retrieved from http://www.ovariancancer.org/2010/09/29/ocna-gives-hope-award-to-congresswoman-rosa-delauro

Balanced Budget Act of 1997, H.R. 2015, 105th Cong.

Bardin, J. (2012, October 1). Medical research funding tied to advocacy, study finds. *Los Angeles Times.* Retrieved from http://articles.latimes.com/2012/oct/01/science/la-sci-sn-medical-research-funding-tied-to-lobbying-study-20121001

Bipartisan Policy Center. (n.d.). Breaking down the Budget Control Act. Retrieved from http://bipartisanpolicy.org/projects/budget-control-act

Breast Cancer Screening Safety Act of 1991, H.R. 3462, 102nd Cong. (1992).

Breast and Cervical Cancer Mortality Prevention Act of 1990, Pub. L. No. 101-354, 101st Cong.

Breast and Cervical Cancer Prevention and Treatment Act of 2000, H.R. 4386, 102nd Cong.

Breast and Cervical Cancer Treatment Act, S. Rep. No. 106-323, 106th Cong., 2nd session (2000).

Budget Control Act of 2011, Pub. L. No. 112-25, 112th Cong.

Campaign for Tobacco-Free Kids. (n.d.). U.S. state and local issues: State tobacco taxes. Retrieved from http://www.tobaccofreekids.org/what_we_do/state_local/taxes

Cancer Leadership Council. (2000, June 7). Cancer Leadership Council applauds Medicare coverage of clinical trials. Retrieved from http://www.cancerleadership.org/policy/clinic_medicare/000607.html

Cancer Network. (1998, July 1). Senate fails to bring McCain tobacco control bill to a vote. Retrieved from http://www.cancernetwork.com/print/173902

Cancer Screening and Prevention Act of 1995. 141 *Cong. Rec.* 134, S12275–S12290 (daily ed. August 10, 1995) (statement of Hon. John Chafee).

Card, R.O. (2005). How to conduct a "Welcome to Medicare" visit. *Family Practice Management, 12*(4), 27–31. Retrieved from http://www.aafp.org/fpm/2005/0400/p27.html?printable=fpm

Centers for Disease Control and Prevention. (1998, March 27). Strategies for providing follow-up and treatment services in the National Breast and Cervical Cancer Early Detection Program—United States, 1997. *Morbidity and Mortality Weekly Report, 47,* 215–218. Retrieved from http://www.jstor.org/stable/23308696

Centers for Disease Control and Prevention. (2009, May 22). Federal and state cigarette excise taxes—United States, 1995–2009. *Morbidity and Mortality Weekly Report, 58,* 524–527. Retrieved from http://www.cdc.gov/mmwr/preview/mmwrhtml/mm5819a2.htm

Centers for Disease Control and Prevention. (2014a). Advisory Committee on Breast Cancer in Young Women. Retrieved from http://www.cdc.gov/cancer/breast/what_cdc_is_doing/young_women.htm

Centers for Disease Control and Prevention. (2014b). Cancer prevention and control. Retrieved from http://www.cdc.gov/cancer

Centers for Disease Control and Prevention, National Breast and Cervical Cancer Early Detection Program. (2013). Breast and Cervical Cancer Mortality Prevention Act of 1990. Retrieved from http://www.cdc.gov/cancer/nbccedp/legislation/law.htm

Centers for Disease Control and Prevention, National Breast and Cervical Cancer Early Detection Program. (2014). About the program. Retrieved from http://www.cdc.gov/cancer/nbccedp/about.htm

Centers for Medicare and Medicaid Services. (n.d.). Your Medicare coverage: Smoking and tobacco use cessation (counseling to stop smoking or using tobacco products). Retrieved from http://www.medicare.gov/coverage/smoking-and-tobacco-use-cessation.html

Centers for Medicare and Medicaid Services. (2009). The guide to Medicare preventive services for physicians, providers, suppliers, and other health care professionals: The screening Pap test. Retrieved from https://www.codemap.com/file/ScreeningPapTests.pdf

Centers for Medicare and Medicaid Services. (2012). Medicare PPS excluded cancer hospitals. Retrieved from http://www.cms.gov/Medicare/Medicare-Fee-for-Service-Payment/AcuteInpatientPPS/PPS_Exc_Cancer_Hospasp.html

Centers for Medicare and Medicaid Services. (2014). Inpatient PPS PC pricer. Retrieved from http://www.cms.gov/Medicare/Medicare-Fee-for-Service-Payment/PCPricer/inpatient.html

Centers for Medicare and Medicaid Services Medicare Learning Network. (2011). Annual wellness visit (AWV), including personalized prevention plan services (PPPS) (MLN Matters No. MM7079). Retrieved from http://www.cms.gov/Outreach-and-Education/Medicare-Learning-Network-MLN/MLNMattersArticles/downloads/mm7079.pdf

Centers for Medicare and Medicaid Services Medicare Payment Advisory Commission. (2003). *Report to the Congress: Medicare payment policy, Appendix B: An introduction to how Medicare makes coverage decisions.* Retrieved from http://www.medpac.gov/publications%5Ccongressional_reports%5CMar03_AppB.pdf

Cimons, M. (1987, January 15). Study may bring smoking ban on planes. *Los Angeles Times.* Retrieved from http://articles.latimes.com/1987-01-15/news/mn-4807_1_smoke-ban-study

Collins, S.R., & Rasmussen, P.W. (2014). New federal surveys show declines in number of uninsured Americans in early 2014. *Commonwealth Fund Blog.* Retrieved from http://www.commonwealthfund.org/publications/blog/2014/sep/new-federal-surveys-show-declines-in-number-of-uninsured-americans-in-early-2014

Congressional Research Service. (1989, November 21). Bill summary and status: 101st Congress (1989–1990): H.R. 3299 CRS summary. Retrieved from http://thomas.loc.gov/cgi-bin/bdquery/z?d102:s.0177:

Congressional Research Service. (1992, October 1). Bill summary and status: 102nd Congress (1991–1992): S. 1777 CRS summary. Retrieved from http://thomas.loc.gov/cgi-bin/bdquery/z?d101:H.R.4790:

Congressional Research Service. (1993, August 4). Library of Congress summary: H.R. 2264 (103rd): Omnibus Budget Reconciliation Act of 1993. Retrieved from https://www.govtrack.us/congress/bills/103/hr2264#summary

Congressional Research Service. (1998, May 14). Bill summary and status: 105th Congress (1997–1998): S. 1415 CRS summary. Retrieved from http://thomas.loc.gov/cgi-bin/bdquery/z?d105:SN01415:

Consolidated Appropriations Act of 2001, Pub. L. No. 106-554, Appendix D, § 152(a)(3) (2000).

Exec. Order No. 13435, 3 C.F.R. 222–223 (2008).

Exec. Order No. 13505, 3 C.F.R. 229–230 (2009).

Family Smoking Prevention and Tobacco Control Act, Pub. L. No. 111-31, 123 Stat. 1776 (2009).

Federal Coverage for Clinical Trials Act of 1996, H.R. 3958, 104th Cong.

Food and Drug Administration Safety and Innovation Act, Pub. L. 112-144, 112th Cong. (2012).

Frontline. (1998a). Inside the tobacco deal: Interviews: Senator John McCain. Retrieved from http://www.pbs.org/wgbh/pages/frontline/shows/settlement/interviews/mccain.html

Frontline. (1998b). Inside the tobacco deal: States' Medicaid lawsuits. Retrieved from http://www.pbs.org/wgbh/pages/frontline/shows/settlement/timelines/medicaid.html

Health Care and Education Reconciliation Act of 2010, H.R. 4872, 111th Cong.

Holm, A.L., & Davis, R.M. (2004). Clearing the airways: Advocacy and regulation for smoke-free airlines. *Tobacco Control, 13,* i30–i36. doi:10.1136/tc.2003.005686

Hughes, V. (2013). The disease olympics. *Nature Medicine, 19,* 257–260. doi:10.1038/nm0313-257

Human embryo research is illegal, immoral, and unnecessary. Hearing on stem cell research: Hearing before the Subcommittee on Labor, Health and Human Services, and Education of the Senate Appropriations Committee, United States Senate, 107th Cong. (2001) (testimony of Richard M. Doerflinger).

Retrieved from http://www.usccb.org/issues-and-action/human-life-and-dignity/stem-cell -research/human-embryo-research-is-illegal-immoral-and-unnecessary.cfm

Institute of Medicine. (1997). *A review of the Department of Defense's program for breast cancer research.* Washington, DC: National Academies Press.

Introduction of the Medicare Preventive Benefits Improvement Act. 144 *Cong. Rec.* 199, E2361 (daily ed. December 14, 1995) (statement of Hon. Benjamin L. Cardin).

Kolata, G. (1990, January 10). Rose Kushner, 60, leader in breast cancer fight. *New York Times.* Retrieved from http://www.nytimes.com/1990/01/10/obituaries/rose-kushner-60-leader -in-breast-cancer-fight.html

Krutz, G.S. (2001). *Hitching a ride: Omnibus legislating in the U.S. Congress.* Columbus, OH: Ohio State University Press.

Lefkowitz, M. (2012). Split 6th Circuit says graphic cigarette pack warnings are constitutional. *Mealey's Litigation Blog.* Retrieved from http://www.lexisnexis.com/legalnewsroom/ litigation/b/litigation-blog/archive/2012/03/19/split-6th-circuit-says-graphic-cigarette -pack-warnings-are-constitutional.aspx

Legacy. (n.d.). Our history. Retrieved from http://www.legacyforhealth.org/about/our-history

Lynch, M.S. (2011). *Statutory budget controls in effect between 1985 and 2002* (CRS Report R41901). Retrieved from http://www.fas.org/sgp/crs/misc/R41901.pdf

Mack (and others) Amendment No. 315. 143 *Cong. Rec.* 68, S4903 (daily ed. May 21, 1997).

Mammography Quality Standards Act of 1992, H.R. 5938, 102nd Cong.

Mammography Quality Standards Act of 1992, S. 1777, 102nd Cong.

Mammography Quality Standards Act of 1992, Pub. L. No. 102-539, 102nd Cong.

Mammography Quality Standards Reauthorization Act of 1998, Pub. L. No. 105-248, 105th Cong.

Mammography Quality Standards Reauthorization Act of 2004, Pub. L. No. 108-365, 108th Cong.

Medicare Cancer Clinical Trial Coverage Act of 1996, S. 1963, 104th Cong.

Medicare Cancer Clinical Trial Coverage Act of 1997, H.R. 1628, 105th Cong.

Medicare Cancer Clinical Trial Coverage Act of 1997, S. 381, 105th Cong.

Medicare Cancer Clinical Trial Coverage Act of 1999, S. 784, 106th Cong.

Medicare Payment Advisory Commission. (2006). *Report to the Congress: Effects of Medicare payment changes on oncology services.* Retrieved from http://www.medpac.gov/documents/Jan06 _Oncology_mandated_report.pdf

Medicare Prescription Drug, Improvement, and Modernization Act of 2003, Pub. L. No. 108-173, 108th Cong.

Mensah, G.A., Goodman, R.A., Zaza, S., Moulton, A.D., Kocher, P.L., Dietz, W.H., ... Marks, J.S. (2004). Law as a tool for preventing chronic diseases: Expanding the spectrum of effective public health strategies. *Preventing Chronic Disease, 1*(2), 1–6. Retrieved from http://www .cdc.gov/pcd/issues/2004/apr/pdf/04_0009.pdf

Mitchell, D. (2010, September 1). HHS expands Medicare coverage of tobacco cessation counseling: Diagnosis requirement no longer barrier to payment. Retrieved from http://www .aafp.org/news-now/health-of-the-public/20100901medicaretobaccouse.html

National Breast Cancer Coalition. (2013a). Legislative accomplishments. Retrieved from http://www.breastcancerdeadline2020.org/get-involved/public-policy

National Breast Cancer Coalition. (2013b). Priority #2: $150 million for the Department of Defense Breast Cancer Research Program for FY 2015. Retrieved from http://www .breastcancerdeadline2020.org/get-involved/public-policy/legislative-and-pp-priorities/ priority-2-150-million-for.html

National Cancer Crusade, H.R. Con. Res. 675, 91st Cong. (1970). Retrieved from http://www .gpo.gov/fdsys/pkg/STATUTE-84/pdf/STATUTE-84-Pg2189.pdf

National Cancer Institute Office of Budget and Finance. (2012). *The NCI annual fact book: The NCI budget in review.* Retrieved from http://obf.cancer.gov/financial/factbook.htm

National Cancer Institute Office of Budget and Finance. (2013). *Plan and budget proposal: The nation's investment in cancer research.* Retrieved from http://obf.cancer.gov/financial/plan.htm

National Cancer Institute Office of Government and Congressional Relations. (n.d.-a). Legislative history. Retrieved from http://legislative.cancer.gov/history

National Cancer Institute Office of Government and Congressional Relations. (n.d.-b). The National Cancer Act of 1971. Retrieved from http://legislative.cancer.gov/history/phsa/1971

National Defense Authorization Act for Fiscal Year 2013, Pub. L. No. 112-239, 126 Stat. 1632, § 1083.

National Institutes of Health. (2013, June 3). Fact sheet: Impact of sequestration on the National Institutes of Health. Retrieved from http://www.nih.gov/news/health/jun2013/nih-03.htm

National Institutes of Health Office of Budget. (n.d.). Mechanism table accompanying FY 2013 operating plan. Retrieved from http://officeofbudget.od.nih.gov/pdfs/FY13/FY%20 2013%20Full-Year%20NIH%20Mechanism%20Table%20Posting%20.pdf

National Institutes of Health Office of History. (n.d.). A short history of the National Institutes of Health. Retrieved from http://history.nih.gov/exhibits/history/index.html

National Library of Medicine. (n.d.). The Mary Lasker papers. Retrieved from http://profiles .nlm.nih.gov/ps/retrieve/Collection/CID/TL

National Library of Medicine. (2007, June 21). Papers of medical philanthropist and NIH benefactor Mary Lasker added to the National Library of Medicine's Profiles in Science web site [Press release]. Retrieved from http://nih.gov/news/pr/jun2007/nlm-21.htm

National Research Council Committee on Airliner Cabin Air Quality. (1986). *The airliner cabin environment: Air quality and safety.* Retrieved from http://www.nap.edu/catalog.php?record _id=913

National Task Force on CME Provider/Industry Collaboration. (n.d.). On-label and off-label usage of prescription medicines and devices, and the relationship to CME. *Fact Sheet,* 2(3). Retrieved from https://cme.wustl.edu/forms/On_Label_and_Off_Label_Usage_of _Prescription_Medicines_and_Devices_and_the_Relationship_to_CME.pdf

National Tobacco Policy and Youth Smoking Reduction Act, S. 1415, 105th Cong. (1998).

New York State Conference of Blue Cross & Blue Shield Plans v. Travelers Insurance Co., 514 U.S. 645, 657 (1995).

Nixon, R. (1971a). Annual message to the Congress on the state of the union, January 22, 1971 [Transcript]. Retrieved from http://www.presidency.ucsb.edu/ws/?pid =3110#axzz2gV0o6bmX

Nixon, R. (1971b). Remarks on signing the National Cancer Act of 1971 [Transcript]. Retrieved from http://www.presidency.ucsb.edu/ws/?pid=3275#axzz2gV0o6bmX

Nixon, R. (1971c). Statement about the National Cancer Act of 1971 [Transcript]. Retrieved from http://www.presidency.ucsb.edu/ws/?pid=3276

Office of Inspector General, Office of Evaluation and Inspections. (2001). Medicare hospital prospective payment system: How DRG rates are calculated and updated. Retrieved from http://oig.hhs.gov/oei/reports/oei-09-00-00200.pdf

Omnibus Budget Reconciliation Act of 1989, H.R. 3299.PP, 101st Cong.

Omnibus Budget Reconciliation Act of 1993, H.R. 2264, 103rd Cong.

O'Sullivan, J., Franco, C., Fuchs, B.C., Lyke, B., Price, R., & Swendiman, K.S. (1997, August 18). *Medicare provisions in the Balanced Budget Act of 1997 (BBA 97, P.L. 105-33)* (CRS Report 97-802). Retrieved from http://greenbook.waysandmeans.house.gov/sites/greenbook .waysandmeans.house.gov/files/2011/images/l97-802_gb.pdf

Pagan, M. (2009, June 11). Lautenberg, longtime Senate leader on anti-tobacco efforts, hails passage of FDA tobacco bill. Retrieved from http://www.politickernj.com/paganm/30554/ lautenberg-longtime-senate-leader-anti-tobacco-efforts-hails-passage-fda-tobacco-bill

Pancreatic Cancer Action Network. (2013, June). The Recalcitrant Cancer Research Act: An important step toward improving pancreatic cancer survival. Retrieved from http://www .pancan.org/wp-content/uploads/2014/04/Recalcitrant-Cancer-Research-Act-Facts-GAA -June-2013-FINAL.pdf

Patient Protection and Affordable Care Act, Pub. L. No. 111-148, 124 Stat. 119 (2010).

Pear, R. (2000, June 7). Clinton to order Medicare to pay new costs. *New York Times.* Retrieved from http://www.nytimes.com/library/politics/060700medicare-clinton.html

Preventive Health Amendments of 1993, H.R. 2202, 103rd Cong. Retrieved from http://www.gpo.gov/fdsys/pkg/BILLS-103hr2202enr/pdf/BILLS-103hr2202enr.pdf

Public Health Law Center. (n.d.). Master Settlement Agreement. Retrieved from http://publichealthlawcenter.org/topics/tobacco-control/tobacco-control-litigation/master-settlement-agreement

Purcell, P., & Staman, J. (2008, April 10). *Summary of the Employee Retirement Income Security Act (ERISA)* (CRS Report RL34443). Retrieved from http://www.nccmp.org/resources/pdfs/other/Summary%20of%20ERISA.pdf

Rettig, R.A. (1978). *Reflections on the "Cancer Crusade."* Santa Monica, CA: RAND Corporation.

Riter, B. (2014). History of breast cancer advocacy. Retrieved from http://www.crcfl.net/content/view/history-of-breast-cancer-advocacy.html

Ryerson, A.B., Benard, V.B., & Major, A.C. (n.d.). *National Breast and Cervical Cancer Early Detection Program: 1991–2002 national report.* Centers for Disease Control and Prevention, National Center for Chronic Disease Prevention and Health Promotion. Retrieved from http://www.cdc.gov/cancer/nbccedp/pdf/national_report.pdf

S. Amdt. 315, 105th Cong. (1998).

Scherer, R. (1989, October 20). Smoking ban is Durbin's crusade. *Christian Science Monitor.* Retrieved from http://www.csmonitor.com/1989/1020/asmok.html

Schultz, D.W. (2014). Campaign to educate young women about breast cancer risks submitted for congressional reauthorization [Press release.]. Retrieved from http://wassermanschultz.house.gov/press-releases/campaign-to-educate-young-women-about-breast-cancer-risks-submitted-for-congressional-reauthorization

Social Security Administration. (n.d.). History of SSA during the Johnson Administration 1963–1968. Retrieved from http://www.ssa.gov/history/ssa/lbjmedicare1.html

Sommers, F. (1984). *Curing nuclear madness.* Toronto, Ontario, Canada: Methuen.

Specter pledges (again) to boost NIH. (1997, January 30). *ScienceNow.* Retrieved from http://news.sciencemag.org/1997/01/specter-pledges-again-boost-nih?ref=hp

Staff of S. Comm. on Commerce, Science, and Transportation. (1998, May 1). *National Tobacco Policy and Youth Smoking Reduction Act: Report of the Committee on Commerce, Science, and Transportation on S. 1415* (S. Rep. No. 105-180). Retrieved from http://www.gpo.gov/fdsys/pkg/CRPT-105srpt180/html/CRPT-105srpt180.htm

State of the Union address by the President of the United States. 143 *Cong. Rec.* 12, H273 (daily ed. February 4, 1997). Retrieved from http://www.gpo.gov/fdsys/pkg/CREC-1997-02-04/pdf/CREC-1997-02-04-pt1-PgH273.pdf

Statement from cochairs of the Joint Select Committee on Deficit Reduction. (2011, November 21). *National Journal.* Retrieved from http://www.nationaljournal.com/supercommittee/statement-from-cochairs-of-the-joint-select-committee-on-deficit-reduction-20111121

Statements on introduced bills and joint resolutions. 149 *Cong. Rec.* S15063 (daily ed. November 18, 2003) (statement of Sen. Barbara Mikulski on S. 1879). Retrieved from http://www.gpo.gov/fdsys/pkg/CREC-2003-11-18/pdf/CREC-2003-11-18-pt1-PgS15062.pdf

Study expected to urge smoking ban on all domestic flights. (1986, August 13). *New York Times.* Retrieved from http://www.nytimes.com/1986/08/13/us/study-expected-to-urge-smoking-ban-on-all-domestic-flights.html

Susan G. Komen Breast Cancer Foundation. (2004). Capitol Hill update: MQSA reauthorized. *Frontline.* Retrieved from http://ww5.komen.org/uploadedFiles/Content_Binaries/frontlineq404.pdf

University of Texas, Ronald Reagan Presidential Library and Museum. (1983). Remarks on signing the Social Security Amendments of 1983: April 20, 1983 [Transcript]. Retrieved from http://www.reagan.utexas.edu/archives/speeches/1983/42083a.htm

U.S. Congress Office of Technology Assessment. (1990, February). *The costs and effectiveness of screening for cervical cancer in elderly women—Background paper* (OTA-BP-H-65). Washington, DC: U.S. Government Printing Office.

U.S. Department of Defense Congressionally Directed Medical Research Programs. (n.d.). Congressionally Directed Medical Research Programs. Retrieved from http://cdmrp.army.mil/pubs/pips/cmlpip.pdf

U.S. Department of Defense Congressionally Directed Medical Research Programs. (2010). Prostate cancer research program. Retrieved from http://cdmrp.army.mil/pcrp/pbks/pcrppbk2012.pdf

U.S. Department of Defense Congressionally Directed Medical Research Programs. (2012a). Lung cancer research program. Retrieved from http://cdmrp.army.mil/lcrp/pbks/lcrppbk2012.pdf

U.S. Department of Defense Congressionally Directed Medical Research Programs. (2012b). Peer reviewed cancer research program. Retrieved from http://cdmrp.army.mil/prcrp/pbks/prcrppbk2012.pdf

U.S. Department of Defense Congressionally Directed Medical Research Programs. (2013a). Breast Cancer Research Program. Retrieved from http://cdmrp.army.mil/bcrp/pbks/bcrppbk2013.pdf

U.S. Department of Defense Congressionally Directed Medical Research Programs. (2013b). Ovarian cancer research program. Retrieved from http://cdmrp.army.mil/ocrp/pbks/ocrppbk2013.pdf

U.S. Department of Defense Congressionally Directed Medical Research Programs. (2014, April). About us: Funding history. Retrieved from http://cdmrp.army.mil/about/fundinghistory.shtml

U.S. Department of Defense Military Health System. (n.d.). Research. Retrieved from http://health.mil/research.aspx

U.S. Department of Labor. (2013). FAQs about Affordable Care Act implementation part XII. Retrieved from http://www.dol.gov/ebsa/faqs/faq-aca12.html

U.S. Food and Drug Administration. (2011). "Off-label" and investigational use of marketed drugs, biologics, and medical devices: Information sheet. Retrieved from http://www.fda.gov/RegulatoryInformation/Guidances/ucm126486.htm

U.S. Food and Drug Administration. (2012). Radiation-emitting products: Mammography Quality Standards Act and Program: About the Mammography Program. Retrieved from http://www.fda.gov/Radiation-EmittingProducts/MammographyQualityStandardsActandProgram/AbouttheMammographyProgram/default.htm

U.S. Food and Drug Administration. (2014a). About the Center for Tobacco Products. Retrieved from http://www.fda.gov/AboutFDA/CentersOffices/OfficeofMedicalProductsandTobacco/AbouttheCenterforTobaccoProducts/default.htm

U.S. Food and Drug Administration. (2014b). Overview of the Family Smoking Prevention and Tobacco Control Act: Consumer fact sheet. Retrieved from http://www.fda.gov/tobaccoproducts/guidancecomplianceregulatoryinformation/ucm246129.htm

U.S. General Accounting Office. (1990). *Screening mammography: Low-cost services do not compromise quality.* Retrieved from http://gao.gov/assets/150/148499.pdf

U.S. Government Accountability Office. (2011, September). *Manufacturer discounts in the 340B program offer benefits, but federal oversight needs improvement* (Report No. GAO-11-836). Retrieved from http://www.gao.gov/assets/330/323702.pdf

U.S. Senate Committee on Labor and Human Resources Subcommittee on Aging. (1992). *Improving the quality of mammography: How current practice fails. Hearing before the Subcommittee on Aging of the Committee on Labor and Human Resources, United States Senate, One Hundred Second Congress, second session, on examining mammography and the growing incidence of breast cancer in American women, February 13, 1991 (Tacoma, WA).* Washington, DC: U.S. Government Printing Office.

Veterans Health Care Act of 1992, Pub. L. No. 102-585, 102nd Cong.

Viebeck, E. (2012, December 25). After long haul, cancer bill passes. *The Hill.* Retrieved from http://thehill.com/blogs/healthwatch/other/274387-after-long-haul-cancer-bill-passes -congress

Wendell H. Ford Aviation Investment and Reform Act for the 21st Century, Pub. L. No. 106-181, 106th Cong. (2000).

White House Office of the Press Secretary. (2000, June 7). President Clinton takes new action to encourage participation in clinical trials [Press release]. Retrieved from http://clinton3 .nara.gov/WH/New/html/20000607.html

Women's Health and Cancer Rights Act of 1997, H.R. 616, 105th Cong.

Women's Health and Cancer Rights Act of 1997, S. 249, 105th Cong.

Women's Health and Cancer Rights Act of 1998, Pub. L. No. 105-277, 105th Cong.

Women's Health Equity Act of 1991, S. 514, 102nd Cong.

Women's Preventive Health Amendments of 1993, H.R. 2158, 103rd Cong.

World Health Organization. (n.d.). Tobacco Free Initiative (TFI): Taxation. Retrieved from http://www.who.int/tobacco/economics/taxation/en/index1.html

CHAPTER 4

The Environment and Cancer

Devra Lee Davis, PhD, MPH, and Brian Bunn, REHS/RS, CPFS-IT, Dual MPH(c)

> *Tragic sins become moral failures only if we should have known better from the outset.*
>
> —Jared Diamond

Introduction

In the summer of 1936, more than 200 of the world's top cancer scientists convened in Brussels to attend the Second International Congress of the Scientific and Social Campaign Against Cancer. The great experimentalist Isaac Berenblum later remembered it as "the most momentous Cancer Congress ever held" (Berenblum, 1977, p. 2). Scientists sailed from Latin America, North America, and Japan, a journey that would have taken close to two weeks. With the world clearly on the brink of war, such a trip required considerable courage and a strong stomach. One of the participants, Wilhelm Hueper, had survived poison gas attacks in the Great War; no doubt several others had had similar experiences. In fact, this historic gathering remained secret for more than 70 years.

At the Brussels meeting, the accomplishments of several centuries of cancer research flashed onto the scene, ready to coalesce into a substantial and coherent body of scientific understanding about the environmental causes of cancer. However, many of these accomplishments were forgotten and their message was ignored. Compelling, conclusive knowledge about the causes of cancer known at that time ended up in the dusty section of the library reserved for books that are never read and papers that are never cited.

Note. Adapted from Devra Davis, The Secret History of the War on Cancer, Basic Books, 2007, with permission of the author.

Today, it is not widely appreciated that in the 21st century we remain locked in ferocious debates about cancer-causing industrial and other exposures that scientists thought they had solved more than three generations ago. When it comes to understanding the causes of cancer, we can rely on experimental studies both in vitro and in vivo, as well as clinical case reports, and ultimately can incorporate epidemiologic studies where such have been generated. But what evidence is deemed sufficient to pass as scientific proof, although founded in methods and measures, also depends on political and economic forces, perhaps more so than on the underlying science itself.

The extraordinary 1936 report from the congress included sections written in several languages: English, Spanish, French, Russian, and German, all presumed to be understood by the multilingual scientific crowd (Fraenkel, 1936). One speaker, Clarence C. Little, famous for creating ways to study the inheritance of cancer in mice, argued that, based on animal studies, most cancer arises from inherited defects. During the conference, however, the view that cancer was dictated by genes was in the clear minority.

William Cramer, of London's Imperial Cancer Research Fund, carefully examined patterns of cancer in people during the previous century. He was able to accomplish this because England had a system for recording deaths and illnesses that dated back more than 300 years. Cramer noted that much of the recorded increase in cancer incidence was nothing more than better record keeping and people living longer lives. However, he developed techniques for evaluating these specific patterns and determined that the number of cancer cases had almost doubled since the turn of the century. He concluded that cancer was about one-third more common than it was at the beginning of the 20th century (Cramer, 1936).

Cramer also noted other evidence that cancer rates had recently grown. He pointed to a profoundly simple and important observation that has been repeatedly confirmed. He looked at cancer rates in "uniovular" twins (more commonly known as identical twins, the result of single fertilized egg splitting into two developing embryos). By 1936, he had already determined that, in most of these genetically identical pairs, if one develops cancer, the other does not. Cramer (1936) concluded that "cancer, as a disease, is not inherited" (p. 17). He urged that patterns of cancer—especially those developed in the workplace—should be tracked to learn how to control and reduce the disease (Cramer, 1936). Like most scientists then and now, Cramer understood that cancer patterns were the result of past exposures. To make progress against cancer, it would be important to rely on experimental animal research to predict and attempt to prevent exposures to cancer-causing factors. Animal tests provide an important way to learn whether chemical or physical agencies that produce cancer in animals also produce cancer in humans. Cramer noted that cancer often develops in the same tissues for rodents and humans. The time between the initial exposure to a chemical and the development of a tumor varies greatly. Tumors can occur within a year in rodents (with their nearly three-year life expectancy) but may not form for many decades in humans. This period of latency is remarkably similar if expressed in fractions of the usual life span in each case. Cramer argued that few diseases existed in which their experimental production so closely simulates the disease in humans. He stated "that cancer in man may, in fact, be considered as an experiment carried out on man by nature" (Cramer, 1936, p. 5).

Cancer specialists of the time understood the importance of experimental studies with animals to predict human health risks. The three volumes of the report from this congress included surprisingly comprehensive laboratory and clinical reports concluding that many widely used agents at that time were known to be cancerous to humans. These cancerous agents included ionizing and solar radiation, arsenic, benzene, asbestos, synthetic dyes, and hormones.

Sunlight and Ionizing Radiation Interacts With Hydrocarbons

In the 1930s, Angel Honorio Roffo, the founding director of the Institute of Experimental Medicine in Buenos Aires, Argentina, described experiments showing that both invisible forms of radiation—ultraviolet and x-ray—could produce cancers in animals. He was one of several experts at the time to demonstrate that these tumors can be removed from one animal and made to grow in another, a method of tumor transplantation still in use today. Roffo's work referenced earlier experiments by Andre Clunet, who had produced sarcomas in rats in 1910, and clinical reports by Bruno Bloch from 1923 finding that radiation induced cancer in animals and in exposed workers (Roffo, 1936).

Roffo's studies of workers showed that those who spent the most time outdoors had the greatest vulnerability to skin cancer. His paper was accompanied by exquisitely detailed drawings of tumors growing from the heads, eyes, ears, and thyroid glands of rats following months of solar or x-ray treatment. He also reported that combining certain hydrocarbons with either sunlight or radiation exacerbated cancer damage compared to the cancer produced from one of these exposures alone. He advised avoiding radiation and sunlight and reducing exposure to hydrocarbons (Roffo, 1936). Unfortunately, the modern world did not begin to take these observations seriously until the 1980s.

Roffo was one of many experts to issue a strong statement against the fashionable view that tanned skin signals good health. At a time when suntanned movie stars and cowboys were idolized, Roffo concluded his presentation by "protesting strongly against excessive sunbathing which exposes the skin to intensive irradiations from the sun, placing individuals, victims of a ridiculous fashion, into a particularly dangerous state of receptivity to the development of skin cancer" (Roffo, 1936, p. 84). The National Toxicology Program of the U.S. government did not formally list ultraviolet light (sunlight) as a definite cause of human cancer until 2002.

Awareness of Hormonal Causes of Cancer

In this 1936 volume, noted researchers J.W. Cook, Edmund L. Kennaway, and others with London's Royal Cancer Hospital reported that more than 30 different studies had found that regular exposure to the hormone estrogen produced mammary (breast) tumors in male rodents (Fraenkel, 1936). As with ultraviolet light, the National Toxicology Program did not identify estrogen as a definite human carcinogen until 2002.

Paths to Understanding Cancer Through Both Experimental Animals and Human Observational Studies

So how did the scientists at this major international meeting in 1936 determine the cause of cancer? They combined autopsies with medical, personal, and workplace histories of people with cancer—ultimately by looking at patients' medical histories. They reasoned that if tar and soot were found in the lungs of individuals who had worked in mining, and if they showed that these same things caused tumors when placed on the skin or in the lungs of animals, that this was sufficient evidence to deem these gooey residues a cause of cancer, and that these substances should be controlled and regulated. These scientists conducted complex laboratory studies with many different animal models: rats, mice, rabbits, monkeys, dogs, and cats, using various physical and chemical agents that left clear marks of cancer. These scientists also established new approaches for observing patterns of cancer in groups of workers. They adjusted their analysis for the age of those being studied and the fact that an older population would equal increased cancer incidence (Fraenkel, 1936).

Before the 20th century, physicians and scientists had an expansive view of what information was required to establish that an agent or substance could be considered a cause of cancer. A broad range of natural experiments, some carried out by researchers on themselves, repeatedly concluded one simple thing—our health is a direct reflection of the sum of our life experiences.

These early scientists appreciated that most cancer arises not because of one's parents or genetic makeup, but because of what occurs to individuals after they are born. Many different factors influence people's health: where and how they live and work, what they eat, how they spend their private time, how they move about. Heat, cold, dust, dirt, radiation, soot, fumes, and myriad natural and synthetic agents combine to affect the chances that anyone will get any disease. Cancer develops not because of one unique circumstance (whether hereditary or environmental) but out of the sum total of the "good and bad" of our lives.

Breast Cancer—An Ancient Disease With Modern Causes

Hippocrates (ca. 460 BCE–ca. 370 BCE) was not the first of the ancient scholars to be fascinated with the uncommon and monstrous growth of cancer, nor was he the earliest to describe a sprawling crab-like tumor of the breast, called *karkinoma*. About a thousand years earlier, one of the first depictions of the disease was recorded on pressed papyrus reeds from Egypt—the world's first preserved paper, the Edwin Smith Papyrus. The paper was named for surgeon and Egyptologist Edwin Smith, who contributed to its translation in the 19th century (Wilkins, 1964), and described eight cases of breast tumors or ulcers in startlingly modern terms. The anonymous author of the papyrus writing records only one treatment for these ancient tumors: repeated use of a "fire drill" to burn out the growths that had broken through the skin. This bears a striking resemblance to contemporary methods that remove all signs of tumors through cauterization (Davis, 2007).

During the Middle Ages, cancerous tumors were sometimes removed successfully. Even then, leading a healthy life—through exercise, nutrition, and avoidance of contaminated environments—was considered to lessen the chance the disease would occur. The 12th-century Jewish polymath Moses Maimonides, who served as chief rabbi of Cairo as well as chief physician to the sultan of Egypt, carefully explained how to remove a cancer and uproot all surrounding tissue. But he warned that this would not work if the tumor contains large vessels or is situated in close proximity to any major organ. To prevent the disease, he counseled patients to stay away from dusty cities and dirty air, eat chicken soup and garlic, and get regular exercise (Rosner, 2002; Yawar, 2008).

Mining Known as a Cause of Cancer in the 16th Century

In the mid-16th century, the geologist and physician Georgius Agricola spent years preparing a massive report on mining that included detailed information on the cancerous lung ailments of miners. He did not just rely on information he heard from others. Instead, Agricola went underground into the Erz Mountains of Central Europe to watch boys and men extracting, preparing, and processing ore. After observing the workers, Agricola was struck by the number of young miners with tumors in their chests.

Agricola's magnum opus, *De Re Metallica*, was published in 1556, one year after the author's death, and included some of the earliest reports on the chronic ailments associated with underground work. Workers who entered the mines at extremely young ages, if they did not perish in gruesome accidents, fared the worst and eventually died from lung diseases and tumors. Agricola's work was printed with 289 remarkable woodcuts and portrayed the brutal work of mining both above and below ground (Davis, 2007).

Sometimes, important scientific work takes a few centuries to make the rounds. In 1912, Herbert Hoover, then one of America's top mining engineers, and his wife, Lou, a Latin scholar, published the first English translation of Agricola's work in *Mining* magazine with the four-century–old woodcuts. In their introductory comments, they explained that they made the translation because this 16th-century work remained relevant to the lives and deaths of 20th-century miners. Agricola's work still proves relevant with the occasional reports of mining disasters in Russia, China, South Africa, and West Virginia. The Hoovers noted that harms to workers were regrettable, although the ways they could be avoided were less apparent than the profitability of the materials (Davis, 2007; Nash, 1983).

Ramazzini Identified 18th-Century Workplace Causes of Cancer

By the turn of the 18th century, the groundbreaking Italian physician Bernardino Ramazzini had documented more than three dozen cancer-prone professions, including mining of coal, lead, arsenic, and iron. At that time, cancer was still uncommon and usually lethal. Ramazzini could not tell which specific part of the job caused which maladies, but he knew that people in many different jobs (e.g., metal gilders, chemists, potters, tobacco workers, blacksmiths, apothecaries, cleaners of privies and cesspits, farmers, fishermen, soldiers) were subject to cancer and other health risks. For each of these trades, Ramazzini explained what particular agents or conditions gave rise to certain classes of illness. Individuals who worked closely with dust and fire, such as miners, blacksmiths, glass workers, printers, bakers, and smelters, tended to suffer from weakened lungs, incurable cough, and, occasionally, suffocating tumors of the lung. When he reached his late 60s, Ramazzini published his major work, *De Morbis Artificum Diatriba* (*Diseases of Workers*), which showed that the tasks performed by men and women at work played a major role in determining what ailments they would develop.

This book laid the foundations for occupational medicine and industrial hygiene in its careful depiction of the importance of the ambient workplace environment (Davis, 2007).

Ramazzini died at age 81 in 1714, in an era when most workingmen did not reach the age of 40. In addition to being adventurous, he was an observant doctor with a penchant for record keeping. He noted that nuns tended to be free of cervical cancer, which was one of the most common fatal tumors in women. Those who lived celibate lives, however, were struck by breast cancer more often compared to other women. Ramazzini speculated that both of these anomalies could be related to the same cause—nuns did not bear children but instead experienced a lifetime of menstrual cycles uninterrupted by pregnancy or nursing. His theory that childbearing affects cancer risk remains a central tenet of cancer research today (Davis, 2007).

One other thing distinguished Ramazzini's work. He believed that individuals who identified workplace hazards had a moral duty to warn workers about the risks and urge them to lower those risks for themselves, their families, and their towns. He offered this modification of Hippocrates' ancient advice:

> When a doctor visits a working-class home he should be content to sit on a three-legged stool, if there isn't a gilded chair, and he should take time for his examination; and to the questions recommended by Hippocrates, he should add one more—"What is your occupation?" (as cited in Davis, 2007, p. 27)

Ramazzini based this advice on his own practice. "I for my part have done what I could and have not thought it unbecoming to make my way into the lowliest workshops and study the mysteries of the mechanical arts" (as cited in Davis, 2007, p. 27).

Industry's Understanding of the Dangers of Benzene in 1936

One fascinating fact about the cancer congress of 1936 that is not well known is that most of the assessments regarding the carcinogenic effects of hormones, arsenic, sunlight, radiation, benzene, and other chlorinated hydrocarbons were not challenged by official industrial sources at that time. Ten years earlier, the American National Safety Council—an industry group—had issued a final report (National Safety Council, 1926) on the hazards of benzol, the German term used to describe benzene. Their document noted (and included 125 different references to) the doses at which narcosis and severe weight loss in animals occurred after exposure to benzene. Highly exposed workers became anemic and sometimes died when overcome by fumes they encountered while cleaning out deep tanks, while workers without lethal exposures developed a range of blood problems (Davis, 2007).

One study of 81 workers by the National Safety Council (1926) reported that nearly one-third of the workforce had benzene toxicity (Davis, 2007):

> 26 gave a blood picture characteristic of benzol [benzene] poisoning; and this ratio of about one man in three affected was maintained even in those workrooms with efficient local ventilation. . . . We were therefore forced to conclude that . . . the use of benzol (except in enclosed mechanical systems) even when the workers are protected by the most complete and effective systems of exhaust ventilation . . . involves a substantial hazard. (National Safety Council, 1926, p. 4)

In response to these reports of serious health problems in men working with benzene, researchers conducted a series of studies using cats, dogs, rabbits, guinea pigs, and rats. These studies, like many carried out in toxicology at that time, chiefly asked how much benzene was needed to anesthetize or kill the animal and how quickly this happened. Animals were observed for minutes, hours, or days to see when they developed jerky tremors, weakness, and muscle contractions, and at what point they dropped dead. Their blood was examined after death for evidence of benzene's effect. Animals that recovered from these exposures looked normal within days. One study decided to inject rats with much smaller amounts of benzene. This study found that it induced an array of symptoms, including loss of appetite, reduction in infection-fighting blood cells, and tremors (Davis, 2007).

Based on this work, the National Safety Council decided that benzene was a highly problematic material in the industrial workforce (Davis, 2007; National Safety Council, 1926).

> We are forced to conclude that the control of the benzol hazard (except where the substance is used in completely closed systems) is exceedingly difficult; that in practice, systems of exhaust ventilation capable of keeping the concentration of benzol in the atmosphere below 100 parts per million are extremely rare; and that, even when this is accomplished, there remains a decreased, but substantial hazard of benzol poisoning. (National Safety Council, 1926, p. 118)

Echoing this work nearly two decades later, the American Petroleum Institute in 1948 conceded that

> it is generally considered that the only absolutely safe concentration for benzene is zero. . . . Skin contact should be avoided. Acute poisoning by benzene should be considered as an acute emergency. . . . Chronic benzene poisoning is extremely refractory to treatment. Practically all therapeutic measures attempted have failed. (American Petroleum Institute, 1948, p. 4)

Today, the American Petroleum Institute takes a radically different position on benzene and is actively working to fund research that it expects will overturn national standards in many countries (American Petroleum Institute, 1948; Center for Media and Democracy, 2014; Davis, 2007). Recent work completed by a team at the University of California, Berkeley, reported that benzene produces toxic metabolites at very low doses (Rappaport et al., 2013).

Scientific American Identified Environmental Carcinogens in 1949

In 1949, a report in *Scientific American* by Groff Conklin featured a list of carcinogenic substances known to be present in the environment. Asbestos was described, along with solar and ionizing radiation, chromates, tar, synthetic dyes, and arsenic, as causing cancer by physically damaging the body or chemically inducing malignant growth. Conklin's article offered a clear statement: "Scientific and technological progress has exposed man to new physical and chemical agents. Some are believed associated with the rise of cancer as a cause of death" (p. 11).

When we look at the leading voices in cancer policy today, we face a tremendous chasm. It took nearly four decades for consensus to overwhelm the tobacco industry's efforts to dismiss the dangers of tobacco. That consensus came only after proof of human harm had become undeniable with growing rates of lung cancer in nations around the world. It is important for those concerned with preventing cancer to recognize that the effort requires a firm foundation in experimental science indicating likely human risks. However, even that foundation will not suffice unless it is tied to political forces that recognize the value of reducing risk.

In the United States, there has been growing recognition lately that regulatory efforts to control toxic chemicals, which began in 1976 with the Toxic Substances Control Act (TSCA), have had limited impact on public health. Discussions to reform TSCA are underway. Our view has been that the act would have been better named the Toxic Substances *Conversation* Act, as it has led to little action but much talking. When it comes to cancer policy overall, the cancer community remains focused on finding and treating the disease (often decades after the cancer began and could have been prevented). The major cancer organizations, such as the American Cancer Society and Susan G. Komen, have made little effort to evaluate environmental causes of cancer, aside from tobacco and obesity, and even less effort to propose policy steps to reduce toxic chemical or radiation exposures. Recently, the Environmental Working Group, Breast Cancer Action, and Breast Cancer Fund, among others, have rallied on the need to provide better labeling and reduce the use of toxic ingredients, especially those used in household products and personal care products. However, these efforts pale when compared to the influence of the manufacturers.

Many legislative attempts to mitigate human exposure to natural and industrial toxic chemicals have occurred during the past 100-plus years. The first major act was the Pure Food and Drug Act of 1906, which was later reformed into the Federal Food, Drug, and Cosmetic Act of 1938, and in 1968, laid the foundation for the creation of the U.S. Food and Drug Administration (FDA). The Federal Meat Inspection Act was codified into law at the same time as the Pure Food and Drug Act.

These laws constituted a political response to Upton Sinclair's (1906) muckraking novel *The Jungle*, which exposed the dark underbelly of the meatpacking industry in Chicago, the exploitation of immigrants, and the unscrupulous nature and function of big business at the time. However, even 100 years later, we still have much contamination in our food, as judged by carcinogenic arsenic contamination in feed given to chickens in the United States (Food & Water Watch, 2010) and levels of arsenic in fruit juices and rice (Navas-Acien & Nachman, 2013).

Numerous other laws have been enacted (see Table 4-1) that regulate practices related to air, water, pesticides, the disposal of toxic wastes, cleanup of those sites, and the aforementioned food, drugs, cosmetics, and other areas involving potential toxic contamination of humans, animals, and the environment. One of the laws hailed for its ability to protect humans and the environment from unsafe business practices was TSCA in 1976.

TSCA mandated that the U.S. Environmental Protection Agency (EPA) protect the public from unreasonable risks related to the manufacture, distribution, importation, and use of potentially toxic substances by creating a list of chemicals. This initial list, called "existing chemicals," grandfathered nearly 62,000 chemicals "in commerce" at that time and has since provided numerous avenues for the exemption of other chemicals for various reasons, including research, development, or because a particular chemical was already regulated under a different act (e.g., food, drugs, cosmetics, pesticides). Thus, many additional chemicals were added to the list without any premarket testing or review. These chemicals now number more than 84,000 (Society of Chemical Manufacturers and Affiliates, n.d.).

Inclusion of a chemical on the list means it can be legally manufactured, imported, distributed, purchased, consumed, or disposed of according to the law. Chemicals not on the list and yet to be imported or manufactured are considered new chemicals and must be submitted to EPA for review via a premanufacture notice (PMN) or a significant new use notice (SNUN, of which there are 160 existing chemicals for which paperwork must be submitted if they are to ever be used in a manner different than the current use), unless it is specifically excluded or exempt (U.S. EPA, 2014).

Most new chemical notifications presented to EPA are quickly approved under TSCA unless an "unreasonable risk to health or to the environment" is found (U.S. EPA, 2012b). If an unreasonable risk exists, the agency can choose to take action. Critics point out that this puts a significant burden on

Table 4-1. Legislative and Regulatory Milestones Relating to the Control of Toxic Chemicals

Year	Act/Agency	Purpose
1906	Pure Food and Drug Act	Precursor to Federal Food, Drug, and Cosmetic Act (1938)
1938	Federal Food, Drug, and Cosmetic Act	Regulates safety of food, drugs, and cosmetics
1948	Federal Water Pollution Control Act (FWPCA)	Precursor to Clean Water Act (1972)
1955	Air Pollution Control Act (APCA)	Precursor to Clean Air Act (1963)
1963	Clean Air Act (CAA)	Requires Environmental Protection Agency to protect human health from known hazardous airborne contaminants
1965	Solid Waste Disposal Act (SWDA)	Precursor to Resource Conservation and Recovery Act (1976)
1969	National Environmental Policy Act	Established research and procedural protocols for determining potential environmental impacts
1970	Environmental Protection Agency	Enacted via executive order (Nixon); write and enforce environmental regulation based on bills signed into law
1970	Clean Air Act (Extension)	Major rewrite of the 1963 legislation
1970	Williams-Steiger Occupational Safety and Health Act	Created the Occupational Safety and Health Administration, an occupational safety administration regulating workplace conditions, and the National Institute for Occupational Safety and Health, a research arm
1972	Clean Water Act (FWPCA Amendments)	Major rewrite and expansion of FWPCA (1948)
1972	Federal Insecticide, Fungicide, and Rodenticide Act (FIFRA)	Established protections for consumers, environment, and applicators from pesticides
1974	Safe Drinking Water Act	Established guidelines for contaminant levels in drinking water
1976	Resource Conservation and Recovery Act	Governs disposal of solid and hazardous waste; amended SWDA (1965)

(Continued on next page)

Table 4-1. Legislative and Regulatory Milestones Relating to the Control of Toxic Chemicals *(Continued)*

Year	Act/Agency	Purpose
1976	Toxic Substances Control Act (TSCA)	Regulates introduction of new or existing chemicals (see REACH, 2006)
1980	Comprehensive Environmental Response, Compensation, and Liability Act (CERCLA)	Created the Superfund program, which remediates abandoned hazardous waste sites
1986	Superfund Amendments and Reauthorization Act	Amended CERCLA (1980)
1990	Clean Air Act Amendments of 1990	Amended Clean Air Act (1963, 1970, etc.)
2006	Registration, Evaluation, Authorization and Restriction of Chemicals (REACH) legislation	European Union law; more expansive than TSCA, but still missing important reforms

the government to disprove two dangerous and unnecessary assumptions made by the legal system, both of which increase risks to public health: (a) most chemicals are presumed "innocent" until otherwise proven "guilty" and only a very few chemicals are ever a risk to public health, and (b) that all chemical manufacturers have a right to manufacture, distribute, and market their products (Guth, 2006). Unless this very high threshold of unreasonable risk is met, EPA cannot restrict the use of a dangerous chemical. Another significant criticism of TSCA is that, unlike the FDA approval process for a drug or medical device, obtaining approval for a PMN for a new chemical requires no safety testing whatsoever.

However, EPA is not the only agency charged with regulating toxic substances. In an unprecedented experiment in 1977, the heads of EPA, the Consumer Product Safety Commission, the Occupational Safety and Health Administration, and FDA joined in an effort called the Interagency Regulatory Liaison Group to create a streamlined and coordinated approach to toxic chemicals. This recognized that such materials could occur in consumer products and workplace conditions and as ingredients in foods, cosmetics, and drugs. The election of Ronald Reagan ended that experiment, leaving behind a patchwork approach with overlapping jurisdictions and frequent gaps in control (National Performance Review, 1993).

Probably one of the most egregious examples of this lapse of regulatory discipline is the failure to ban the use of the lipophilic, toxic, organochlorine gamma-hexachlorocyclohexane (γ-HCH) for the treatment of head lice in the United States. Reflecting the curious fact that this chemical is banned in most modern nations but not in the United States (Vijgen et al., 2011), the Centers for Disease Control and Prevention (CDC) website advises the following:

Although lindane shampoo 1% is approved by the FDA for the treatment of head lice, it is not recommended as a first-line treatment. Overuse, misuse, or accidentally swallowing lindane can be toxic to the brain and other parts of the nervous system; its use should be restricted to patients for whom prior treatments have failed or who cannot tolerate other medications that pose less risk. Lindane should not be used to treat premature infants, persons with HIV, a seizure disorder, women who are pregnant or breast-feeding, persons who have very irritated skin or sores where the lindane will be applied, infants, children, the elderly, and persons who weigh less than 110 pounds. (CDC, 2013)

In fact, the American Academy of Pediatrics has long advised against the use of lindane (CDC, 2013). The question is, why is this chemical still approved by FDA? The answer is straightforward: American companies have successfully lobbied for its continued approval, despite the growing consensus of scientists that it poses a danger to public health. Much of the regulatory process is similarly encumbered by outdated thinking and intense political jockeying.

Growing efforts to directly intimidate government research and evaluations have been underway for the past few years. For more than three decades, the U.S. National Toxicology Program has issued regular reports on suspected carcinogens based on reviews of experimental, clinical, and epidemiologic evidence and its own laboratory studies. Costly and heated battles have taken place to try to remove any number of high-volume commercial chemicals from the list. Well-paid expert consultants are used to argue that, while the evidence looks problematic on any given substance, in fact, there are special reasons why this is not the case. Detailed discussion on the political conflicts over the evaluation of vinyl chloride and several other major industrial chemicals can be found in my earlier work, *When Smoke Ran Like Water* (Davis, 2002). The bottom line remains that policy makers were mistaken to believe they merely needed the resources to study problems in order to prevent future harm from occurring. At this point, growing numbers of those involved in formulating policy recognize that studying problems can become an excuse for not acting to change current practices. Case in point: EPA released its draft review of dioxin toxicity in 1994. After years of review and revision, the noncancer portion of the report was issued in early 2012 (U.S. EPA, 2012a). Congressional attacks on the National Toxicology Program are mounting, with threats to defund much of the work, as special chemical interests seek to strip the National Toxicology Program of its capacity to conduct research and review evidence on modern toxic substances.

The protracted history of efforts to regulate toxic chemicals makes it worthwhile to look at Conklin's half-century–old views from *Scientific*

American (Conklin, 1949). The ideas expressed at that time are remarkably contemporary, and subsequent efforts by the modern chemical industry have effectively undermined many of them. It is a reminder that what has been lacking in cancer policy is not scientific evidence on avoidable causes of cancer, but rather the political will to act on knowledge already at hand:

> It has been established that certain agents to which people are exposed in industrial occupations cause cancer if the exposure to them is sufficiently intense and prolonged. As an example, over 75 per cent of the miners in the Schneeberg cobalt-uranium mines of Germany die of lung cancer. . . . In the 18th century it was learned that among chimney sweeps exposed to intense concentrations of soot, deaths from cancer were between three to four times as high as those in the general population. . . .
>
> Although these are special cases of intense exposure, they naturally suggest speculation as to whether the average human being's relatively mild but long-continued exposure to new substances in a contaminated atmosphere, in processed foods, in cosmetics and in other elements of our environment may be a contributory cause of cancer. (Conklin, 1949, p. 11)

Conklin further emphasized the role of physicians and medical professionals in identifying possible workplace and environmental exposures contributing to cancer:

> Generally speaking, however, employers are no more responsible for the lack of information about industrial cancer than are the many thousands of physicians who have cancer patients in industrial areas or who actually are associated with factories. It is an unquestionable fact that an appreciable number of occupational cancers slip through the hands of doctors unidentified. This is due in a great degree to a general ignorance of the occupational aspects of cancer. Physicians have never been adequately informed of the basic symptomatic and sociological factors involved in identifying occupational carcinogenesis.
>
> The medical profession should be better educated about the need for exhaustive case histories which carry the individual's job record in detail back as far as 25 years, about the urgency of checking medical suspicions of industrial cancer hazards against careful epidemiological studies of all workers in a plant, and about the paramount importance of impressing plant management with the seriousness of the problem. (Conklin, 1949, p. 14)

Conklin's conclusion was posited more than 60 years ago and yet is still salient today: "It is obvious, therefore, that the control of occupational carcinogenesis . . . is a public health problem of considerable magnitude" (p. 14).

The Toxic Substances Control Act Today

Since 1976, TSCA has helped inventory more than 84,000 chemicals. These are subcategorized as "existing" chemicals, numbering approximately 62,000, and some 22,000 "new" chemicals inventoried since its passage. Of the initial 62,000, EPA has restricted the production, importation, or use of only five existing chemicals: polychlorinated biphenyls (PCBs), dioxin, asbestos, hexavalent chromium (chromium VI), and chlorofluorocarbons (known as CFCs, an environmental contaminant) (Congressional Digest, 2010).

However, finding these five chemicals in any authoritative document was quite a chore for an able researcher and likely would be extremely difficult for anyone among the general public. This is because the EPA's web pages and materials relating to the TSCA have been quite cryptic, misleading, and frustrating, as documented by Bill Chameides, dean of the Duke University Nicholas School of the Environment (Chameides, 2011a).

The removal of lead from paints and some gasolines is regularly hailed by many as a success of chemical regulation. The ingestion of lead has been understood to be toxic for more than 2,000 years (its use predates the historically documented dates of toxicity), when lead from vessels used in the production of wine to boil unfermented grape juice leached into the product during the early period of the Roman Empire (Nriagu, 1983). Despite this knowledge of toxicity among Western cultures and EPA's inclusion of the Lead-Based Paint Disclosure Rule on one of its own TSCA pages (U.S. EPA, 2013b), "there appear to be no TSCA regulations on lead or lead-based products at this time" (Chameides, 2011a).

Asbestos is also hailed as modern success of TSCA, and, to be sure, TSCA has regulated asbestos in part. Like lead, the inhalation of asbestos has long been known to be toxic. In the Middle Ages, soiled tablecloths made from asbestos fibers would be cleaned by throwing them into the fire where food and drink residues would burn off. Asbestos fibers would dislodge regularly, though, during this process, often causing harm to those in the area (Unger, 2010).

Despite this, however, asbestos has been only partially restricted with respect to its manufacture and use (under TSCA), while existing applications using these chemicals were allowed to remain (U.S. EPA, 2012b). There is some wisdom in not disturbing an extremely toxic product in many applications, although at some point their continued and unaddressed presence will likely create significant future health risks, cancerous and otherwise.

The legal fight over asbestos regulation proved protracted and limited in effectiveness.

Asbestos was first regulated in schools and in public and commercial buildings via the Asbestos Hazard Emergency Response Act added to Title II of TSCA by Congress in 1986. In 1989, EPA issued a more comprehensive ban on asbestos-containing products under TSCA's Section 6. However, in 1991 a federal court overturned most of these regulations—ruling that EPA had not met the "unreasonable risk" threshold. As a result, TSCA's regulation of asbestos pertains only to "flooring felt, rollboard, and corrugated, commercial, or specialty paper" as well as new uses. (Chameides, 2011b)

In 1991, the Fifth Circuit Court of Appeals ruled in *Corrosion Proof Fittings v. EPA* that, in regard to "unreasonable risk," regulators must take the "least burdensome" (to companies trying to market their products) approach, thereby overturning EPA's TSCA rule and ultimately making TSCA enforcement practically impossible (Stadler, 1993). In short, it ensured that asbestos was not banned and would only apply to the aforementioned uses described by Chameides. More importantly, it severely constrained TSCA review and restriction of existing chemicals to the "least burdensome" manner.

In fact, most of the chemicals regulated under TSCA are only partially controlled. Thus, the family of fire-resistant cooling fluids used in electrical capacitors, known collectively as PCBs, are mostly banned under TSCA (Chameides, 2011b), which unequivocally benefits human health. However, they remain important public health and environmental threats for several reasons. They exist in old transformers and other devices that can release large amounts of contaminants during fires, demolition, and even vandalism. They are also still regularly produced as by-products during the manufacture of other approved chemicals (e.g., pesticides, herbicides) and diarylide yellow pigments, which contaminate U.S. watersheds and are used in many consumer applications such as clothes, paints, paper, and other products (Rodenburg, Guo, Du, & Cavallo, 2010). Warnings of such contaminations are not disclosed on product labels or safety data sheets. PCBs are also produced during the incineration of many types of waste as a result of the heating and cooling process in the presence of a particular few chemicals.

Perhaps most important is that wherever PCBs are found, dioxin-like compounds (DLCs) and polychlorinated dibenzo-p-dioxins and dibenzofurans (commonly referred to as PCDD/Fs) are also found. Dioxins and furans are two different chemical families containing more than 200 chemicals between them, including 17 chemicals known to be toxic to humans and the environment (Winters, 2002). Dioxins are included on EPA's TSCA list of regulated existing chemicals (U.S. Government Accountability Office, 2005). They contaminated Agent Orange, a chemical manufactured by Dow Chemical and Monsanto and used by the U.S. military in Southeast Asia during the Vietnam War as a defoliant (Schecter et al., 1995).

PCDD/Fs and PCBs may continue to be an issue in the current production of the newly approved use of one of Agent Orange's two major chemical components, the pesticide 2,4-dichlorophenoxyacetic acid (2,4-D), as it will be even more widely distributed as a major component of a chemical herbicide salt and weed control system (Dow AgroSciences, 2014). The problem is that the chemical reactions that occur during the manufacture of many intermediate chemicals used as reagents to make phenoxy pesticides and herbicides, such as 2,4-D, inadvertently create dioxins (and thus PCBs, furans, and other DLCs), as well as other toxic chemical by-products (Carey, 2006). A recent study suggested that current levels of PCDD/F contamination of 2,4-D products "may increase the risk for the human and environmental health," although they are much higher in the production of 2,4,5-trichlorophenoxyacetic acid (known as 2,4,5-T, the other major component of Agent Orange) (Liu, Li, Tao, Li, Tian, & Xie, 2013). In some countries, 2,4-D is not being regulated as one of the 17 toxic congeners of dioxin, illustrating that selective regulation of toxic chemicals is not an exclusively U.S. problem.

Dioxins in water can be toxic to humans at levels millions of times lower than other known carcinogens. For instance, according to EPA, eating less than a quarter pound of Shiner surfperch from the San Francisco Bay increases one's lifetime risk of developing cancer to more than 1 in 1,000 (U.S. EPA, 2013a). So although dioxins may have been added to the list of existing chemicals in TSCA, this does not suggest that dioxin risks are minimal for humans, wildlife, the food web, or the environment.

The use of hexavalent chromium is also only partially restricted, limited to commercial applications but not those pertaining to industry. While trivalent chromium is an essential nutrient, hexavalent is a known carcinogen (Chameides, 2011b).

Perhaps more concerning than the partial regulation of these chemicals is that toxicologists do not fully understand the health impacts of these toxic chemical families, especially the potential synergistic (interactions between two or more of these chemicals that result in effects which exceed additive or multiplicative impacts) health effects of more than 400 of these compounds or their interactions with many other widely available toxic compounds. Yet, at least 29 PCBs, dioxins, and furans are known to be toxic (Winters, 2002).

So, TSCA regulates five "existing" chemicals, four of which are very toxic to humans (CFCs are restricted because of their role in ozone depletion), but only partially—leading to present-day contamination of humans, consumer products, the food web, and the environment. EPA regulates four "new" chemicals, all of which are used in metalworking fluids (U.S. Government Accountability Office, 2005).

However, even many of these partial regulations and restrictions are on shaky legal ground, as a U.S. appeals court overturned many of them in 1991. Other court rulings have made it quite difficult for EPA to regulate specific chemicals, while new chemicals are presumed safe until and unless they are found to be harmful (U.S. Government Accountability Office, 1994).

Much of the public and even many in the scientific community are surprised to find that industry is not required to test any of these chemicals for safety before manufacture, distribution, importation, or use. Instead, companies merely must submit a PMN saying insufficient data are available to determine safety (the criticisms of this process by both industry and many health advocates may be suggestive of its failure as well).

EPA, under TSCA, has only required testing on approximately 200 (0.24%) chemicals out of the more than 84,000. From a safety standpoint, not much is known about the potential health risks of nearly all the remaining 84,000 chemicals in high-volume use in commerce (Congressional Digest, 2010). This is because of the controversial "unreasonable risk" threshold, which essentially requires EPA regulators to presume a chemical to be nontoxic unless this difficult threshold is met. This is the exact opposite approach from the precautionary principle, sometimes used in public health, which states that if there are concerns about safety, it is better to exclude such unsafe products, chemicals, etc., and err on the safe side if reasonable to do so.

According to EPA's Chemical Hazard Data Availability Study (U.S. EPA, 2010), of the more than 3,000 chemicals that are considered *high production volume* (produced or imported at more than one million pounds per year), merely 7% have full Screening Information Data Set (SIDS) testing completed, and some of these chemicals have been produced for decades. SIDS tests are the standard for basic testing as established by the Organisation for Economic Co-operation and Development and include six basic toxicity tests: acute toxicity, chronic toxicity, developmental/reproductive toxicity, mutagenicity, ecotoxicity, and environmental fate (U.S. EPA, 2010). The estimated cost to close the data gap was 0.2% of a single year's revenues from the top 100 chemical-producing companies (U.S. EPA, 2010). Many view this as a failing of EPA and a disinterest in regulating the chemical industry. *Regulatory capture* (whereby, over time, a regulatory agency becomes more and more influenced by the industry it is supposed to regulate) is a serious issue for nearly every industry and regulatory agency, but in this case, judicial findings and linguistic loopholes have also made enforcement of TSCA extremely difficult.

Some industry advocates, such as the Society of Chemical Manufacturers and Affiliates, have correctly noted that not all 84,000 of these chemicals are "in commerce," and no chemical can ever be deleted from the inventory, so, they argue, the list just continues to grow. They have stated that approximately 25,000 are currently "in commerce" and that exempted chemicals are not likely to reach even 15,000 in number. They also acknowledge, however, that there is no way to truly know exact numbers (Society of Chemical Manufacturers and Affiliates, n.d.).

A recent study on bottled water in Germany found 24,520 detectable chemicals in bottled water (Wagner, Schlüsener, Ternes, & Oehlmann, 2013). Bottled water manufacturing is highly standardized and quite centralized, suggesting that water distributed in the United States using similar plastic materials and production methods would likely have similar concentrations and types of chemicals as the ones tested in Germany. This study looked at chemical health effects that are more insidious than cancer (e.g., those resulting from endocrine-disrupting chemicals) and at doses lower by, at times, nearly a dozen orders of magnitude. Of course, not all of these detected chemicals are toxic, but the fact that they can be detected now indicates the extent to which we live in a "chemical soup"—making regulation and evaluation of the health impact of individual chemicals all the more challenging.

Irrespective of how many chemicals are officially deemed to be in commerce, many, such as the very toxic persistent organic pollutants (POPs), PCBs, and dioxins, are ubiquitous today in humans, animals, and the environment. These lipophilic (fat-seeking) chemicals bioaccumulate, bioconcentrate, and biomagnify (i.e., they move up the food chain and can be found in mammals and humans that consume diets high in animal fats). Thus, even if many old and new POPs were banned, as an international treaty requires (Ditz, Tuncak, & Wiser, 2011), their residues will be with this planet for decades to centuries.

In that same regard, although lead-based paints are no longer "in commerce," they are still very much a problem in decaying housing stock. In developing countries, lead is still used in glazing and in fuels. Similarly, although the pesticide DDT was banned more than 40 years ago (1972) in the United States, it can still be detected in the tissues of most humans because its biologic half-life, or the time it takes for half of its physiologic effect to be reduced in the body, is estimated at anywhere from six to nine years. For many lipophilic agents and people, fat remains a natural hazardous waste site.

Considering all of these loopholes, failures, court rulings, interpretations, and gaps in testing and review, significant toxics reform legislation is widely regarded as a major priority in efforts to reduce and prevent a wide range of chronic illnesses (Chameides, 2011a; Landrigan & Goldman, 2011; Society of Chemical Manufacturers and Affiliates, n.d.). As of this writing, cancer is without question one of the most serious diseases, affecting one out of every two males and one of every three females in their lifetimes. Yet, exposures to toxic chemicals also create many other diseases that—irrespective of their magnitude relative to cancer—are just as preventable. Specifically, endocrine-disrupting chemicals and various neurodevelopmental chemicals can produce powerful epigenetic transformations that can persist in organisms for several generations. Other classes of chemicals also need to be properly regulated, including persistent, bioaccumulative and toxic substances (known as PBTs), POPs, and benzene, toluene, ethylbenzene, and xylenes (known as BTEX) from liquid natural gas extraction processes, heavy metals, and many others.

The diseases that these unregulated chemicals are believed to cause, in addition to the extremely tiny doses that are being implicated in their genesis, have prompted some experts to advocate for all chemicals to be suspected as neurodevelopmental toxicants (Landrigan & Goldman, 2014). The problem of toxics reform is beyond the realm of just looking at ways to prevent cancer. Meaningful TSCA reform is considered essential to protecting our most sensitive and vulnerable populations, as well as future generations, from all of these exposures and preventable diseases (Landrigan & Goldman, 2011).

Despite this backdrop and universal agreement on the necessity of reform, what form it should take remains hotly contested. Nearly 20 years ago, Colborn, Dumanosky, and Myers wrote a book ushering in a new era of recognition about the broad range of health impacts of toxic chemicals, titled *Our Stolen Future.* The advice they proffered then remains quite relevant today:

* Place the burden of proof on the chemical manufacturers.
* Focus on prevention of exposure.
* Establish standards to protect vulnerable populations, particularly children and the unborn.
* Consider cumulative exposure from air, water, food, and other sources.
* Amend trade secret laws to enable people to prevent unwanted exposure to themselves while still preserving any genuine need for trade-related confidentiality.
* Require sellers, especially of food, to monitor their products for contamination.
* Expand the concept of the Toxic Release Inventory database to encompass deliberate release (e.g., pesticides, detergents, plastics).
* Mandate notice and full disclosure in settings where pesticides are used and may come in contact with the public.
* Reform health data systems so that they contain the information necessary for the development of sound, protective policies.

Since that time, many of the most respected toxics researchers have stated that any new standard should be health-based (instead of a cost-balanced method, which must use the "least burdensome" approach) (Landrigan & Goldman, 2011).

If, as previously suggested, all chemicals should be suspected as neurodevelopmental toxicants (causing diseases such as autism spectrum disorders, attention-deficit/hyperactivity disorder, dyslexia, speech pathologies, and genetic disorders, like Down syndrome) (Grandjean & Landrigan, 2014; Landrigan & Goldman, 2011), new legislation would need to ensure not only basic SIDS testing but also a mandatory program with more robust testing. This would ensure that toxic chemicals (whether new or existing) remain out of commerce and less toxic or nontoxic chemicals in the same class could be substituted.

A new standard is needed to protect society's most vulnerable populations (infants and children specifically, as well as nursing mothers, pregnant women, and more generally women of childbearing age), as found in the 1993 National Academies report *Pesticides in the Diets of Infants and Children* (National Research Council, 1993). Furthermore, 1997 Executive Order No. 13045 stated that "proposed federal rules must be evaluated for the effect of the rules on children's environmental health and safety and an explanation provided as to why the planned rule is the most preferable alternative" (Minnesota Department of Health, 2003).

Potential health endpoints to be considered for assessment before a chemical might enter commerce could comprise carcinogenicity, mutagenicity and genotoxicity, reproductive toxicity, developmental toxicity, endocrine activity, acute toxicity, systemic toxicity and organ effects, neurotoxicity, skin and respiratory sensitization, skin and eye irritation, acute and chronic aquatic toxicity, other ecotoxicity, biologic persistence, and bioaccumulation, as well as reactivity and flammability.

The National Institute of Environmental Health Sciences and EPA both possess newer technologies and techniques that can help assess for these (and other) endpoints. Tests could be performed using any of the following advances in technologic toxicity testing: quantum dots for measuring sensitive biomarkers, physiologically based pharmacokinetic modeling using data on the absorption, distribution, metabolism, and excretion of a particular chemical, in vitro neural stem cells, in silico (computer-based testing) and clinical methods, and other advanced toxicologic testing (Balls, Combes, & Bhogal, 2012; Grandjean & Landrigan, 2014). Additional approaches might rely on continuous epidemiologic surveillance monitoring (Grandjean & Landrigan, 2014; Landrigan & Goldman, 2011), such as pharmacoepidemiologic approaches that assess potential health effects related to potential exposures. It also might be possible to create a chemical equivalent of the Vaccine Adverse Event Reporting System.

Other important issues related to TSCA reform include replacing the vague or restrictive language (e.g., phrases like *unreasonable risk* and *least burdensome*) that led to courts interpreting these terms so that the United States functionally had an industry-based law. Additionally, creating a standard that can be applied in a relatively swift manner, yet does not compromise its primary function of being health-based, would be fair to industry and would not undermine protection of current and future generations. It could be modeled upon the FDA process for regulating pharmaceutical drugs or devices.

Finally, one of the most important aspects of TSCA reform relates to the issue of preemption, that is, whether states have the right to require higher standards than an enacted federal law. States such as California took action in the vacuum left after TSCA was judicially neutralized, enacting laws that were more protective of human and environmental health. Industry, on the other hand, dislikes having to adapt to numerous state standards and prefers a federal law (although deregulation is almost always the preferred option). But, in this case, industry was feeling not only "bottom-up" pressure from states but also "top-down" pressure from international and European movement on these issues—the European Union passed the Registration, Evaluation, Authorisation and Restriction of Chemicals (REACH) legislation (Bach, 2014).

Senator Frank Lautenberg (D-NJ) proposed a series of amendments to TSCA from 2005 until his death in June 2013. The goal of his bills was to ensure that chemicals were made as safely as possible (Bach, 2014). The Safe Chemicals Act of 2011 (S. 847) was a bill undesirable to industry groups and more desirable to consumer, medical, health, conservation, and environmental groups. Lautenberg's bills sought a "reasonable certainty" standard that would limit "aggregate exposure to a no more than 1 in 1,000,000 risk of adverse effects in the population of concern" (Bach, 2014, p. 507). None of the early Lautenberg bills were enacted.

Just before Lautenberg died, the Chemical Safety Improvement Act (CSIA) of 2013 was introduced. Although touted as bipartisan, the proposed bill reflects the massive divide between industry and public health scientists, consumer groups, and environmental groups. For example, the CSIA bill still uses the term *unreasonable risk*, despite its being one of the more subjective phrases in the previous TSCA legislation that is widely credited with weakening the enforcement opportunities.

The CSIA more closely resembles a "TSCA II" than the spirit and language of Lautenberg's earlier proposed legislation. For successful reform to take place that incorporates more proactive approaches, it would need to address a number of major issues that are unlikely to be considered in the current antiregulatory congress, including the scope of EPA's authority in reviewing new and existing chemicals; the form that risk assessment and management might take; the need for greater transparency of chemicals reviewed; states' rights to preemption; the protection of vulnerable populations; the problem of synergistic and interactive chemical effects and aggregate exposures; cumulative risk; the cost burden for testing; the necessity of basic and more advanced safety, health, and environmental testing before chemicals are produced, distributed, and sold; the process of restricting such chemicals if found to be dangerous; timeliness of the process; recent issues that have yet to gain traction in the public sphere, such as the potentially toxic effect of nanomaterials; and, possibly most important, the elimination of vague, nonspecific language (Bach, 2014). Overall, the presumption of the CSIA remains that chemicals are safe until proven otherwise.

Critics of CSIA further contend that while the bill does make a few very small overtures to the failings of TSCA, the bill does not address the biggest defects of TSCA and affirms the previous weak standard set forth by TSCA. First, it still contains the phrase *unreasonable risk*, which has been one of the biggest issues with TSCA. Thus, manufacturers would likely be afforded legal and financial immunity once a chemical was determined not to be an unreasonable risk. It prohibits states from enacting stricter reforms to protect its own citizens, fails to protect vulnerable populations (e.g., pregnant/nursing women, children, older adults, immunocompromised individuals), and does not protect workers, economically disadvantaged communities, or "hot spots." It lacks the ability to examine cumulative risk or interactive/synergistic effects from aggregate exposures, and all costs of regulation would be borne by taxpayers, not the corporations seeking to put a product on the market. Premarket testing would not be a necessary condition for manufacture, distribution, and sale. Yet, if EPA were to find problems with a particular dangerous chemical, it would face mountains of costs and obstacles in enacting a ban or restriction. The bill would still not require basic safety testing (e.g., SIDS testing, or even the more necessary tests beyond those) for new or existing chemicals. It would not offer special protections from especially pernicious classes of chemicals such as PBTs. Finally, it uses nonspecific phrases regarding time frames for regulatory action (Andrews, 2013).

The lessons of the TSCA failures and other major environmental statutes are clear. Laws state the intentions and values of society. However, few laws can be crafted that will withstand well-organized efforts to undermine it, no matter how well intentioned the drafters of laws may be. Even with a good start, important reform is a lengthy and expensive process and requires participation and a cautious eye to watch how the players attempt to support or thwart implementation of significant reform. This process will ultimately determine whether risks to humans, animals, and the environment are prevented, mitigated, or intensified. And as always, the devil is in the details and how those details are later interpreted by regulatory agencies, lawyers, and courts.

Figure 4-1 lists interested organizations and businesses that are concerned about risks from products containing toxic chemicals in homes, yards, and occupational environments (Safer Chemicals, Healthy Families, n.d.). These groups actively support revisions to TSCA, and they fall along predictable lines. The details of any specific proposal will change as bills move through the political and legislative process and are interpreted afterward by regulators. However, the bottom line is that consumer advocacy and environmental groups tend to seek greater transparency and a more health-protective approach where thorough testing of chemicals is done *prior* to their introduction into commerce, whereas industry groups generally support less testing beforehand and taking regulatory actions only *after* risks have been suggested or demonstrated.

Yet it is important to note that legislation and regulatory policy is only one way that people can mitigate their risk of exposure to toxic chemicals. Consumers and businesses can become more conscious of the potential toxic chemicals they use and seek alternatives. A discussion of the myriad ways of substituting with less toxic products and chemicals and practicing safer use of those without easy substitutions is beyond the scope of this

Figure 4-1. Organizations and Businesses That Support Revisions to the Toxic Substances Control Act

Healthcare Providers/Research Institutions
- Mount Sinai Children's Environmental Health Center
- National Medical Association
- Physicians for Social Responsibility
- Science and Environmental Health Network
- Yale School of Medicine, Environmental Health Group

Public Health Organizations
- Agent Orange Legacy—Children of Vietnam Veterans
- American Public Health Association—Public Health Nursing Section
- Association of State and Territorial Directors of Nursing
- Breast Cancer Action
- Breast Cancer Fund
- Consumers Union
- Endometriosis Association
- Institute for Agriculture and Trade Policy
- National Center for Environmental Health Strategies
- National Disease Clusters Alliance
- Oregon Public Health Association
- Women's Health and Environmental Network
- Women's Voices for the Earth

Nursing Organizations
- Alliance of Nurses for Healthy Environments
- American Holistic Nurses Association
- American Nurses Association
- Association of Women's Health, Obstetric and Neonatal Nurses
- Developmental Disabilities Nurses Association
- National Association of Hispanic Nurses
- Nurses for Global Health
- Washington State Association of Occupational Health Nurses

Labor Organizations
- United Automobile Workers
- United Steelworkers

National Environmental Organizations
- Center for Health, Environment and Justice
- Center for International Environmental Law
- Chlorine Free Products Association
- Environmental Defense Fund
- Environmental Health Fund
- Environmental Working Group
- Jean-Michel Cousteau's Ocean Futures Society
- Natural Resources Defense Council
- Pesticide Action Network North America
- Rachel's Network

(Continued on next page)

Figure 4-1. Organizations and Businesses That Support Revisions to the Toxic Substances Control Act *(Continued)*

- Sierra Club
- Union of Concerned Scientists
- U.S. Public Interest Research Group

Environmental Justice Organization
- Indigenous Environmental Network

Parent Organizations
- Children's Environmental Protection Alliance (Children's EPA)
- Healthy Child Healthy World
- Holistic Moms Network
- National Organization for Women

Reproductive Health Organizations
- American Fertility Association
- Association of Reproductive Health Professionals
- National Asian Pacific American Women's Forum
- National Latina Institute for Reproductive Health
- Physicians for Reproductive Health
- Planned Parenthood Federation of America

Learning and Developmental Disabilities Organizations
- American Association on Intellectual and Developmental Disabilities
- Arc of the United States
- Association for Children's Mental Health
- Children and Adults With Attention-Deficit/Hyperactivity Disorder
- Learning Disabilities Association of America
- National Institute of Neurological Disorders and Stroke

Note. Based on information from Safer Chemicals, Healthy Families, 2014.

---

chapter but is ubiquitous within the realm of more "green" and less contaminated options for food, cosmetic and grooming products, clothing, and so on.

EPA, the University of California, San Francisco, the Center for Environmental Research and Children's Health, and the California Department of Pesticide Regulation (2013) have developed materials identifying opportunities to limit toxic exposures of children in early childhood and educational settings. EPA also has attempted to create a list of products that are safer for the environment in its Design for the Environment initiative (see www .epa.gov/dfe). Other organizations, government agencies, and initiatives, such as the Healthier Hospital Initiative and the Environmental Health Trust (which focuses on limiting radiation due to cell phone use), provide opportunities for our society to begin to think about how to live less toxic lives in ways that many are just beginning to consider.

The Modern Failure to Control Cancer

Four centuries ago, some observant physicians laid the basic foundations of public health research. By the 1950s, scientists had developed a program aimed at training physicians to recognize and reduce risks from workplace and environmental hazards. How do scientists today determine the health hazards at work or in the world around us? They basically do what Agricola, Ramazzini, and Roffo did: They look around. They visit and talk to people who are going through natural experiments of their own sort to learn about the good and bad in their life histories that may account for their health.

In classic scientific experiments, results are contrasted between two groups that ideally differ in only one way (Davis, 2007). In public health research, we rely on our ability to compare groups that may differ in many ways to conclude whether some of those differences account for why some are healthier or sicker than others. For workplace hazards, such as those that first fascinated Ramazzini, we compare various measures of well-being of those in some jobs with those in other jobs. Scientists also ask and count what types and numbers of illnesses arise in those who work directly with certain agents. Where possible, researchers measure residues in air, water, blood, and urine and contrast this information with what happens to those who are not exposed to such substances (Davis, 2007).

We are left to wonder what happened to derail cancer prevention efforts that began in the last century. The top scientists from around the world understood in 1936 that much cancer came from the workplace, nutrition, hormones, sunlight, radiation, and other external sources. By 1949, the National Cancer Institute had begun a program to train doctors to look for signs of these health risks and to promote their reduction (Conklin, 1949). Why were these efforts stymied? What happened to undermine programs to reduce the burden of cancer? Why have we spent so much effort treating cancer and so little on understanding how to keep the disease from happening?

In the run-up to World War II, as well as in its aftermath, science could not remain an abstract matter carried out because of the inherent curiosity of lone geniuses. Instead, scientific investigations became part and parcel of vital national efforts to conduct and carry out warfare. During the various early-19th century French revolutions, the philosophers had boasted—at least until some of them were beheaded for doing so—of the value of pursuing cross-national exchanges (Davis, 2007).

For humanity, the specter of death and national conflict that began to course around the world in the second quarter of the 20th century concentrated the imagination, but seldom in a way that inspired clear thinking about the future. The future was shorted by those who looked solely at the present. Thanks to the many good works of Stanton Glantz at the University of California, Berkeley, Robert Proctor at Stanford, Allan Brandt at Harvard, and their young colleagues, we have ample understanding of the extent to which the tobacco industry used science and scientists as part of an insidiously effective public relations strategy that sustained their poisonous and highly profitable product. David Michael's (2008) work *Doubt Is Their Product*, Markowitz and Rosner's (2013) *Deceit and Denial*, and my *Secret History of the War on Cancer* (Davis, 2007) and *Disconnect: The Truth About Cell Phone Radiation, What the Industry Has Done to Hide It, and How to Protect Your Family* (Davis, 2010) have amply documented that the strategy of deceit, denial, and delay continue to characterize all modern cancer-causing hazards.

The example of cell phones and other wireless transmitting devices is but the latest instance of a highly profitable, widespread technology where evidence of danger has been dismissed and undermined by well-paid experts, many of whom do not appreciate the extent to which they and their findings have become part of a huge industrial operation. Without more independent funding to support the investigation of these and other hazards, we remain committed to a pattern where action to prevent future harm cannot take place until evidence of current human damage has mounted. This effectively means that we mortgage the health of the future against that of the present. We may well be able to afford this economically, but history will have to judge the moral legacies of such efforts (Davis, 2007).

The Legacy of World War II

As we have come to know, the august cancer congress was held in Brussels in 1936, during an era of mounting hostility and widespread militarization of the most common aspects of life. As a committed Unitarian, the biologist Walter B. Cannon saw international scientific collaboration as a moral duty. He resisted nationalistic impulses to pull back from working and meeting with scientists from other nations. He journeyed to Leningrad, Russia—then in the grip of its own revolutionary violence—to meet his colleague Ivan Pavlov, the pioneering behavioral psychologist, in 1935. His address to this 1936 congress foretold the lapse of long-term interest in scientific matters, including the ability of chemicals and various forms of radiation to damage human life:

> During the last few years how profoundly and unexpectedly the world has changed. Nationalism has become violently intensified until it is tainted with bitter feeling. The world-wide economic depression has greatly reduced the material support for scholarly efforts. What is the social value of the physiologist or biochemist? (as cited in Davis, 2007, p. 39)

Cannon is known today for coining the term "fight or flight" to describe the physical response of living beings to life-threatening terrors. A chance finding of what made cats arch their backs when under duress led him to his life's work of examining the complex physical ways that bodies deal with danger, and he collaborated across oceans and national borders to do so (Cannon, 1994). When facing danger, the body mobilizes. A surge of hormones turns on the ability to fight or run harder, faster, longer. The heart beats more power-fully, energy surges throughout the body, and the hair stands on end; every organ system is marshaled in defense against the perceived threat (Davis, 2007).

Nations do much the same. The prospect of massive, unrestrained global conflict fundamentally changed public priorities and altered the way science was supported and used by those who underwrite its efforts. The immediate need to defend against the threats of the Axis conquest trumped consideration of the longer-term results of leading crisis-driven lives. To be concerned with preventing cancer requires planning and consideration about what will happen in a few decades. A world facing highly uncertain, potentially cataclysmic prospects was not inclined to ponder the future (Davis, 2007).

Once the war was over (and a slower, colder war took its place), the old knowledge about cancer hazards fell victim to enthusiasm for modern industrial advances and the social and economic forces that lay behind them. A combination of optimism about the industrial future, bona fide improvements in the ability to see and grasp the basic biology of disease, and darker forces fueling that optimism guaranteed that the burden of proving that any modern activity caused cancer would become impossibly heavy. Contemporary discussions about TSCA must be seen in this same context: demands for proof of human harm can stymie efforts to prevent or restrict suspect agents from becoming widely used in commerce. Today, as in the aftermath of World War II, the search for more scientific information easily morphs into a reason to reject what had once been known (Davis, 2007). In the discussions of how to reform TSCA, the insistence for strong evidence of definitive human harm before acting to avoid future harm fundamentally subverts public health principles that seek to prevent disease and promote health by identifying and reducing toxic chemicals and other risks.

References

American Petroleum Institute. (1948). *API toxicological review: Benzene.* Retrieved from http://www.hobsonbradley.com/articles/pdf/pdffile.pdf

Andrews, D. (2013). Why EWG opposes the Chemical Safety Improvement Act. *Enviroblog.* Retrieved from http://www.ewg.org/enviroblog/2013/06/why-ewg-opposes-chemical-safety-improvement-act

Bach, T. (2014). Better living through chemicals (Regulation)? The Chemical Safety Improvement Act of 2013 through an environmental public health law lens. *Vermont Journal of Environmental Law, 15,* 490–537. Retrieved from http://vjel.vermontlaw.edu/files/2014/04/Bach_FORPRINT.pdf

Balls, M., Combes, R.D., & Bhogal, N. (Eds.). (2012). *New technologies for toxicity testing.* New York, NY: Springer Science + Business Media.

Berenblum, I. (1977). Cancer research in historical perspective: An autobiographical essay. *Cancer Research, 37,* 1–7.

Cannon, B. (1994). Walter Bradford Cannon: Reflections on the man and his contributions. *International Journal of Stress Management, 1,* 145–158. doi:10.1007/BF01857608

Carey, F.A. (2006). *Organic chemistry* (6th ed.). Boston, MA: McGraw-Hill.

Center for Media and Democracy. (2014). American Petroleum Institute. *SourceWatch.* Retrieved from http://www.sourcewatch.org/index.php/American_Petroleum_Institute#Concerns _about_API-funded_research

Centers for Disease Control and Prevention. (2013). Parasites: Lice: Head lice: Treatment. Retrieved from http://www.cdc.gov/parasites/lice/head/treatment.html

Chameides, B. (2011a, June 13). In search of the toxic five. Retrieved from http://blogs .nicholas.duke.edu/thegreengrok/insearchoftsca5

Chameides, B. (2011b, June 14). The Toxic Substances Control Act's toxic baddies. Retrieved from http://blogs.nicholas.duke.edu/thegreengrok/tscatoxics

Chemical Safety Improvement Act of 2013, S. 1009, 113th Cong.

Colborn, T., Dumanoski, D., & Myers, J.P. (1996). *Our stolen future: Are we threatening our fertility, intelligence, and survival? A scientific detective story.* New York, NY: Dutton.

Congressional Digest. (2010). Controlling toxic substances. Retrieved from http://congressionaldigest.com/issue/controlling-toxic-substances

Conklin, G. (1949). Cancer and environment. *Scientific American, 180*(1), 11–15. Retrieved from http://www.scientificamerican.com/article/cancer-and-environment

Cramer, W. (1936). The importance of statistical investigations in the campaign against cancer. In M. Fraenkel (Ed.), *Report of the Second International Congress of Scientific and Social Campaign Against Cancer.* Brussels, Belgium: Ligue Nationale Belge Contre Le Cancer.

Davis, D. (2010). *Disconnect: The truth about cell phone radiation, what the industry has done to hide it, and how to protect your family.* New York, NY: Penguin.

Davis, D.L. (2002). *When smoke ran like water: Tales of environmental deception and the battle against pollution.* New York, NY: Basic Books.

Davis, D.L. (2007). *The secret history of the war on cancer.* New York, NY: Basic Books.

Ditz, D., Tuncak, B., & Wiser, G. (2011). U.S. law and the Stockholm POPs Convention: Analysis of treaty-implementing provisions in pending legislation. Retrieved from http://www.ciel .org/Publications/US_Law_and_Stockholm_POPs.pdf

Dow AgroSciences. (2014). Dow AgroSciences announces launch of Enlist Duo™ herbicide in the U.S. Retrieved from http://www.enlist.com/~/media/enlist/pdf/dowagrosciencesannounces launchofenlistduoherbicideintheus.ashx

Food & Water Watch. (2010). Poison-free poultry: Why arsenic doesn't belong in chicken feed. Retrieved from https://www.foodandwaterwatch.org/tools-and-resources/poison-free -poultry

Fraenkel, M. (Ed.). (1936). *Report of the Second International Congress of Scientific and Social Campaign Against Cancer* (Vols. 1–3). Brussels, Belgium: Ligue Nationale Belge Contre Le Cancer.

Grandjean, P., & Landrigan, P.J. (2014). Neurobehavioural effects of developmental toxicity. *Lancet Neurology, 13,* 330–338. doi:10.1016/S1474-4422(13)70278-3

Guth, J.H. (2006). Introduction to Toxic Substances Control Act of 1976. Retrieved from http://sehn.org/lawpdf/TSCASummary.pdf

Landrigan, P.J., & Goldman, L.R. (2011). Children's vulnerability to toxic chemicals: A challenge and opportunity to strengthen health and environmental policy. *Health Affairs, 30,* 842–850. doi:10.1377/hlthaff.2011.0151

Landrigan, P.J., & Goldman, L.R. (2014). Chemical safety, health care costs and the Affordable Care Act. *American Journal of Industrial Medicine, 57,* 1–3. doi:10.1002/ajim.22268

Liu, W., Li, H., Tao, F., Li, S., Tian, Z., & Xie, H. (2013). Formation and contamination of PCDD/Fs, PCBs, PeCBz, HxCBz and polychlorophenols in the production of 2,4-D products. *Chemosphere, 92,* 304–308. doi:10.1016/j.chemosphere.2013.03.031

Markowitz, G., & Rosner, D. (2013). *Deceit and denial: The deadly politics of industrial pollution.* Berkeley, CA: University of California Press.

Michaels, D. (2008). *Doubt is their product: How industry's assault on science threatens your health.* New York, NY: Oxford University Press.

Minnesota Department of Health. (2003). Children's environmental health: National initiatives. Retrieved from http://www.health.state.mn.us/divs/eh/children/national.html#executive

Nash, G.H. (1983). *The life of Herbert Hoover: The engineer, 1874–1914.* New York, NY: W.W. Norton.

National Performance Review. (1993). Create an interagency regulatory coordinating group. Retrieved from http://www.ai.mit.edu/ARCHIVE/org/npr/documents/commentable/npr.ovp.eop.gov.us/1993/9/6/378.html

National Research Council. (1993). *Pesticides in the diets of infants and children.* Retrieved from http://www.nap.edu/catalog/2126/pesticides-in-the-diets-of-infants-and-children

National Safety Council. (1926). *Final report of the Committee, Chemical and Rubber Sections, National Safety Council, on benzol, May 1926.* New York, NY: National Bureau of Casualty and Surety Underwriters.

Navas-Acien, A., & Nachman, K.E. (2013). Public health responses to arsenic in rice and other foods. *JAMA Internal Medicine, 173,* 1395–1396. doi:10.1001/jamainternmed.2013.6405

Nriagu, J.O. (1983). Saturnine gout among Roman aristocrats: Did lead poisoning contribute to the fall of the Empire? *New England Journal of Medicine, 308,* 660–663. doi:10.1056/NEJM198303173081123

Rappaport, S.M., Kim, S., Thomas, R., Johnson, B.A., Bois, F.Y., & Kupper, L.L. (2013). Low-dose metabolism of benzene in humans: Science and obfuscation. *Carcinogenesis, 34,* 2–9. doi:10.1093/carcin/bgs382

Rodenburg, L.A., Guo, J., Du, S., & Cavallo, G.J. (2010). Evidence for unique and ubiquitous environmental sources of 3,3'-dichlorobiphenyl (PCB 11). *Environmental Science and Technology, 44,* 2816–2821. doi:10.1021/es901155h

Roffo, A.H. (1936). La etiologia fisica-quimica del cancer (sobre todo en relacion con las irradiaciones solares). In M. Fraenkel (Ed.), *Ponencias Congreso International de Lucha Cientifica y Social Contra el Cancer.* Brussels, Belgium: Ligue Nationale Belge Contre Le Cancer.

Rosner, F. (2002). The life of Moses Maimonides, a prominent medieval physician. *Einstein Quarterly Journal of Biology and Medicine, 19,* 125–128. Retrieved from http://www.einstein.yu.edu/uploadedFiles/EJBM/19Rosner125.pdf

Safe Chemicals Act of 2011, S. 847, 112th Cong. (2012).

Safer Chemicals, Healthy Families. (n.d.). Who we are. Retrieved from http://saferchemicals.org/who-we-are

Safer Chemicals, Healthy Families. (2014). Coalition. Retrieved from http://saferchemicals.org/coalition

Schecter, A., Dai, L.C., Thuy, L.T., Quynh, H.T., Minh, D.Q., Cau, H.D., … Baughman, R. (1995). Agent Orange and the Vietnamese: The persistence of elevated dioxin levels in human tissues. *American Journal of Public Health, 85,* 516–522. doi:10.2105/AJPH.85.4.516

Sinclair, U. (1906). *The jungle.* New York, NY: Doubleday, Page & Co.

Society of Chemical Manufacturers and Affiliates. (n.d.). Myth versus fact about chemicals in commerce. Retrieved from http://www.socma.com/GovernmentRelations/index.cfm?subSec=26&articleID=3259

Stadler, L. (1993). Corrosion Proof Fittings v. EPA: Asbestos in the Fifth Circuit—A battle of unreasonableness. *Tulane Environmental Law Journal, 6,* 423. Retrieved from http://heinonline.org/HOL/LandingPage?handle=hein.journals/tulev6&div=20&id=&page

Toxic Substances Control Act of 1976, 15 U.S.C. §§ 2601–2629.

Unger, S.H. (2010). Pioneer killer products: Asbestos, lead, and tobacco. *Ends and Means Blog.* Retrieved from http://www1.cs.columbia.edu/~unger/articles/killerProducts.html

U.S. Environmental Protection Agency. (2010). HPV Chemical Hazard Data Availability Study. Retrieved from http://www.epa.gov/hpv/pubs/general/hazchem.htm

U.S. Environmental Protection Agency. (2012a). *EPA's reanalysis of key issues related to dioxin toxicity and response to NAS comments, volume 1* (CAS No. 1746-01-6). Retrieved from http://www.epa.gov/iris/supdocs/dioxinv1sup.pdf

U.S. Environmental Protection Agency. (2012b). Toxic Substances Control Act (TSCA). Retrieved from http://epa.gov/agriculture/lsca.html

U.S. Environmental Protection Agency. (2013a). Dioxins in San Francisco Bay: Questions and answers. Retrieved from http://www.epa.gov/region9/water/dioxin/sfbay.html

U.S. Environmental Protection Agency. (2013b, March 28). Lead paint. Retrieved from http://www.epa.gov/compliance/monitoring/programs/tsca/leadpaint.html

U.S. Environmental Protection Agency. (2014). TSCA chemical substance inventory: Basic information. Retrieved from http://www.epa.gov/oppt/existingchemicals/pubs/tscainventory/basic.html

U.S. Environmental Protection Agency, University of California, San Francisco, Center for Environmental Research and Children's Health, & California Department of Pesticide Regulation. (2013). *Green cleaning, sanitizing and disinfecting: A toolkit for early care and education.* Retrieved from http://www2.epa.gov/sites/production/files/2013-11/documents/green_cleaning.pdf

U.S. General Accounting Office. (1994). *Toxic Substances Control Act: Legislative changes could make the act more effective* (Report No. GAO/RCED-94-103). Washington, DC: Author.

U.S. Government Accountability Office. (2005). *Chemical regulation: Options exist to improve EPA's ability to assess health risks and manage its chemical review program* (Report to Congressional Requesters). Retrieved from http://www.gao.gov/assets/250/246667.pdf

Vijgen, J., Abhilash, P.C., Li, Y.F., Lal, R., Forter, M., Torres, J., ... Weber, R. (2011). Hexachlorocyclohexane (HCH) as new Stockholm Convention POPs—A global perspective on the management of lindane and its waste isomers. *Environmental Science and Pollution Research, 18*, 152–162. doi:10.1007/s11356-010-0417-9

Wagner, M., Schlüsener, M.P., Ternes, T.A., & Oehlmann, J. (2013). Identification of putative steroid receptor antagonists in bottled water: Combining bioassays and high-resolution mass spectrometry. *PLoS One, 8*(8), e72472. doi:10.1371/journal.pone.0072472

Wilkins, R.H. (1964). Neurosurgical Classic—XVII. *Journal of Neurosurgery, 21*, 240–244. doi:10.3171/jns.1964.21.3.0240

Winters, D. (2002). *Conceptual model for dioxin in the environment* [Slide presentation]. Retrieved from http://www.epa.gov/pbt/presentations/dioxin.ppt

Yawar, A. (2008). Maimonides' medicine. *Lancet, 371*, 804. doi:10.1016/S0140-6736(08)60365-7

Other Suggested Reading

Castleman, B.I. (2005). *Asbestos: Medical and legal aspects* (5th ed.). New York, NY: Aspen.

Denison, R.A. (2013, May). How the Chemical Safety Improvement Act of 2013 (S. 1009) addresses key flaws of TSCA, along with key tradeoffs. Retrieved from http://blogs.edf.org/health/files/2013/06/EDF-TSCA-vs.-CSIA-analysis-v2.pdf

Environmental Working Group. (2013, June 11). EWG side-by-side comparison: Safe Chemicals Act vs. Chemical Safety Improvement Act. Retrieved from http://static.ewg.org/pdf/EWG-SCA-CSIA-Comparison-Chart-6-11-13.pdf

Epstein, S.S. (2000). The politics of cancer. *JAMA, 284*, 442. Retrieved from http://jama.jamanetwork.com/article.aspx?articleid=1030878

CHAPTER 5

The Role of Professional and Voluntary Organizations

Brenda Nevidjon, MSN, RN, FAAN

Introduction

Numerous organizations focused on health care, and more specifically cancer care, expend significant human and financial capital advocating for their policy agenda. Healthcare professionals can promote and influence legislative policies both individually and as part of a collective voice when they join a professional or voluntary organization. Depending on the organization's structure, advocacy ranges from informing elected officials about an issue to lobbying on an issue. Before joining a cancer organization, cancer care professionals should know the organization's mission, health policy agenda, and legal rules regarding lobbying. With cancer being a leading cause of death in the United States (Centers for Disease Control and Prevention, 2014), cancer care professionals have a powerful voice in shaping policy that affects their practice and the care of their patients. This chapter provides an overview of the types of organizations that engage in policy making and the basics of many oncology-related organizations, alliances, and coalitions.

Federal Definitions of Tax-Exempt Organizations

The tax structure of professional and voluntary organizations is complex, as seen in the headlines in 2013 about the variety of organizations seeking tax-exempt status that had delayed approval. The following designations are only a few of the possibilities, but ones that nurses most likely need to know.

501(c) Organizations

Per the Internal Revenue Service (IRS) tax code, more than twenty 501(c) organization types exist, each with a specific definition (IRS, 2013a). The three that are important for nurses to differentiate are 501(c)(3), 501(c)(4), and 501(c)(6).

A 501(c)(3) organization is a public charity or foundation, and individuals who donate to the organization can claim a federal tax deduction(IRS, 2013a). Confirming an organization's nonprofit status can be done through the IRS website. Examples include the American Cancer Society, Robert Wood Johnson Foundation, Association of Oncology Social Work, ONS Foundation, Susan G. Komen, and American Nurses Foundation.

A 501(c)(4), or social welfare, organization provides for and promotes the interests of its members, and its earnings go to charitable, educational, or recreational purposes. They can participate in limited political activities as long as their aim is social welfare (IRS, 2013a). The IRS is seeing increased applications for and political activity by 501(c)(4) organizations (IRS, 2013b). Contributors to these organizations cannot claim a deduction for donations. An example is the American Cancer Society Cancer Action Network.

501(c)(6) organizations include business leagues, which are associations of people having a common interest, and are not organized for profit (IRS, 2013a). These organizations may lobby as long as it is related to the organization's purpose. Examples include the Oncology Nursing Society (ONS) and American Society for Radiation Oncology.

Other

527 groups are groups that may raise money for political activities such as issue advocacy, but not for the expressed purpose of electing or defeating a candidate. Typically run by special interest groups that can raise unlimited money from individuals, corporations, and unions, 527 organizations often advertise their position on an issue. During election campaigns, they may develop television ads that, although not candidate specific, promote an issue that can be related to a particular candidate's platform. The purpose is to influence the viewers' perception of the candidates and mobilize them to vote. An example is the Swift Boat 2 ad from 2004 (see www.youtube.com/watch?v=6HXEQD54204) sponsored by a group named Swift Vets that was speaking out against claims made by 2004 presidential candidate John Kerry.

Political action committees (PACs) raise funds specifically to elect or defeat candidates in an election and will distribute funds to candidates accordingly. Organizations that raise money for issue advocacy can also establish a PAC. Regulations govern how much an individual may give to a

PAC and how much a PAC can give to candidates or a political party. In addition to distributing money to candidates or political parties, PACs can and do offer publicized support for them. PACs must register with the Federal Election Commission and comply with its regulations. Table 5-1 shows selected healthcare PACs and their contributions in the 2012 election. The two examples from nursing may look impressive, but compared to the other contributors shown, the amounts are far less. Although this may put nursing at a disadvantage for shaping policy, it is somewhat offset by nursing being the most highly trusted profession as measured in Gallup surveys (Gallup, 2013) and the size of the profession. Thus, endorsement by nursing does carry influence (Bowers-Lanier, 2012). Other examples of PACs are the American Nurses Association PAC; the 21st Century Oncology, Inc. PAC; and the US Oncology Inc. Network PAC.

Since 2010, Super PACs have emerged and grown rapidly. The rules are different for these organizations, as they may raise and spend unlimited money to support or oppose a candidate, but may not give it directly to a candidate. The Center for Responsive Politics provides a list of the top Super PACs and, for many, identifies which candidate is supported or opposed (see www.opensecrets.org/pacs/superpacs.php).

Types of Advocacy Organizations

Many types of organizations advocate for legislation and policies at the federal and state levels, including cancer care professionals' employers. This

Table 5-1. Healthcare PACs' Contributions in the 2012 Federal Election

PAC	Democrats	Republicans
American Medical Association	$655,500	$966,700
American Society of Anesthesiologists	$511,150	$892,500
Pfizer	$560,000	$563,950
American Physical Therapy Association	$569,850	$463,000
Amgen	$462,500	$539,500
American Association of Nurse Anesthetists	$343,300	$338,500
American Nurses Association	$445,500	$89,000

PAC—political action committee
Note. Based on information from Center for Responsive Politics, 2014.

chapter will discuss three main groups: professional associations, voluntary interest and advocacy groups, and coalitions and alliances.

Professional Associations

All healthcare professions have member organizations; some professions, particularly medicine and nursing, have many. Resource lists with more than 70 nursing organizations have been published (see "Guide to Nursing Organizations," 2013; Romano, 2011). Matthews (2012) identified several categories of professional organizations by their specialty focus. Using Matthews' categories, healthcare professions organizations can be grouped as follows.

- Setting specific: American Academy of Ambulatory Care Nursing, American Academy of Urgent Care Medicine, Association of Community Cancer Centers, Association of periOperative Registered Nurses
- System-specific disorders or conditions: American College of Gastroenterology, American Society of Hematology, American Academy of Pain Medicine
- Age periods: American Academy of Pediatrics, American Geriatrics Society, National Association of Neonatal Nurses, Society of Pediatric Nurses
- Ethnic and cultural: American Assembly for Men in Nursing, Association for Academic Minority Physicians, Association of Black Women Physicians, National Black Nurses Association
- Advanced practice: American Association of Legal Nurse Consultants, National Association of Clinical Nurse Specialists
- Roles: American Association of Diabetes Educators, American Medical Directors Association, American Organization of Nurse Executives, National Association of Advisors for the Health Professions
- Education, professional development, and regulatory: American Medical Association, American Association of Colleges of Nursing, American Nurses Association, National Council of State Boards of Nursing, ONS, Physician Assistant Education Association

Many of these listed organizations have state and/or local level affiliates or chapters. In addition, there are many local organizations with no national parent. Depending on the legal structure of the professional organizations, they may or may not be able to use funds to support a candidate directly, but can lobby or educate candidates.

Professional organizations will identify advocacy as central to their mission by having it as a value or in their strategic plan. Somewhat unique is the American Nurses Association's *Code of Ethics for Nurses* (Fowler, 2010) outline of the advocacy role of nursing associations: "The profession of nursing, as represented by associations and their members, is responsible for articulating nursing values, for maintaining the integrity of the profession and its practice, and for shaping social policy" (p. 13). Associations should and do educate legislators and their staff about an issue and advocate for a specific position on the issue. Their focus is generally on national issues; these organizations rarely get involved with state-level advocacy. For example, many healthcare professional organizations have had tobacco control as a national policy priority. In 2009, Congress passed and President Obama signed the Family Smoking Prevention and Tobacco Control Act, which gives the U.S. Food and Drug Administration the authority to regulate the tobacco industry. Representatives from numerous professional and voluntary organizations were present in the Rose Garden when the president signed the bill. The breadth of this audience demonstrated the importance of advocacy by so many organizations in passing the legislation.

Another major focus of professional organizations is the education and preparation of members to engage in policy activities. For example, the Nurse in Washington Internship (NIWI) is offered annually by the Nursing Organizations Alliance and available to any nurse (see www.nursing-alliance .org/content.cfm/id/niwi). NIWI includes advocacy training and visits to the participants' elected representatives and demonstrates the power that a nurse's voice can have in discussing health policies. Many organizations will hold Hill Day visits when their national meeting is in Washington, DC. The Association of Community Cancer Centers has a priority to schedule its annual national meeting in the greater Washington, DC, area to coordinate Capitol Hill visits for their attendees. Most organizations highlight their advocacy activities on their websites, showcasing how members have engaged in the policy process by speaking with members of Congress and recognizing those who have championed cancer care. Most of the major oncology-related professional organizations have health policy resources available on their websites (see Table 5-2).

Voluntary Interest and Advocacy Groups

The earliest definition of interest groups is seen in Madison's Federalist Papers (1787): "By a faction, I understand a number of citizens, whether amounting to a majority or a minority of the whole, who are united and actuated by some common impulse of passion, or of interest, adversed to the rights of other citizens, or to the permanent and aggregate interests of the community." Simply defined, interest groups are people with a common interest or view who unite to influence the political process and policy (Longest, 2010). Within the cancer care community, innumerable groups exist; Table 5-3 shows only a selected few national ones. At the local level, many interest groups develop because of someone's personal experience with cancer, and some, such as Susan G. Komen, have grown to a national presence. There is redundancy in cancer interest groups, though, and many have similar names, as can be seen in Table 5-3. Thus, it is impor-

Table 5-2. Selected Organizations for Oncology Professionals

Organization	Mission Statement/Purpose	Advocacy Resources
Academy of Oncology Nurse and Patient Navigators www.aonnonline.org Cranbury, NJ Approximately 3,000 members	To advance the role of patient navigation in cancer care and survivorship care planning by providing a network for collaboration and development of best practices for the improvement of patient access to care, evidence-based cancer treatment, and quality of life during and after cancer treatment	None listed
American Association for Cancer Research www.aacr.org Philadelphia, PA More than 34,000 members who work in laboratories, clinics, universities, medical centers, government, and industry	To prevent and cure cancer through research, education, communication, and collaboration	Yes
American College of Surgeons Commission on Cancer (CoC) www.facs.org/quality-programs/ cancer/coc Chicago, IL Composed of 98 individuals who are surgeons representing the American College of Surgeons or representatives from the 50 national professional organizations affiliated with the CoC	To improve survival and quality of life for patients with cancer through standard-setting, prevention, research, education, and the monitoring of comprehensive quality care	Yes
American Psychosocial Oncology Society www.apos-society.org Charlottesville, VA Membership information not available	To advance the science and practice of psychosocial care for people affected by cancer	None listed
American Society for Radiation Oncology www.astro.org Fairfax, VA More than 10,000 radiation oncologists, medical physicists, dosimetrists, radiation therapists, radiation oncology nurses and nurse practitioners, biologists, physician assistants, and practice administrators	To improve patient care through education, clinical practice, advancement of science, and advocacy	Yes

(Continued on next page)

Table 5-2. Selected Organizations for Oncology Professionals *(Continued)*

Organization	Mission Statement/Purpose	Advocacy Resources
American Society of Clinical Oncology www.asco.org Alexandria, VA More than 30,000 oncology professionals, encompassing all oncology subspecialties	A professional oncology society committed to conquering cancer through research, education, prevention, and delivery of high-quality patient care	Yes
Association of Community Cancer Centers www.accc-cancer.org Rockville, MD Approximately 20,000 cancer care professionals from 1,900 hospitals and practices nationwide	To provide improved cancer care at the community level by implementing present knowledge and technology relating to cancer detection, cancer diagnosis, cancer treatment, and cancer rehabilitation, so that it is made available to the greatest number of patients possible	Yes
Association of Oncology Social Work www.aosw.org Philadelphia, PA More than 1,000 members	To advance excellence in the psychosocial care of patients with cancer, their families, and caregivers	Yes
Hematology/Oncology Pharmacy Association www.hoparx.org Glenview, IL More than 2,000 members	To support pharmacy practitioners and promote and advance hematology/oncology pharmacy to optimize the care of individuals affected by cancer	Yes
National Coalition of Oncology Nurse Navigators Rockville, MD Membership information not available	To promote excellence in oncology patient care by fostering collaborative relationships and professional development among oncology nurse navigators and all healthcare disciplines locally, regionally, and nationally	None listed
Oncology Nursing Society www.ons.org Pittsburgh, PA More than 35,000 RNs and other healthcare providers	To promote excellence in oncology nursing and quality cancer care	Yes

Table 5-3. Selected Oncology Voluntary Organizations

Organization	Mission Statement/Purpose	Advocacy Resources
American Breast Cancer Foundation www.abcf.org Towson, MD	To provide financial assistance for breast cancer screenings and diagnostic tests for uninsured and underserved individuals, regardless of age or gender	No
American Cancer Society www.cancer.org Atlanta, GA	To eliminate cancer as a major health problem by preventing cancer, saving lives, and diminishing suffering from cancer through research, education, advocacy, and service	Yes
Breastcancer.org www.breastcancer.org Ardmore, PA	To help women and their loved ones make sense of the complex medical and personal information about breast cancer so that they can make the best decisions for their lives	No
Fight Colorectal Cancer http://fightcolorectalcancer.org Alexandria, VA	To empower survivors to raise their voices, train advocates around the country, and educate lawmakers and push them for better policies	Yes
Kidney Cancer Association www.kidneycancer.org Washington, DC	To eradicate death and suffering from renal cancers	Yes
Leukemia & Lymphoma Society www.lls.org White Plains, NY	To cure leukemia, lymphoma, Hodgkin disease, and myeloma, and improve the quality of life of patients and their families	Yes
Livestrong Foundation www.livestrong.org Austin, TX	To improve the lives of people affected by cancer	Yes
Lung Cancer Alliance www.lungcanceralliance.org Washington, DC	To end injustice and save lives through an alliance of advocacy, education, and support	Yes
Lung Cancer Foundation of America www.lcfamerica.org New Ulm, MN	To accomplish dramatic improvement in survivorship of patients with lung cancer through the funding of transformative science with the ultimate goal of curing the disease	No
National Breast Cancer Foundation www.nationalbreastcancer.org Frisco, TX	To save lives by increasing awareness of breast cancer through education and by providing mammograms for those in need	No

(Continued on next page)

Table 5-3. Selected Oncology Voluntary Organizations *(Continued)*

Organization	Mission Statement/Purpose	Advocacy Resources
Pancreatic Cancer Action Network www.pancan.org Manhattan Beach, CA	To advance research, support patients, and create hope for those affected by pancreatic cancer	Yes
Prostate Cancer Foundation www.pcf.org Santa Monica, CA	To identify and invest in the most promising research programs and channel resources to the world's top scientific minds—cutting red tape and encouraging collaboration to speed breakthroughs	No
Scott Hamilton CARES Foundation www.scottcares.org Cleveland, OH	To advance toward the cure of cancer through research and education and to improve the quality of life and support for people affected by cancer	No
Sisters Network www.sistersnetworkinc.org Houston, TX	To increase local and national attention to the devastating impact of breast cancer in the African American community	No
Stupid Cancer http://stupidcancer.org New York, NY	To empower young adults affected by cancer by building community, improving quality of life, and providing meaningful survivorship	Yes
Susan G. Komen www.komen.org Dallas, TX	To end breast cancer in the United States and throughout the world through groundbreaking research, community health outreach, advocacy, and programs in more than 50 countries	Yes (Advocates in Science)

tant to research an organization prior to joining as a volunteer or donating. Likewise, professional organizations often establish criteria to determine partnerships with other organizations or whether to join a coalition.

The American Cancer Society, which celebrated its 100-year anniversary in 2013, has the broadest scope of the cancer interest organizations. It not only advocates for the elimination of cancer but also performs a myriad of other activities including public education, research funding, patient services, and fund-raising. Other groups are specific to a type of cancer, such as the Bladder Cancer Advocacy Network or the Leukemia & Lymphoma Society. Still others may focus on an age group, such as Critical Mass: The Young Adult Cancer Alliance and Stupid Cancer, or on a specific service, such as Locks of Love or Ronald McDonald Houses. Not all will have advocacy and policy shaping as part of their mission, but all will have philanthropy needs and thus compete with those organizations that do commit resources to advocacy and policy.

Coalitions and Alliances

Coalitions and alliances are organizations of organizations. Like interest groups, innumerable coalitions and alliances exist, and individual organizations must choose carefully which to join, as participation necessitates both fiscal and personnel resources. Usually coalitions develop as a strategy to strengthen voice and influence for an issue or policy agenda or because they have a common goal (Bowers-Lanier, 2012). A few may be temporary, but most seem to continue to address ongoing problems or issues. Some are formalized with a defined leader, board, dues, and employed staff support, whereas others operate from a shared leadership model, have no dues, and have staff donated from member organizations. Coalitions may be of professional organizations, such as the Nursing Organizations Alliance, or disease-related and include professional organizations and voluntary interest groups, such as One Voice Against Cancer. Table 5-4 lists a selection of coalitions. Not all will have a policy agenda. The Nursing Organizations Alliance, for example, clearly states on its website that it does not have authority to speak for nursing, but it does oversee the NIWI program as noted previously.

Coalitions arise for the specific purpose of influencing policy and do not offer other services as professional organizations and voluntary interest groups do. For organizations with limited resources, joining a coalition can

Table 5-4. Selected Alliances and Coalitions

Organization	Mission Statement/Purpose	Advocacy Resources
Health Professions and Nursing Education Coalition www.aamc.org/advocacy/hpnec Informal alliance of more than 60 organizations representing a variety of schools, programs, health professionals, and students	To advocate for adequate and continued support for the health professions and nursing education programs authorized under Titles VII and VIII of the Public Health Service Act	Yes
National Cancer Policy Forum www.iom.edu/Activities/Disease/ NCPF.aspx Washington, DC Governmental and nongovernmental sponsors plus distinguished experts from the cancer community	To identify emerging high-priority policy issues in the nation's effort to combat cancer and to examine those issues by convening activities that promote discussion about potential opportunities for action	No

(Continued on next page)

Table 5-4. Selected Alliances and Coalitions *(Continued)*

Organization	Mission Statement/Purpose	Advocacy Resources
National Coalition for Cancer Survivorship www.canceradvocacy.org Silver Spring, MD Survivors, caregivers, healthcare professionals, and advocates who care about survivorship issues	To advocate for quality cancer care for all people touched by cancer	Yes
National Comprehensive Cancer Network www.nccn.org Fort Washington, PA Not-for-profit alliance of 25 of the world's leading cancer centers	To improve the quality, effectiveness, and efficiency of cancer care so that patients can live better lives	No
National Patient Advocate Foundation www.npaf.org Washington, DC Has a working relationship with more than 100 organizations	To provide the patient voice in improving access to and reimbursement for high-quality health care through regulatory and legislative reform at the state and federal levels	Yes
Nursing Community www.thenursingcommunity.org 58 nursing organizations representing approximately 1 million nurses	To improve the health and health care of the nation by collaborating to support RNs and advanced practice RNs	Yes
Nursing Organizations Alliance www.nursing-alliance.org Lexington, KY Approximately 60 specialty nursing organizations	To provide a forum for identification, education, and collaboration building around issues of common interest to advance the nursing profession	Yes (Nurse in Washington Internship)
One Voice Against Cancer www.ovaconline.org Washington, DC A collaboration of national nonprofit organizations representing millions of Americans	To deliver a unified message to Congress and the White House on the need for increased cancer-related appropriations	Yes

help them achieve goals that they could not on their own. Like individual organizations, coalitions will prepare environmental scans on issues, attend meetings and hearings, and publish position papers. They also will organize a united response to an issue identifying all members of the coalition in a show of strength. Coalitions can be effective and energizing, but they can have challenges too, such as distrust among member organizations, poor decision making, inactivity, and lack of resources. Ultimately, the characteristics of successful organizations apply to and must be instilled in coalitions.

How Individuals and Associations Influence Policy

The most direct way an individual can influence policy is by voting for candidates who share the person's perspectives on issues at the national, state, and local levels. Policy makers want to know what their constituents think, regardless of whether they agree or disagree. Donating to campaigns, attending local events for candidates, and communicating with elected officials elevate an individual's engagement in influencing policy. More healthcare professionals are running for office, some successfully. The American Medical Association PAC (www.ampaconline.org) conducts a candidate workshop for members contemplating running for office. Twenty physicians and six nurses are serving in the 113th U.S. Congress, and more serve at the state and local levels.

Associations offer many strategies for influencing policy. Knowledge of the various types of organizations and the implications of common tax statuses provides a foundation for these strategies. Whether a professional association, voluntary interest or advocacy group, or coalition, all groups usually establish a policy agenda or priorities that reflect the organization's mission, values, and resources. The latter is critical in determining how involved an organization can be. Once established, the agenda guides the activities of the leadership and members of the organization.

Development of Advocates

Education

Professional associations, in particular, have education as part of their mission. Educating members on policy issues encompasses passive activities, such as having resources on the website or tweeting updates, to more active methods, such as offering workshops and scheduled visits to congressional offices. As referenced previously, NIWI has oriented nurses for many years on the legislative process and how to be an advocate. Central to NIWI and other similar workshops is the visit to legislative offices. Many are state-based programs, but all require resources to deliver the workshop and coordinate visits. Primomo and Björling (2013) evaluated the effectiveness of a legislative day, which includes training and visits, on participants' political astuteness. Their findings suggested that legislative days seem to be a useful strategy.

Integral to any education program is training in how to communicate effectively verbally, in writing, and electronically. Cancer care professionals have compelling stories to tell that can put a human face on the issue and enliven the data. Face-to-face meeting opportunities in public forums or in legislators' offices typically are short, and developing a 60-second pitch is essential.

Grassroots Campaigns

Periodically, organizations will mobilize members to address a specific issue through physical or virtual presence. "Hill Day" is a common event often scheduled to coincide with a cause's designated day, week, or month, such as October as National Breast Cancer Awareness Month. Identifying T-shirts, hats, or buttons creates recognition of the whole, as individuals or smaller groups visit offices. Prior to September 11, 2001, organizations would provide draft language for letter-writing campaigns. However, given security procedures and increased electronic access, the draft language is used for emails or submissions through the elected official's website. Telephone calls are another approach to communicating on an issue. However, staff will log the topic and the caller's position on the matter, but do not take extensive notes. Thus, in-person visits with printed materials or electronic methods are better options for more effective communication.

Coalition Letters

As a member of a coalition or alliance, an organization will be asked to sign on to position papers or letters that will be sent to congressional committees or key leaders.

Testimony

Occasionally, the opportunity will arise to give in-person testimony to a committee or government group. An organization generally will have the president of the board or chief executive officer be the spokesperson, but individual members, because of their expertise, may have the opportunity to testify. Written testimony is also accepted by committees and other government agencies. Organizations will notify members of testimonies through usual communication methods and often will send a press release about the testimony.

Rules Setting

After a law is passed, the rule making begins by the implementing organizations. In health care, a frequent implementing organization is the Centers for Medicare and Medicaid Services (CMS). This is another juncture where associations and interest groups can exert influence. This can be in the form of meetings to discuss the formulation of the rules, as well as how they would be implemented and managed. For example, the nursing profession has lobbied for changes in CMS rules that regulate reimbursement for advanced practice nurses.

Propose Legislation

Associations and interest groups can and occasionally do propose legislation. This is a lengthy process that begins with drafting the details of the legislation and finding bipartisan sponsors to introduce it in either the House or Senate; eventually both are needed. In 2008, ONS reached a seminal moment in its history when it developed draft legislation proposing Medicare reimbursement for treatment education provided by RNs to patients with cancer. Upon finding a primary sponsor to introduce it as a bill, ONS worked with congressional offices to obtain bipartisan support. The bill has been introduced in consecutive sessions of Congress and was again introduced in the first session of the 113th Congress as the Improving Cancer Treatment Education Act of 2013.

Conclusion

Shaping cancer health policy is integral to professional and voluntary cancer organizations. Many have clearly and succinctly written policy agendas supported by materials to use when communicating with elected officials. Educating members on how to advocate and facilitating their communication with elected officials are core activities for many of these organizations. Members of the organization have a responsibility to stay current on the organization's priorities and to use their individual voices as well as support the organization.

References

Bowers-Lanier, R. (2012). Coalitions: A powerful political strategy. In D.J. Mason, J.K. Leavitt, & M.W. Chaffee (Eds.), *Policy and politics in nursing and health care* (6th ed., pp. 626–632). St. Louis, MO: Elsevier Saunders.

Center for Responsive Politics. (2014). Super PACs. Retrieved from http://www.opensecrets.org/pacs/superpacs.php?cycle=2014

Centers for Disease Control and Prevention. (2014, July 14). FastStats: Leading causes of death. Retrieved from http://www.cdc.gov/nchs/fastats/lcod.htm

Family Smoking Prevention and Tobacco Control Act, Pub. L. No. 111-31, 123 Stat. 1776 (2009).

Fowler, M.D.M. (Ed.). (2010). *Guide to the Code of Ethics for Nurses: Interpretation and application.* Silver Spring, MD: American Nurses Association.

Gallup. (2013, December 5–8). Honesty/ethics in professions. Retrieved from http://www.gallup.com/poll/1654/honesty-ethics-professions.aspx

Guide to nursing organizations [Online exclusive]. (2013). *Nursing, 43*(2). Retrieved from http://journals.lww.com/nursing/Fulltext/2013/02001/Guide_to_nursing_organizations.11.aspx

Improving Cancer Treatment Education Act of 2013, H.R. 1661, 113 Cong.

Internal Revenue Service. (2013a, March 20). Federal tax code—Exempt organizations. Retrieved from http://www.irs.gov/Charities-&-Non-Profits/Federal-Tax-Code-Exempt-Organizations

Internal Revenue Service. (2013b, May 15). Questions and answers on 501(c) organizations. Retrieved from http://www.irs.gov/uac/Newsroom/Questions-and-Answers-on-501%28c%29-Organizations

Longest, B.B., Jr. (2010). *Health policymaking in the United States* (5th ed.). Chicago, IL: Health Administration Press.

Madison, J. (1787). Federalist No. 10. The same subject continued: The union as a safeguard against domestic faction and insurrection. Retrieved from http://thomas.loc.gov/home/histdox/fed_10.html

Matthews, J.H. (2012). Role of professional organizations in advocating for the nursing profession. *Online Journal of Issues in Nursing, 17*(1), Manuscript 3. Retrieved from http://nursingworld.org/MainMenuCategories/ANAMarketplace/ANAPeriodicals/OJIN/TableofContents/Vol-17-2012/No1-Jan-2012/Professional-Organizations-and-Advocating.html

Primomo, J., & Björling, E.A. (2013). Changes in political astuteness following nurse legislative day. *Policy, Politics, and Nursing Practice, 14,* 97–108. doi:10.1177/1527154413485901

Romano, C. (2011). Guide to nursing organizations. *Nursing, 111,* 1–5. doi:10.1097/01.NAJ.0000392864.75060.33

CHAPTER 6

Contributions of the Federal Advisory Boards

Karen Meneses, PhD, RN, FAAN

Introduction

Advisory committees composed of experts from the public sector have contributed a significant amount of work to the federal government. An advisory committee was first used in the early days of our nation when President George Washington appointed one to help him deal with the Whiskey Rebellion (Federal Advisory Committee, n.d.). Thereafter, formal advisory committees were created for the purpose of providing expertise from private citizens to aid in policy making. Over the years, advisory committees grew substantially, based on initiatives of both the executive and legislative branches. In 1962, President John F. Kennedy issued an executive order (11007) to establish regulations for advisory committee use. In 1972, President Richard Nixon issued another executive order (11671) to establish a centralized management system, with subsequent approval of the Federal Advisory Committee Act (Public Law [P.L.] 92-463) by Congress. The President's Cancer Panel was one of the 1,439 advisory committees in existence in 1972 (Federal Advisory Committee, n.d.). The National Cancer Advisory Board within the Department of Health, Education, and Welfare was established in 1972 (Federal Advisory Committee, n.d.).

The overarching goal of this chapter is to acknowledge the sustained contributions of the distinguished advisory boards to cancer. The aims of this chapter are to (a) provide an overview of the charge and activities of three key cancer advisory groups: the National Cancer Policy Board (NCPB), the National Cancer Advisory Board (NCAB), and the President's Cancer Panel (PCP), (b) discuss the role of these boards and panels in shaping cancer healthcare policy, and (c) describe the implications for cancer care.

Federal Cancer Advisory Groups

The 74th Congress of the United States established the National Cancer Institute (NCI) through the National Cancer Institute Act of 1937 (P.L. 75-244). NCI was created to "conduct and support research with respect to the cause, diagnosis, prevention, and treatment of cancer, rehabilitation from cancer, and the continuing care of cancer patients and also the families of cancer patients" (NCAB Ad Hoc Working Group, 2010). Since that time, NCI has been the lead agency for the conduct of cancer research for the federal government. Three federal cancer advisory groups, NCPB (later changed to the National Cancer Policy Forum), NCAB, and PCP, have reported their work and findings to NCI. The following is a discussion of each of the three federal cancer advisory boards, their charters, and contributions.

National Cancer Policy Board (1997–2005)

NCPB was established in March 1997 as a shared board between the Institute of Medicine (IOM) and the National Research Council's Board of Life Sciences. With support from NCI and the Centers for Disease Control and Prevention, the major focus of NCPB was cancer policy (Herdman, McGuire, & Simone, 2006).

The function of NCPB was to address broad policy issues affecting cancer and to make recommendations to advance efforts against cancer in the United States. NCPB brought together prominent scientists, healthcare providers, third-party payers, social scientists, advocates, and others from the cancer community to identify and conduct studies and other activities that contribute to cancer research, prevention, treatment, and public awareness (IOM, 2005). The multidisciplinary expertise from basic, clinical, public health, consumer, and advocacy combined with support from NCI and the Centers for Disease Control and Prevention served to improve knowledge and develop public policy.

NCPB was established in 1997 in response to requests from NCI, National Institutes of Health, and PCP to examine ongoing research, technology, and problems faced by all sectors engaged in the nation's battle against cancer. Since its launch, NCI and Centers for Disease Control and Prevention have provided core funding support with contributions from the American Cancer Society and contributions or funding for specific studies from various agencies or organizations. Formal appointments to the 21-member board were made by the National Research Council chair and IOM president.

During the eight years of its existence, NCPB issued 28 peer-reviewed reports and 21 studies covering a broad and diverse range of cancer topics, including (Herdman et al., 2006)

- Tobacco control
- Cancer quality care
- Reimbursement for clinical trials
- Development of mammography technologies
- Improvement in breast cancer detection and diagnosis
- Breast cancer psychosocial care
- Pediatric quality care
- Cancer survivorship
- Improvement in palliative care
- Death in America.

Several key NCPB reports led to a fundamental shift in cancer health policy development. For example, one major public policy the NCPB tackled was tobacco control (Smigel, 1997a, 1997b). The board issued its report in 1998 to take action to reduce tobacco use (NCPB, 1998). The report highlighted a three-point plan to prevent new smokers from starting, to get current smokers to quit, and to reduce environmental exposure from secondhand smoke (Reh, 1998). Historically, NCPB recommended raising the price of tobacco products to reduce its use among current smokers and to deter new smokers. Further, NCPB suggested that the revenue generated could be used to support tobacco control and treatment programs and fund tobacco control research. Third, NCPB issued a subsequent tobacco control report near the time that state governors and legislatures were deliberating on the distribution of the tobacco settlement funds (NCPB, 2000).

Herdman et al. (2006) further examined NCPB's impact on cancer policy. Two landmark NCPB reports, *Ensuring Quality Cancer Care* (Hewitt & Simone, 1999) and *Enhancing Data Systems to Improve the Quality of Care* (Hewitt & Simone, 2000), recommended the development of clinical guidelines and a core set of cancer quality measures, better data systems, and high-quality palliative care. These reports prompted NCI to start the Quality of Cancer Care Initiative to develop a working model for quality care research and application. In addition, the Department of Health and Human Services established the Quality of Cancer Care Committee to support the development of a national cancer data system (Herdman et al., 2006).

A second example is the NCPB report, *Improving Breast Imaging Quality Standards*, which was requested by the Congress during its deliberations evaluating the reauthorization of the federal Mammography Quality Standards Act (MQSA) (Nass & Ball, 2005). The MQSA was enacted in 1993 to provide a general overarching guide for national quality standards in mammography screening through accreditation, certification, and annual inspection. The 2005 follow-up MQSA report recommended changes in U.S. Food and Drug Administration regulations and in policies to improve breast imaging interpretations (Nass & Ball, 2005). This report had a major impact on federal policy concerning mammography to revise MQSA regulations and enforce inspections. Moreover, the 2005 report strongly recommended that an adequate workforce be trained in breast cancer screening and diagnosis through improved mammography and the development of newer breast imaging techniques.

Palliative care is the third example of cancer policy relevance. The IOM report *Improving Palliative Care for Cancer* directed attention to palliative care at the national policy level. This report had the following 10 recommendations (Foley & Gelband, 2001).

- NCI should designate cancer centers of excellence in symptom control and palliative care.
- NCI should require research in palliative care and symptom control for designation as a comprehensive cancer center.
- The Health Care Financing Administration (now known as the Centers for Medicare and Medicaid Services) should fund demonstration projects for service delivery and reimbursement that integrate palliative care.
- Private insurers must provide compensation for end-of-life care.
- Cancer organizations and pharmaceutical companies should revise patient materials to include accurate information about palliative care.
- Best available practice guidelines should dictate the standard of palliative care.
- Best available practice guidelines should enhance data systems to improve the quality of palliative care.
- NCI should convene a state of the science meeting on palliative care and symptom control.
- NCI should establish an appropriate institutional locus on palliative care.
- NCI should review membership of advisory bodies to ensure representation of experts in cancer pain and palliative care.

Herdman et al. (2006) provided a comprehensive listing of peer-reviewed reports issued by the NCPB (available in the online appendix at http://content.healthaffairs.org/content/25/3/800).

National Cancer Policy Forum (2005–Present)

In 2005, IOM established the National Cancer Policy Forum (NCPF) to replace NCPB to continue to provide a cancer focus within the National Academies to examine issues in science, clinical medicine, public health, and public policy relevant to the goals of preventing and treating cancer (IOM, 2005). The focus changed from policy making to policy advising using a broader constituency of both federal and nonfederal groups. NCPF accomplished its mandate by holding forums and meetings among federal and nonfederal sponsors to increase interaction among government, industry, academic, consumer, and other representatives. NCPF was organized as a forum rather than a board so that all members can bring ideas and requests for deliberations. In addition, members (both federal and nonfederal) can take an active part in discussions. Thus, NCPF identifies and explores policy concerns, but does not issue IOM advisory reports as did the previous NCPB (Herdman et al., 2006).

The convening activities of NCPF result in published reports that are available to the public and that can provide input to planning formal IOM consensus committee studies. Ideas for committee studies that emerge from the forum's deliberations are given to the appropriate ad hoc committee appointed by IOM. Forum sponsors can pursue activities to facilitate implementation of the recommendations from the consensus reports (IOM, 2005). For example, NCPB and IOM commissioned a report to examine the role of oncology nursing to ensure quality care for cancer survivors (Ferrell, Virani, Smith, & Juarez, 2003). The authors conducted a content analysis of data from textbooks, journals, Oncology Nursing Society documents, oncology nursing programs, and externally funded grants. They synthesized the critical content of the data and examined quality care specific to cancer survivors. They further identified significant contributions by oncology nursing to ensure quality cancer care and identified eight specific recommendations to NCPB and IOM. The recommendations focused on increasing support for basic and continuing education in cancer survivorship, increasing support for pilot studies on cancer survivorship and joint research in conjunction with clinical trials, and increasing the focus of professional organizations, such as the Oncology Nursing Society, in support of cancer survivorship care.

NCPF continues to hold an extensive number of workshops that have subsequently led to cancer policy at the regional and national level. Figure 6-1 lists a selection of NCPF reports issued since 2006 for further reading and examination of specific cancer problems and issues that contributed to changes in health policy.

National Cancer Advisory Board (1971–Present)

NCAB is a presidentially appointed panel that was established with the authorization of the National Cancer Act of 1971 (P.L. 92-218), empowering NCAB to hold hearings and to evaluate the National Cancer Program and provide an annual report to Congress (U.S. Department of Health and Human Services, 2004). NCAB's primary purpose is to advise and assist the NCI director with respect to the National Cancer Program.

NCAB consists of 18 members appointed by the president and 12 nonvoting ex officio members across various federal departments. Appointed members are selected from the health and scientific disciplines in basic, behavioral, social, and public health, and with no more than six members from the general public, including leaders in public policy, law, health policy, economics, and management (NCI, 2013). While the NCAB membership is interdisciplinary, it has had oncology nursing representation, starting in 1991 with the appointment of Deborah K. Mayer (1991–1996) and then Sandra

---

Figure 6-1. Selected Reports From the National Cancer Policy Forum at the Institute of Medicine

---

- *Effect of the HIPAA Privacy Rule on Health Research: Proceedings of a Workshop Presented to the National Cancer Policy Forum* (September 2006)
- *Implementing Cancer Survivorship Care Planning: Workshop Summary* (December 2006)
- *Cancer Control Opportunities in Low- and Middle-Income Countries* (February 2007)
- *Cancer Biomarkers: The Promises and Challenges of Improving Detection and Treatment* (March 2007)
- *Cancer in Elderly People: Workshop Proceedings* (March 2007)
- *Cancer-Related Genetic Testing and Counseling—Workshop Proceedings* (August 2007)
- *Improving the Quality of Cancer Clinical Trials—Workshop Summary* (May 2008)
- *Implementing Colorectal Cancer Screening—Workshop Summary* (December 2008)
- *Multi-Center Phase III Clinical Trials and NCI Cooperative Groups—Workshop Summary* (January 2009)
- *Ensuring Quality Cancer Care through the Oncology Workforce: Sustaining Care in the 21st Century—Workshop Summary* (April 2009)
- *Assessing and Improving Value in Cancer Care—Workshop Summary* (November 2009)
- *A National Cancer Clinical Trials System for the 21st Century: Reinvigorating the NCI Cooperative Group Program* (April 2010)
- *A Foundation for Evidence-Driven Practice: A Rapid Learning System for Cancer Care—Workshop Summary* (June 2010)
- *Extending the Spectrum of Precompetitive Collaboration in Oncology Research—Workshop Summary* (July 2010)
- *Nanotechnology and Oncology—Workshop Summary* (February 2011)
- *The National Cancer Policy Summit: Opportunities and Challenges in Cancer Research and Care* (February 2011)
- *Patient-Centered Cancer Treatment Planning: Improving the Quality of Oncology Care—Workshop Summary* (June 2011)
- *Implementing a National Cancer Clinical Trials System for the 21st Century—Workshop Summary* (July 2011)
- *Facilitating Collaborations to Develop Combination Investigational Cancer Therapies—Workshop Summary* (October 2011)
- *The Role of Obesity in Cancer Survival and Recurrence—Workshop Summary* (April 2012)
- *Informatics Needs and Challenges in Cancer Research—Workshop Summary* (July 2012)
- *Reducing Tobacco-Related Cancer Incidence and Mortality—Workshop Summary* (November 2012)
- *Delivering Affordable Cancer Care in the 21st Century—Workshop Summary* (February 2013)
- *Implementing a National Cancer Clinical Trials System for the 21st Century—Second Workshop Summary* (July 2013)

Note. Reports are available through the Institute of Medicine at http://www.iom.edu/reports.

Millon-Underwood (1996–2002), Karen Meneses (2006–2012), and Victoria Champion (2008–2014).

NCAB has three major functions (NCI, 2013), which are to

- Recommend acceptance of conditional gifts to support research, training, health information dissemination, and other programs related to the cause, diagnosis, prevention, and treatment of cancer, rehabilitation from cancer, and the continuing care of patients with cancer and their families.
- Review applications for grants and cooperative agreements for research and training.
- Collect information about studies conducted in the United States or other countries and make this information available for public and private health entities, scientists, and the general public.

Figure 6-2 lists selected NCAB Working Group reports and supplementals. A complete listing of the meeting agendas, minutes, and presentations from 2010 to the present can be accessed at http://deainfo.nci.nih .gov/advisory/ncab/ncabmeetings.htm. Archived meeting information from 1980 to 2000 is also available through the same link. The NCAB website also contains the orientation book for NCAB appointees (see http:// deainfo.nci.nih.gov/advisory/ncab/OrientationBook.pdf), which provides an excellent overview of the Health and Human Services mission and organization.

In 1996, in honor of the 25th anniversary of the signing of the 1971 National Cancer Act, Jonathan Rhoads, the first chair of NCAB, and Walter Lawrence, NCAB board member, published their reflections on NCAB in a special issue of *Cancer* (Lawrence, 1996; Rhoads, 1996). Rhoads began his essay with the acknowledgment that his recollection "at age 89 years of events taking place 25 years ago may not be precise" (p. 2594).

Figure 6-2. National Cancer Advisory Board Working Group Reports and Supplementals

- *Decade of Discovery: Advances in Cancer Research 1971–1981* (1981)
- *A Review of the Intramural Program at the National Cancer Institute: A Report by the Ad Hoc Working Group of the National Cancer Advisory Board* (1995)
- *Recruitment and Retention of Minority Participants in Clinical Cancer Research: Conference Summary* (1996)
- *Advancing Translational Cancer Research: A Vision of the Cancer Center and SPORE Programs of the Future—Ad-Hoc P30-P50 Working Group* (2003)
- *Report of the Clinical Trials Working Group of the NCAB: Restructuring the National Cancer Clinical Trials Enterprise* (2005)
- *Report to National Cancer Advisory Board: Working Group on Biomedical Technology* (2005)
- *To Create a Strategic Vision for the National Cancer Program and Review Progress of the National Cancer Institute* (2010)

However, Rhoads wove a fascinating and clear description of discussions concerning collaborations among organizations and cancer champions in shaping public policy. As president of the American Cancer Society in 1970, he was asked to serve on an advisory committee created by the U.S. Senate under the leadership of Senator Ralph W. Yarborough (D-TX). It was their vision that "a sharply increased effort in cancer research might yield dramatic results paralleling those of the Manhattan Project in atomic energy" (Rhoads, 1996, p. 2594). The advisory committee report contained a large majority of the elements that eventually became the National Cancer Act, which was signed into law by President Nixon in 1971, and the creation of the NCAB.

Lawrence served on the board from 1988 to 1994. In his view, NCAB was the major administrative mechanism for assisting in the implementation of the goals of the National Cancer Program. According to Lawrence, during the early years, NCAB started a wide range of initiatives that had significant impact. These included (Lawrence, 1996)

• Establishing cancer centers as NCI-designated comprehensive cancer centers
• Establishing an organ site program
• Expanding research funding considered vital to cancer research and training programs.

Another highly important early innovation of NCAB was its further delineation of a "new" area of science: cancer control (Lawrence, 1996). These initiatives remain a significant example of cancer policy changes that continue to influence the National Cancer Program today.

Several major policy outcomes occurred between 1971 and 1996. The first was the landmark report evaluating the NCI intramural program (Calabresi, 1996), which led to substantial reorganization and improvement of this program. The second was an initiative hosting a conference on minority recruitment and retention into clinical trials, which resulted in a broader understanding about minority participation in clinical research and produced a guide on recruitment and retention of minority participants in clinical cancer research that was distributed across the country (NCAB, 1996).

NCAB also requested a review of behavioral research at NCI with subsequent recommendations to increase behavioral research funding. It led the process of examining the controversies surrounding screening mammography in women younger than age 50 every one to two years. At a consensus conference convened by the National Institutes of Health, the members could not reach consensus on screening mammography; however, NCAB recommended that mammography should be provided to women younger than age 50 (Freund & Pastorek, 1998), leading to marked, polarizing public reaction (Sackett, 1997). Nevertheless, NCAB influenced public health policy changes, resulting in NCI's revised mammography guidelines in 1997.

President's Cancer Panel (1972–Present)

The PCP is a federal advisory committee that reports directly to the president on activities of the National Cancer Program. It was established by the Public Health Service Act (42 U.S.C. 285a-4, § 415, as amended) (NCI Division of Extramural Activities, n.d.). The PCP consists of three members, including the chair, who are appointed by the president and who by virtue of their training, experience, and background are exceptionally qualified to appraise the National Cancer Program. Of the three members, at least two must be distinguished scientists or physicians. The third individual may be from the lay public. All nonfederal members serve as special government employees. The PCP monitors the development and execution of the activities of the National Cancer Program and reports directly to the president (NCI Division of Extramural Activities, n.d.).

In addition to distinguished service from scientists, service from members of the lay public has helped galvanize public interest and support of cancer in unique and colorful ways. For example, Hill Harper currently serves on the PCP. He is a cancer survivor and *New York Times* best-selling author, actor, and philanthropist. Lance Armstrong, another previous PCP lay member, provided dedicated service to promoting healthy lifestyles through physical activity and nutrition.

Topics discussed at PCP meetings, which are held in different parts of the country and are open to the public, cover a wide variety of areas, including
• Cancer survivorship
• Reducing the burden of cancer
• Challenges in translating research
• Promoting healthy lifestyles to reduce cancer risk
• Maximizing the nation's investment in cancer
• Environmental factors in cancer
• Demographic and cultural implications for cancer.

A complete listing of meeting agendas, minutes, and presentations from 2003 to the present can be accessed at http://deainfo.nci.nih.gov/advisory/pcp/pcpmeetings.htm. Archived meeting information from 1996 to 2002 is also available through the same link.

Implications for Cancer Care

Each of the three cancer advisory boards and panels created shortly after the National Cancer Act were highly instrumental in developing research, reporting the evidence, and taking a stand on a wide variety of advocacy issues, leading to public forums and discussions and finally to public policy. The implications of these boards on cancer care and health policy are several. The first is that cancer care professionals, within and outside of federal agencies, along with the lay public, have made significant direct and indirect contributions and service to the NCPB, NCAB, and PCP. Second, oncology professionals throughout the country have attended PCP meetings and provided testimony and statements, both informal and formal.

Cancer professionals often wonder how they can contribute to public policy. They may not always consider that cancer health policy is a process that involves many steps; it is not an event. The actual signing into law is the last step of a long process by which cancer health policy is shaped. The first step in contributing to health policy is to be aware of the issues. Readers are strongly encouraged to access the numerous links and websites noted throughout this chapter. Read and review the summary of reports and papers on a wide variety of cancer issues and problems during the past 50 years. Select one or a few of the reports and examine the evidence surrounding the issues. NCPB, NCAB, and PCP hold public meetings at various times throughout the year. Attend a meeting, or listen in on a podcast.

Finally, it is vital to give reasoned voice to the issues, whether that occurs in documenting and submitting views; participating in public forums; writing letters to the editor, op-ed columns, or letters to public officials; or informally through social networking. Cancer professionals must be willing to step up to the plate to get involved through professional organizations and collectively join others in voicing their views.

Conclusion

In the first session of the 112th Congress in December 2011, the U.S. Senate passed a resolution recognizing the 40th anniversary of the National Cancer Act (see Figure 6-3) and the more than 12 million cancer survivors alive today because of the commitment of the United States and its citizens to cancer research and advances in cancer prevention, detection, diagnosis, and treatment. In the intervening years since the passage of the National Cancer Act of 1971, the resolution recognized that cancer touches everyone, either directly through personal diagnosis or indirectly through a family member or friend. For every person touched by cancer, there has been an oncology professional at the bedside, in the clinic, and in the community; at the cutting edge of research; and at the administrative level who has also been touched by cancer and has contributed in rich ways to determining cancer policy.

Figure 6-3. Resolution Recognizing the 40th Anniversary of the National Cancer Act

In the Senate of the United States
December 13, 2011
Mr. Brown of Ohio (for himself, Mr. Moran, Mr. Kerry, Mrs. Feinstein, Mr. Cardin, Ms. Stabenow, Mr. Lautenberg, Mr. Levin, Mr. Tester, Mr. Casey, Mr. Inouye, Mrs. Murray, Mr. Harkin, Mrs. McCaskill, Mr. Begich, Mr. Sanders, Ms. Mikulski, Mr. Franken, Mr. Blumenthal, Mr. Durbin, Mr. Nelson of Nebraska, Mr. Whitehouse, Mr. Merkley, Ms. Landrieu, Mr. Coons, Mr. Menendez, Mrs. Gillibrand, Mr. Johnson of South Dakota, Mrs. Boxer, Mr. Reed, Mr. Bennet, Mr. Wyden, Ms. Klobuchar, Mr. Kohl, Mr. Brown of Massachusetts, Mr. Roberts, Mr. Blunt, Mr. Cochran, Mr. Boozman, Mr. Heller, Mrs. Hutchison, Mr. Wicker, Mr. Burr, Mr. Kirk, Mr. Reid, and Mr. Grassley) submitted the following resolution; which was referred to the Committee on Health, Education, Labor, and Pensions
December 15, 2011
Committee discharged; considered and agreed to

RESOLUTION

Recognizing the 40th anniversary of the National Cancer Act of 1971 and the more than 12,000,000 survivors of cancer alive today because of the commitment of the United States to cancer research and advances in cancer prevention, detection, diagnosis, and treatment.

Whereas 40 years ago, with the passage of the National Cancer Act of 1971 (Public Law 92-218; 85 Stat. 778), the leaders of the United States came together to set the country on a concerted course to conquer cancer through research;

Whereas the passage of the National Cancer Act of 1971 led to the establishment of the National Cancer Program, which significantly expanded the authorities and responsibilities of the National Cancer Institute, a component of the National Institutes of Health;

Whereas the term "cancer" refers to more than 200 diseases that collectively represent the leading cause of death for people in the United States under the age of 85, and the second leading cause of death for people in the United States overall;

Whereas cancer touches everyone, either through a direct, personal diagnosis or indirectly through the diagnosis of a family member or friend;

Whereas, in 2011, cancer remains one of the most pressing public health concerns in the United States, with more than 1,500,000 people in the United States expected to be diagnosed with cancer each year;

Whereas the National Institutes of Health estimated the overall cost of cancer to be greater than $260,000,000,000 in 2010 alone;

Whereas approximately 1 out of every 3 women and 1 out of every 2 men will develop cancer in their lifetimes, and more than 570,000 people in the United States will die from cancer this year, which is more than 1 person every minute and nearly 1 out of every 4 deaths;

Whereas the commitment of the United States to cancer research and biomedical science has enabled more than 12,000,000 people in the United States to survive cancer, 15 percent of whom were diagnosed 20 or more years ago, and has resulted in extraordinary progress being made against cancer, including—

(1) an increase in the average 5-year survival rate for all cancers combined to 68 percent for adults and 80 percent for children and adolescents, up from 50 percent and 52 percent, respectively, in 1971;

(2) average 5-year survival rates for breast and prostate cancers exceeding 90 percent;

(3) a decline in mortality due to colorectal cancer and prostate cancer; and

(Continued on next page)

Figure 6-3. Resolution Recognizing the 40th Anniversary of the National Cancer Act *(Continued)*

(4) from 1990 to 2007, a decline in the death rate from all cancers combined of 22 percent for men and 14 percent for women, resulting in nearly 900,000 fewer deaths during that period;

Whereas the driving force behind this progress has been support for the National Cancer Institute and its parent agency, the National Institutes of Health, which funds the work of more than 325,000 researchers and research personnel at more than 3,000 universities, medical schools, medical centers, teaching hospitals, small businesses, and research institutions in every State;

Whereas the commitment of the United States to cancer research has yielded substantial returns in both research advances and lives saved, and it is estimated that every 1 percent decline in cancer mortality saves the economy of the United States $500,000,000,000 annually;

Whereas advancements in understanding the causes and mechanisms of cancer and improvements in the detection, diagnosis, treatment, and prevention of cancer have led to cures for many types of cancers and have converted other types of cancers into manageable chronic conditions;

Whereas continued support for clinical trials to evaluate the efficacy and therapeutic benefit of promising treatments for cancer is essential for translating new knowledge and discoveries into tangible benefits for patients, especially because all standard cancer therapies began as clinical trials;

Whereas, despite the significant progress that has been made in treating many cancers, there remain those cancers for which the mortality rate is extraordinarily high, including pancreatic, liver, lung, multiple myeloma, ovarian, esophageal, stomach, and brain cancers, which have a 5-year survival rate of less than 50 percent;

Whereas research advances concerning uncommon cancers, which pose unique treatment challenges, provide an opportunity for understanding the general properties of human cancers and curing uncommon cancers as well as more common cancers;

Whereas crucial developments have been achieved in cancer research that could provide breakthroughs necessary to address the increasing incidence of, and reduce deaths caused by, many forms of cancer;

Whereas research into the effect of certain forms of cancer on different population groups offers a significant opportunity to lessen the burden of the disease, because many population groups across the country suffer disproportionately from certain forms of cancer; and

Whereas a sustained commitment to the research of the National Institutes of Health and the National Cancer Institute is necessary to improve the entire spectrum of patient care, from cancer prevention, early detection, and diagnosis, to treatment and long-term survivorship, and to prevent research advances from being stalled or delayed: Now, therefore, be it

Resolved, That the Senate—

(1) recognizes the 40th anniversary of the National Cancer Act of 1971 (Public Law 92-218; 85 Stat. 778); and

(2) celebrates and reaffirms the commitment embodied in the National Cancer Act of 1971, specifically, that support for cancer research continues to be a national priority to address the scope of this pressing public health concern.

Note. From *Senate Resolution 347,* 112th Congress, 1st Session (2011). Retrieved from https://www.govtrack.us/congress/bills/112/sres347/text/ats.

References

Calabresi, P. (1996). Results of the National Cancer Advisory Board evaluation of the National Cancer Program. *Cancer, 78,* 2607–2608. doi:10.1002/(SICI)1097-0142(19961215)78:12<2607::AID-CNCR30>3.0.CO;2-Y

Federal Advisory Committee. (n.d.). The annual report of the president on federal advisory committees: Printed annual reports 1972–1998. Retrieved from http://fido.gov/facadatabase/PrintedAnnualReports.asp

Federal Advisory Committee Act, Pub. L. 92-463, 86 Stat. 770 (1972).

Ferrell, B.R., Virani, R., Smith, S., & Juarez, G. (2003). The role of oncology nursing to ensure quality care for cancer survivors: A report commissioned by the National Cancer Policy Board and Institute of Medicine [Online exclusive]. *Oncology Nursing Forum, 30*(1), E1–E11. doi:10.1188/03.ONF.E1-E11

Foley, K.M., & Gelband, H. (Eds.). (2001). *Improving palliative care for cancer: Summary and recommendations.* Retrieved from http://www.nap.edu/catalog.php?record_id=10147

Freund, K.M., & Pastorek, J.G., 2nd. (1998). Perspective on women's health: Editors' 1997–1998 year in review. *Medscape Women's Health, 3*(1), 2.

Herdman, R., McGuire, W., & Simone, J. (2006). Influencing cancer policy. *Health Affairs, 25,* 800–807. doi:10.1377/hlthaff.25.3.800

Hewitt, M., & Simone, J.V. (Eds.). (1999). *Ensuring quality cancer care.* Retrieved from http://www.nap.edu/catalog.php?record_id=6467

Hewitt, M., & Simone, J.V. (Eds.). (2000). *Enhancing data systems to improve the quality of cancer care.* Retrieved from http://www.nap.edu/catalog.php?record_id=9970

Institute of Medicine. (2005). National Cancer Policy Board. Retrieved from http://www.iom.edu/About-IOM/Leadership-Staff/Boards/National-Cancer-Policy-Board.aspx

Lawrence, W., Jr. (1996). The National Cancer Advisory Board: 25 years later. *Cancer, 78,* 2603–2606. doi:10.1002/(SICI)1097-0142(19961215)78:12<2603::AID-CNCR29>3.0.CO;2

Nass, S.J., & Ball, J. (Eds.). (2005). *Improving breast imaging quality standards.* Retrieved from http://www.nap.edu/catalog.php?record_id=11308

National Cancer Act of 1971, Pub. L. 92-218, 85 Stat. 778.

National Cancer Advisory Board. (1996). *The recruitment and retention of minority participants in clinical cancer research: Transcripts.* Washington, DC: Author.

National Cancer Advisory Board Ad Hoc Working Group. (2010, December). *To create a strategic scientific vision for the National Cancer Program and review progress of the National Cancer Institute.* Retrieved from http://deainfo.nci.nih.gov/advisory/ncab/workgroup/StrategicVisionWG/SVfinalReport.pdf

National Cancer Institute. (2013). National Cancer Advisory Board: Charter summary. Retrieved from http://deainfo.nci.nih.gov/advisory/ncab/ncab-charter-summary.pdf

National Cancer Institute Act of 1937, Pub. L. 75-244, ch. 565, 50 Stat. 559.

National Cancer Institute Division of Extramural Activities. (n.d.). President's Cancer Panel: Charter summary. Retrieved from http://deainfo.nci.nih.gov/advisory/pcp/charterSummary.pdf

National Cancer Policy Board. (1998). *Taking action to reduce tobacco use.* Retrieved from http://www.nap.edu/catalog.php?record_id=6060

National Cancer Policy Board. (2000). *State programs can reduce tobacco use.* Retrieved from http://www.nap.edu/catalog.php?record_id=9762

Reh, M. (1998). Policy board recommends raising prices to cut tobacco use. *Journal of the National Cancer Institute, 90,* 190–192. doi:10.1093/jnci/90.3.190

Rhoads, J.E. (1996). Recollections of the first chairman of the National Cancer Advisory Board at the National Institutes of Health. *Cancer, 78,* 2594–2596. doi:10.1002/(SICI)1097-0142(19961215)78:12<2594::AID-CNCR25>3.0.CO;2-Q

Sackett, D.L. (1997). A science for the art of consensus. *Journal of the National Cancer Institute, 89*, 1003–1005. doi:10.1093/jnci/89.14.1003

Smigel, K. (1997a). National Cancer Policy Board adds its voice to tobacco issues. *Journal of the National Cancer Institute, 89*, 1097–1098.

Smigel, K. (1997b). National Cancer Policy Board hears pleas for priority at first public forum. *Journal of the National Cancer Institute, 89*, 613–614. doi:10.1093/jnci/89.9.613

S. Res. 347, 112th Cong., 157 Cong. Rec. S8690 (2011).

Selected Topics in Cancer Policy

CHAPTER 7

Biospecimen Collection and Cancer Genomics

Ellen Giarelli, EdD, RN, CRNP

Introduction

There is unequivocal acceptance across disciplines and lines of inquiry that empirical data are needed to support hypotheses and justify clinical interventions and approaches to care. Studies in basic sciences with animal models are early steps in identifying treatment options. Studies of human cell lines might coincide or follow this work. At this time, genomic cancer research using human cell lines, and ultimately human participants, is an irreplaceable step in the sequence toward validating treatments. Until there are other ways to conduct cancer research, the scientific community must ensure that the utmost care and consideration is given to the technical, ethical, legal, and social issues and challenges associated with cancer genomics research. This chapter will discuss policy aspects of biospecimen collection, storage, and use in the context of developing and testing genomic cancer therapeutics. It begins with an overview of the role of genetics and genomics in cancer care.

Genetics and Cancer

Scientists have observed that cancer develops as a consequence of changes, either inherited or acquired, in the underlying mechanisms of cellular replication and repair. These two functions are controlled by genes found in the nucleus of every cell. Some types of cancer are familial; that is, they occur in some families at a higher rate than among the general population. These cancers may be associated with specific genetic disorders or with inherited genetic mutations that predispose an individual to develop cancer.

Most cancers are not clearly linked to the genes that one inherits from one's parents; rather, they are linked to environmental factors that cause changes to nuclear genetic material (chromosomes, genes, and surrounding structures). These changes, called *somatic mutations*, will accumulate or worsen over time and eventually result in cancer (Greenman et al., 2007). Whether caused by inherited or acquired defects, all cancers have a genetic component (Fearon, 1997; Guttmacher & Collins, 2002; Kinzler & Vogelstein, 2002).

According to the World Health Organization (2002), *genetics* is the study of heredity, including the molecular structure and function of genes, gene behavior in the context of a cell or organism, gene distribution, and variation and change in populations (see Figure 7-1 for definitions). Genetics explains cellular reproduction, repair, and the inheritance and expression of traits. *Genomics* addresses all genes and their interrelationships in order to identify their combined influence on the growth and development of the organism. Moreover, genomics applies principles of recombinant DNA, DNA sequencing methods, forensics, and bioinformatics to sequence, assemble, and analyze the function and structure of genomes (Lockhart & Winzeler, 2000; Mardis, 2008; Pagon, 2004; Weedn, 1996). The field of genomics involves uncovering the sequence of base pairs in the DNA of humans and other organisms. These sequences are then called maps because they can be used by scientists and clinicians to navigate the complex network of genes contained in chromosomes. Genomics research is continually lead-

---

Figure 7-1. Definitions

- **Bioinformatics:** "Research, development, or application of computational tools and approaches for expanding the use of biological, medical, behavioral or health data, including those to acquire, store, organize, archive, analyze, or visualize such data." (National Institutes of Health, 2000)
- **DNA sequencing:** "A detailed description of the order of the chemical building blocks, or bases, in a given stretch of DNA." (National Human Genome Research Institute, 2011b)
- **Genetic mapping:** Also called *linkage mapping*, genetic mapping "can offer firm evidence that a disease transmitted from parent to child is linked to one or more genes. It also provides clues about which chromosome contains the gene and precisely where it lies on that chromosome." (National Human Genome Research Institute, 2012b)
- **Genome:** "An organism's complete set of DNA." (National Human Genome Research Institute, 2011a)
- **Molecular genetics:** Identifies "genes associated with specific functions, diseases, and disorders." (National Human Genome Research Institute, n.d.)
- **Population genetics:** "A field of biology that studies the genetic composition of biological populations, and the changes in genetic composition that result from the operation of various factors, including natural selection." (Okasha, 2012)
- **Recombinant DNA:** Joins together DNA molecules "from two different species that are inserted into a host organism to produce new genetic combinations." ("Recombinant DNA Technology," 2014)

---

ing to progress in research in biotechnology. This field of research has contributed to the development of socioeconomic applications, such as tests for determining an individual's risk for developing cancer, and drug discovery, such as monoclonal antibodies and targeted therapies (Druker, 2002; Risch, 2000).

The first and most familiar example of genomics research was the international Human Genome Project, completed in 2003, which determined and deposited in international, publicly available, and online databanks the complete DNA sequence of the human genome—hence the name *genomics* (Hartl & Jones, 2011; Peters & Hadley, 1997). The project inspired a number of other projects, such as proteomics and metabolomics, which deal with different molecules or molecular interactions but share a systematic, high-throughput approach. *High-throughput research* is defined as the automation of experiments that require large-scale repetition, such as sequencing of long strands of genetic material. The sources of samples for high-throughput analysis and genetic and genomic research are biospecimens.

Because all cancers have a genetic component, continual and growing interest exists in assessing the genetic determinants of this disease. In cancer research, biospecimens are assessed for their genetic and genomic information, including DNA sequences, RNA sequences, epigenetic factors, mitochondrial DNA, and protein products.

In 2012, the National Human Genome Research Institute (NHGRI) of the National Institutes of Health (NIH) identified as part of its long-range strategic plan the goal of systematically studying the structure of genomes, the biology of genomes, the biology of diseases, such as cancer, and the effectiveness of genomic health care (NHGRI, 2013b). In the NHGRI, the Division of Genomic Medicine was established to "promote the institute's efforts to advance the application of genomics to medical science and clinical care" (NHGRI, 2013b). Cancer genomics is a significant component, and the mission of the Cancer Genetics and Comparative Genomics Branch of NHGRI is to develop and use state-of-the-art genomic-based technologies and apply these advances to cancer-related questions of public health concern. The primary focus is to identify the genetic contribution to the processes of cancer susceptibility, tumor initiation, progression, treatment response, and long-term outcomes (NHGRI, 2014). To accomplish this, researchers must have the ability to systematically study biospecimens.

Biospecimens are materials that are taken from the human body, such as tissue, blood, plasma, saliva, and urine, that can be used for diagnosis and analysis. When patients have a biopsy, surgery, or other procedure, a small amount of the bodily material may be removed and stored for later research. After these samples have been processed and stored, they are known as *human biospecimens*. These products may be used to confirm the presence or absence of disease and are data sources that may be useful to physicians and researchers.

Each sample may contain DNA, proteins, and other molecules important for understanding disease progression (National Cancer Institute [NCI], 2013c).

NHGRI has also established a Division of Policy, Communications, and Education to maintain and foster the instrumental link between the work of geneticists and research clinicians and the public that they ultimately serve. Policy development requires the engagement of the broad community of stakeholders. Policy regarding genomic health care should reflect the outcome of the dialogue among the general public, patients, physicians, nurses, scientists, politicians, and educators (NHGRI, 2013a). Ongoing debates about policy issues related to biobanking take place within the Division of Policy, Communications, and Education. The main topics of the debate are the regulatory issues associated with biospecimen acquisition and retention.

Biospecimens and Biobanking

Regulatory issues are primarily under the purview of the National Cancer Institute (NCI) Office of Biorepositories and Biospecimens Research (OBBR). Legislative actions might follow this office's recommendations. Healthcare providers practicing in cancer care also can influence regulations and legislation. The first step in garnering such influence is to fully understand biospecimen and biobanking practices. Knowledgeable healthcare providers may then add their voices to the national discussion of best practices.

Biobanking is the collection, storage, and distribution of human body materials. The process was developed in the context of clinical trials and as a by-product of clinical activities. Biobanking is regarded as a tool for producing scientific knowledge (Rial-Sebbag & Cambon-Thomsen, 2012). NCI describes a biorepository (or biobank) as a "library" in which the actual biospecimens or information about them are stored and made available for clinical or research purposes. According to the NCI Biorepositories and Biospecimen Research Branch, "there are thousands of biorepositories in the United States, which vary widely by size, the type of biospecimens collected, and purpose" (NCI, 2013c).

Purpose of Policy in Genomic Cancer Research

Policies assist in decision making. They are principles or rules, statements of intent, protocols and procedures, and other instructions designed to assist stakeholders to achieve reasoned outcomes. Underlying every policy is a presumption of what is a "right" or "good" outcome. The ethical or moral premise of any policy originates from deliberations among stakeholders. Typically, policies are generated and adopted by regulatory boards or governing bodies within organizations or groups of individuals with the same or complementary interests (Rowe & Frewer, 2005). Therefore, the membership of policy-making bodies should be as diverse and honestly representative of the stakeholder group as possible (Tutton, 2007).

Policies can also be understood as mechanisms that are political, managerial, financial, or administrative and arranged to reach explicit goals. The intended effects of policies are the accomplishment of goals deemed "worthy" or "good." Policies may have unintended effects or consequences because of the complex nature of organizations and social aims. At the onset, those who develop policies should attempt to assess as many areas of potential impact as possible to lessen the chance that a given policy will have unexpected or unintended consequences (Horlick-Jones, Rowe, & Walls, 2007). In the case of an emerging science, such as cancer genomics, it may not be possible to predict and account for all the potential effects of a given policy. However, policy issues will correspond with ethical, legal, and social implications.

Any policy governing the collection, storage, or use of biospecimens in cancer genomics is considered a science policy, which is a type of public policy that addresses the responsibilities of scientists and/or clinicians in the conduct of securing, storing, or using biologic samples for the study of the genetics and genomics of cancer (Rial-Sebbag & Cambon-Thomsen, 2012). This type of policy is also concerned with how other public policies might be affected as a consequence of research with biospecimens. The underlying "good" is the well-being of the people and how biospecimen collection, in the process of cancer genomics research, can ultimately serve the public.

Policies are an important means by which biobankers are held accountable to the public and their peers. They are the means to establishing and maintaining public trust.

Biospecimen Research

Biospecimen research involves the analysis of tissue samples and is divided into genomics, proteomics, and metabolomics. These are approaches to findings from molecular research using human analytes or substances undergoing chemical and biochemical analysis. They are the methods to identify the biologic targets to be used for cancer detection, therapy, and prevention. *Genomics* is the study of genes and their functions, including all or a substantial portion of the genes of an organism, over time to determine how those genes interact and influence biologic pathways, networks, and physiology (Eiseman, Bloom, Brower, Clancy, & Olmsted, 2003). *Proteomics* is the study of the full set of proteins encoded by a genome, including the study of identities, quantities, structures, and the biochemical and cellular functions of all proteins in an organism (Eiseman & Haga, 2009). *Metabolomics* is the study of the "unique chemical fingerprints that specific cellular processes leave behind" (Daviss, 2005, para. 3) and the study of their small-molecule metabolite profiles (Preti, 2005).

Many institutions, especially those that are research oriented, derive most of their biospecimens for cancer genomic research from their clinical partners' surgical pathology services (McDonald et al., 2011). As a result of emerging genomic, proteomic, and metabolomic techniques, tissue banking is evolving from primarily a research activity to a direct clinical activity. The resources and processes needed to support successful procurement of samples are complicated but are becoming integral parts of patient care. As is often the case, the distinction between research and clinical care is not clear. Therefore, both researchers and clinicians must be mindful of possible confusion and misunderstanding by patients who are asked to donate biospecimens.

Generally, biosamples in a genomics repository may comprise preserved tissues, stored RNA, and stored DNA from 50 tissue groups and 900 postmortem donors, many of whom were diagnosed with cancer. In addition to the biospecimens, future researchers would also have access to molecular data, standard operating procedures, histopathologic interpretations, laboratory processing variables (e.g., complementary DNA, library preparation methods), and sex and age at death for each donor.

Once biobanks are established and collection and storage standardized, research can proceed within a policy structure that facilitates collaboration. For example, in 2012, NIH announced a request for information (RFI) to gauge interest in using stored biospecimens collected in the Genotype-Tissue Expression (GTEx) Project of the NIH Common Fund. In the interest of making maximal use of unique biospecimen resources with rich clinical and genomic information, the RFI was solicited in anticipation of announcing a funding opportunity to support future studies using these biosamples (NIH, 2012). This RFI clearly illustrates NIH's efforts to distribute high-quality data among researchers. Figure 7-2 shows the life cycle of a biosample.

National Cancer Institute Biospecimen Research Network

In the interest of advancing cancer research, the NCI OBBR created the NCI Biospecimen Research Network in 2006 (Moore, 2012). Its formation was prompted by concern about the issue of biospecimen biology and the potential for specimens of poor or unknown quality. The network's purpose is to conduct, sponsor, and collaborate on research to examine the effects of

Figure 7-2. Life Cycle of a Biosample

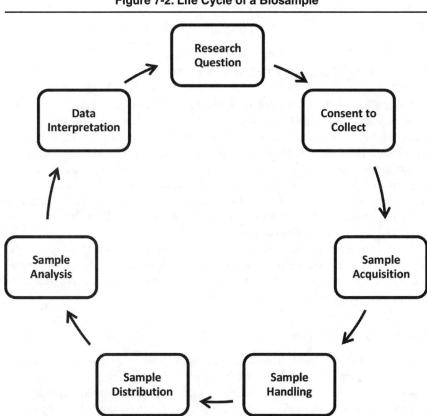

different biospecimen collection methods on downstream molecular analysis (Moore, 2012).

According to Moore (2012), there is a three-pronged best practice approach to enhancing the quality of biospecimens. The first approach provides guidance for biobanking in order to standardize and integrate procedures for collecting, processing, storing, and distributing biospecimens (NCI, 2013b). The second effort will develop procedures for sponsoring active research on how pre-analytic variables affect the molecular integrity of biospecimens (NCI, 2013a). The OBBR's third major effort is to design ways to integrate best practice guidelines and biospecimen research into a set of operating procedures to promote and facilitate cancer research.

Policies and procedures on biobanking can never be completely removed from ethical, legal, and social considerations (Hawkins & O'Doherty, 2011). The intersection of ethical issues with genomic cancer research and policy must be addressed with regard to the rights of donors. A full discussion of these ethical issues is beyond the scope of this chapter.

Biobanking Policies for Cancer Care

Biobanking policies should cover definitions and the use of biobanks, how they are established, and the processes for collecting, storing, distributing, and dissolving. NCI has published the *NCI Laboratory of Pathology Policy Manual* (NCI Center for Cancer Research, 2013). The policies included in the manual are designed to expand the scope of cancer scientists' expertise and incorporate the newest tools of diagnosis, training, and research. Among the values articulated in the manual are the need to promote excellence in patient care, work output and collaboration, and research methodology (NCI Center for Cancer Research, 2013).

The categories of instruction include requests for human biologic materials for research; patient privacy; specimen collection, handling, and transportation; infection control; and emergency management plans (NCI Center for Cancer Research, 2013).

Policies on Collection

Quality cancer research that uses human biospecimens must be based on quality biospecimens that have been obtained using rigorous procedural standards with consideration of the ethical, legal, and social implications. The reliability of the findings depends on the methodology. Varying methods of collection, processing, and storage can alter the physical or biologic state of the specimen. This, in turn, alters the possibility of accurate, useful results from analyses. A pure biosample is essential to an accurate diagnosis. When the quality of biospecimens varies, several effects on clinical outcomes result. Morphologic artifacts in a sample may result in a missed or incorrect diagnosis. A therapy may be linked to the result of a molecular diagnostic test on a biosample. If the biosample is impure, the test may be inaccurate. This can potentially result in incorrect therapy or treatment, or worse, no treatment at all (Watson, Kay, & Smith, 2010). Logically, standardization of the collection of biospecimens would be one way to ensure high quality and utility in cancer research and clinical application translation.

Definition of Cancer Biobanks

Several types of cancer biobanks exist, including population, disease, and clinical trials based. The type of biobank is defined by its statement of purpose and goals, which subsequently determine the types of samples collected. A clear definition of the biobank's scope is essential and must be incorporated into the consenting process (Vaught, Rogers, Carolin, & Compton, 2011). In addition to clarity, flexibility is vital, in part to respond to new technologies and new understandings of cancer's complexity.

Operating Procedures

The day-to-day operations and specifications for conducting the business of biobanking must be well and carefully documented. The principle purpose is to guarantee that data generated from the samples are valid and reproducible. These procedures must be standardized, and these standards must be applied across multiple biobanks. Standards prevent variations in collection, storage, and use that could compromise findings. NCI defined these standards in its *Best Practices for Biospecimen Resources* (NCI, 2013b). When these standards are not applied or are applied incorrectly, the result is less productive cancer research. Several organizations have been established to address issues of standardization (see Figure 7-3). They have all prioritized the need for quality assurance systems that are operational across sites and borders. The process of collaboration and systematization of standards is ongoing.

Technical Aspects

The life cycle of a biospecimen begins with the asking of research or clinical questions, then proceeds to analysis of data generated from the study of the biosample (see Figure 7-2). It also involves careful consideration of all variables that affect the purity and integrity of a specimen. These are called *pre-analytic variables* and are divided into pre-acquisition and post-acquisition phases (De Cecco et al., 2009; Engel & Moore, 2011).

Pre-Acquisition Factors

Pre-acquisition variables are factors that affect the actual sample and its collection. Any patient-centered event affects the sample. A variety of pre-analytic factors have contributed to poor specimen quality, including patient therapy, such as type and number of pharmaceuticals; medical procedures in the vicinity of the sample; and the patient's physiology. Pre-acquisition factors also include the handling of the instruments used during sample collection, including inconsistent use of instruments, inconsistencies or inadequacies in the collection, and storage devices (Wolff et al., 2007). Standard operating procedures outlined in policies will address the use of collection tube additives, such as ethylenediaminetetraacetic acid (commonly known as EDTA) and heparin, and how they can affect analyses (Vaught, 2006).

An example of a policy and procedure related to a pre-acquisition variable is the Fresh Frozen Tissue Protocol developed by the Cancer Control and Population Sciences section of NCI. This protocol describes the proce-

---

Figure 7-3. Biobanks and Repositories

- Canadian Tumour Repository Network: www.ctrnet.ca
- European Biobanking and Biomolecular Resources Research Infrastructure: http://bbmri.eu
- European Network to Promote Research into Uncommon Cancers in Adults and Children: Pathology, Biology and Genetics of Bone Tumours: http://eurobonet.pathobiology.eu/cd/index.php
- Frederick National Laboratory for Cancer Research Repositories: http://frederick.cancer.gov/Services/Repositories.aspx
- Global Directory of Biobanks, Tissue Banks, and Biorepositories (see this site for a current list of all tissue banks and biorepositories by state and country, including university-based repositories): http://specimencentral.com/biobank-directory.aspx
- National Comprehensive Cancer Network: www.nccn.org/index.asp
- National Institute on Aging's Aging Cell Repository: https://catalog.coriell.org/0/Sections/Collections/NIA/?SsId=9
- National Institutes of Health and National Cancer Institute (NCI)
  – Biorepositories and Biospecimen Research Branch: http://biospecimens.cancer.gov/default.asp
  – Cancer Human Biobank: http://cahub.cancer.gov
  – Chemical Carcinogenesis Research Information System (provides historical information from 1985 to 2011; is no longer updated): http://toxnet.nlm.nih.gov/newtoxnet/ccris.htm
  – Common Fund's Genotype-Tissue Expression Project: https://commonfund.nih.gov/GTEx
  – Cooperative Human Tissue Network: www.chtn.nci.nih.gov
  – Developmental Therapeutics Program: http://dtp.nci.nih.gov/index.html
  – National Cancer Informatics Program: http://cbiit.nci.nih.gov/ncip/about-ncip
  – National Center for Biotechnology Information's Database of Genotypes and Phenotypes: www.ncbi.nlm.nih.gov/gap
  – National Heart, Lung, and Blood Institute's Biologic Specimen and Data Repository: https://biolincc.nhlbi.nih.gov/home
  – Residual Tissue Repository Program: http://seer.cancer.gov/biospecimen
  – Specimen Reference Sets: NCI Early Detection Research Network: http://edrn.nci.nih.gov/resources/sample-reference-sets
    * Breast Cancer Reference Set
    * Colon Cancer Reference Set
    * Liver (Hepatocellular Carcinoma) Reference Set
    * Lung Cancer Reference Set
    * Ovarian and Breast Cancer Reference Sets
    * Prostate Cancer Reference Set
- Organisation of European Cancer Institutes' TuBaFrost database: www.tubafrost.org/research/index.php
- Spanish National Cancer Research Centre Biobank: www.cnio.es/ing/grupos/plantillas/presentacion.asp?grupo=50004308

---

dure for collection, storage, and distribution of colorectal cancer tissue in the Cancer Family Registry frozen tissue biorepository. The protocol provides investigators with access to optimally preserved tissue that is linked to relevant epidemiologic, genetic, and clinical data (NCI, 2013d).

Another example of a pre-acquisition factor is arterial clamp time. This is defined as how long a sample of tissue has been without oxygen during surgery and before it is removed from the body. Von Elm et al. (2008) reported that changes in gene expression occur as a result of changes in clamp time, rather than disease. This pre-acquisition variable will interfere with accurate analysis of the genome. In another example, Rai et al. (2005) reported that the lack of standardization of biospecimens leads to the lack of reproducibility of protein biomarkers.

Post-Acquisition Factors

Post-acquisition factors include any and all variables after the sample is collected, such as all aspects of sample handling (time at room temperature, time to fixation, speed of fixation with formalin, size of sample) (Khoury et al., 2009). Variables of time are also applied to sample storage and distribution. For example, sample integrity is affected by the consistency of the temperature of the storage facility and the speed of handling of the sample by technicians who process or distribute the sample (NCI, 2013b). In another example, standard operating policies and procedures might state that storage in liquid nitrogen temperatures is preferred for long-term cell viability and that specimens such as DNA will be stable for most analyses if stored at temperatures of $-80°C$ (NCI, 2013b).

Labeling of Specimens

The labeling of specimens is a fundamental and highly important issue. NCI (2010) issued a white paper titled *Labeling of Biological Specimens*, which aims to provide the necessary technical and product-related information to enable standardization of labels used on various types of biologic specimens collected by NCI and its collaborators for NCI-directed studies. This white paper presents information for optimized label configuration and supplies and equipment needed for specimen storage vessels or devices at different temperatures commonly used by NCI. NCI recognized a need to provide investigators, study managers, and repositories associated with NCI-directed studies with a convenient, centralized location for label-relevant information in an effort to standardize all specimen labels, with regard to size, readable information, two-dimensional barcode encryption, supplies, and equipment. This white paper is a superior example of how cancer biobanking procedures can be standardized and translated into policies that can be used by many or all repositories. It is extraordinarily detailed, technical, comprehensive, and sufficiently descriptive to be applicable in any laboratory setting.

Information Technology

An important aspect of policy development in biobanking is creating a system for acquiring samples for research. Information technology management systems are being considered to track, store, and search the data stored in biobanks. These data include the kinds of samples; the quantity and sources of samples; the associated cancers, symptoms, and therapies; the demographic of the sources; and health and medical histories of the sources (patients) and family members. Such clinical data is especially relevant when studying familial cancer syndromes and relationships between phenotype and genotype. Comprehensive databases are difficult to maintain and update; the difficulty of these tasks is compounded when multiple databases are combined. In addition to creating an easy-to-use search mechanism, these databases must keep a high level of security to protect confidentiality and privacy. Biobanking information management is becoming an important driver of medical economies. According to the Biobanking Global Summit of 2011 website, "An estimated $1 billion has been invested in the biobanking industry within the last ten years. With biobank collections increasing in value by medical researchers and drug developers worldwide, the biobank market is enjoying rapid growth" (Appel Consulting, 2011).

Biobanks for cancer research, whether clinical or research in focus, require resources to maintain infrastructure, support personnel, and continue operations. Economic considerations are taking a higher priority in policy making for biobanking, primarily because of the high cost to institutions and investigators who collect, store, and test biospecimens. The larger the collection, the higher the cost. Policies include recommendations for facilities personnel and their qualifications, costs of equipment maintenance, cost of informatics, and quality assurance. Personnel costs are a major component, and a large, long-term biobank requires a variety of specially trained technicians and scientists who maintain their expertise (Vaught et al., 2011).

Specimen procurement and biobanking is being viewed as the same as any other technology (McDonald, Velasco, & Ilasi, 2010). Many sources of financial support for infrastructure and operations exist, including philanthropic, third-party payer, and, in some cases, research sponsorship.

Along with the costs of biobanking come economic benefits, mostly in the form of intellectual property rights and liability or warranty. These may be negotiated using material transfer agreements or other means of documenting the relationship (responsibility or fiduciary) between the biobank and the end user. Prior to using biospecimens, researchers should examine biologic material agreements if they exist and clarify any issues of liability or warranty. Samples of such agreements are available for comparison (NIH Office of Technology Transfer, n.d.; Stanford University, 1995). Policies governing access and levels of security are being developed with consideration for the interchangeability between biobanks and language differences across cultures (Watson et al., 2010).

Policies on Access

When biosamples are made available to researchers, several policy issues should be considered, including the process for transfer. For example, will the researcher receive a physical sample or summary data? If a physical sample is delivered, procedures must be in place to ensure that the sample is used only for the stated purpose and that it is not shared with others. If data about the sample are transferred, the biobank must ensure that these data are coded or encrypted (if personalized data are included). A policy must include provisions for the verification of appropriate institutional approvals prior to release of the data or the sample (Salter & Jones, 2005).

Quality Assurance

The issue of quality assurance cannot be overstated. It must be a priority when developing and updating policies. Policies on quality assurance and quality control for cancer biospecimen banking are similar to those for laboratories and other organizations that require this kind of monitoring. The policies should address equipment maintenance, calibration, and repair; training and monitoring of staff; data management plans; record keeping; and the systematic review and revision of standard operating procedures. According to Vaught and Lockhart (2012), additional quality control policies for biobanks include

- Biospecimen handling
- Laboratory processing
- Shipping and receiving protocols
- Material transfer agreements
- Record management systems
- Building, personnel, and biospecimen security
- Safety and waste disposal
- Procedures to investigate, document, and report staff injuries or incidents.

Prior to requesting data or samples from a biobank, researchers should request information on the policies and practices of the biobank with respect to these issues, especially quality assurance and control.

Ethical Issues: The Rights of the Source-Persons

Biobanks of various kinds are proliferating with a trend toward expanding highly institutionalized, broad population-based biobanks that collect and store blood or tissue. The research and ethical challenges are gaining attention and drawing public interest, especially since the publication of the best-selling book *The Immortal Life of Henrietta Lacks* (Skloot, 2010). Lacks' tissue was stored without her or her family's knowledge and later used by thousands of researchers, generating millions of dollars in profits for the biologics industry. One main response has been to apply principles of informed consent to biobanking, thereby treating the process as if it were a research endeavor.

In the context of biobanking, two ethical considerations are paramount: consent and a guarantee of confidentiality. These are called the *rights of the source-person*. Two different sets of expectations apply, one for patients and another for research participants. When samples are collected during the course of clinical treatment, the source-person is protected by patients' rights. However, when samples are gathered from research participants, these individuals are considered donors of body elements and are specifically protected by rules guiding donation. According to Gottweis and Zatloukal (2007), the two are very different. The ethical considerations become less clear when samples collected from patients are then used in research. People from whom these samples are collected may not know their change of status from patient to donor. In the case of research, source-persons should be given the right to claim control over the future uses of their biosamples. This is often an option contained in research consent documents. Rial-Sebbag and Cambon-Thomsen (2012) asserted that it is unrealistic and impractical to expect that there will be an accurate and consistent trace (or lack of one) between the person and the biosample once it is added to a biobank for research. This is because it will likely be used by various researchers, for different reasons, and coded in many different ways.

The kind and extent of oversight at this level raises legal and ethical questions that need to be addressed continually (Hakimian & Korn, 2004). One should ask whether the donor is protected if he or she is asked and gives permission to allow broad future use of his or her sample (Hansson, Dillner, Bartram, Carlson, & Helgesson, 2006). Other considerations include the following: What type of governance will offer the best oversight? What should be the level and kind of regulatory response? What role should decision makers play? How should responsibilities be distributed? What should be the ongoing reevaluation of the effectiveness and comprehensiveness of oversight as technology improves and science advances?

Withdrawal of Samples

When biobank policies are developed for cancer biospecimens, policy makers should consider whether donors should have the right to withdraw their samples. This is in the spirit of the Nuremberg Code and the Declaration of Helsinki (Hansson et al., 2006). Two questions arise from this option: what can be withdrawn and when? No consensus exists on the answers to these questions, except for the agreement that they must be considered when writing policy. An option often is presented to donors that satisfies the concerns of the donor for anonymity and of the researcher for continued access. A participant might be offered the right to have the sample completely depersonalized such that there can be no link to the source. According to Gertz (2008), this is a particularly important provision in the event that samples are shared across biobank networks.

Donor Consent

Within policies for obtaining consent from biosample donors, certain information is essential to include. A consent document must contain information on (a) the circumstances of sampling, (b) the aims of storage, (c) the future use (e.g., transfer, destruction) of samples, (d) fate of samples if the biobank closes, (e) use of samples for commercial purposes, and (f) possible consequences of sharing biosamples. This information is in addition to statements that should be included in any consent documents, such as (a) the measures taken to ensure confidentiality, (b) the voluntary nature of participation, (c) the type of consent (research or clinical care), (d) the disclosure of data, and (e) the risks and benefits to the participant.

A governance plan that addresses ethical issues will include consideration for the legacy of the database. This is needed in the event that sponsorship ends, budgets are depleted, research is accomplished, or other events occur that result in the need to terminate the biobank. Such policies should consider a possible transfer of ownership, management, and items across responsible parties. Any transfer of biospecimens must comply with human subject regulations and honor the consent documents (Yassin et al., 2010).

A brochure on biospecimen donation, titled *How You Can Help Medical Research: Donating Your Blood, Tissue, and Other Samples*, is available from the Biorepositories and Biospecimen Research Branch, which is now part of the Cancer Diagnosis Program of the Division of Cancer Treatment and Diagnosis of NCI (see NCI, 2012). This resource was written for sourcepersons and provides information on uses of biosamples, how they might be collected, and examples of positive medical outcomes as a result of access to biosamples, privacy, rights, and risks, along with a link for accessing additional information. It was written for patients to help them understand the purpose and process of sample donation. The brochure provides a simple and thorough explanation that is suitable for adult patients. It is available in English only. Investigators might wish to study how patients who do not speak English could receive the information and react to a translation of the brochure.

Williams, Schepp, McGrath, and Mitchell (2010) reported that programs have been established to linked biobanks in order to cull samples. Some of these include the Canadian Tumour Repository Network, the Data Schema and Harmonization Platform for Epidemiological Research (known as DataSHaPER), and the Public Population Project in Genomics and Society (known as P3G) (see Figure 7-4).

Public Perceptions of Biobank Research

The success of cancer biobanking will depend on public opinion of the process and whether the public perceives there will be a benefit. Pullman et al. (2012) tested the assumption that the public would value biobanking. After collecting responses from 330 participants (approximately 60:40 ratio of women to men), they reported that this cohort viewed biobanks as a public good. The majority consistently ranked privacy and confidentiality as the least important of the variables to consider when evaluating biobanking. The potential beneficiary of research was ranked as the highest value. The authors concluded that the manner in which the consent form described the disposition and ultimate use of the biospecimen could affect value preferences, that is, willingness to be donors. This study points to the need to reconsider the approach to soliciting donors. The primary concern for the protection of personal health information, confidentiality, and privacy, while important, is perhaps the wrong focus (Murphy et al., 2009).

Similar findings were reported by Simon et al. (2011), who interviewed and surveyed 48 and 751 participants, respectively. When asked about willingness to contribute samples to biobanks, the majority preferred an opt-in rather than an opt-out consent approach. However, within this model, most preferred broad, unspecified consent over categorical, study-specific consent. These findings suggest that most

---

Figure 7-4. Research Collaboratives Related to Biobanking

- Data Schema and Harmonization Platform for Epidemiological Research: www.datashaper.org
- European, Middle Eastern and African Society for Biopreservation and Biobanking: http://esbb.org
- European Prospective Investigation into Cancer and Nutrition: http://epic.iarc.fr
- National Cancer Institute Center to Reduce Cancer Health Disparities: http://crchd.cancer.gov
- Promoting Harmonisation of Epidemiological Biobanks in Europe: www.fhi.no/artikler/?id=73793
- Public Population Project in Genomics and Society: http://p3g.org
- Telethon Network of Genetic Biobanks (Italy): http://biobanknetwork.org

individuals (at least in this study) prefer more personal control of the process of consent but were not necessarily interested in the details of the research.

Surrogacy Model

Current ethical considerations of biosampling and biobanking presume that issues may be sufficiently resolved by applying principles of informed consent to steps in the process. However, biobanking is an emerging biotechnology that may require a different approach to guarding the public interest. Mongoven and Solomon (2012) proposed the alternative analogy of clinical surrogacy. They advocated that, instead of giving informed consent, biosampling should be informed by the "designation of surrogate decision makers for incapacitated patients, informed by advance directives expressing patients' basic values" (Mongoven & Solomon, 2012, p. 185). According to the surrogacy model (Sulmasy & Snyder, 2010), the first responsibility of a surrogate is to become familiar with the patient's values instead of merely providing vague information on possible future uses of samples. In this model, community engagement allows individuals and groups (e.g., ethnic, racial, or family cohorts) to participate in the dialogue regarding their values and the potential uses of specimens in cancer care. This approach may best serve the mission of the Division of Policy, Communications, and Education of the NHGRI. In this model, the biobank will need to consider the donor's values and the values of the research initiative (Caulfield, Einsiedel, Merz, & Nicol, 2006).

Stewardship Model

Jeffers' stewardship model (Jeffers, 2001) can be applied to the process of procuring biospecimens for cancer genomic research. Williams et al. (2010) astutely applied this model to biobanking. The model establishes a relationship between parties that must consider both intent and expectations. Like the surrogacy approach, the stewardship model considers the responsibility of the investigator who uses the sample to the contributor of the sample. In both models, the relationship between or among parties is the crucial factor in determining what constitutes "consent." The relationship should be considered when defining and designing policies.

With regard to the best approach to obtaining donations, the only consensus among policy makers is that the rights of donors must continue to have a prominent role in policy development. The form of honoring these rights remains controversial. Indeed, Master, Nelson, Murdoch, and Caulfield (2012) reviewed the literature on biobanking and consents and concluded that, while many take a broad approach, there is no evidence of consensus on the best way to obtain donor permission.

Legislative and Regulatory Milestones

The major milestones with regard to biospecimen regulations can be reviewed on the OBBR website (see http://biospecimens.cancer.gov/default .asp). The systematic and structured review of biospecimen collection and handling practices began in earnest more than a decade ago (see Figure 7-5). In 2002, NCI conducted an internal and external review of its biospecimen resources using surveys and several community forums. The outcome was the statement that biospecimen resources were and will continue to be critically important to genomic cancer research. This was followed in 2003 by the publication of a National Biospecimen Network blueprint (Friede, Grossman, Hunt, Li, & Stern, 2003). This important step drew attention to the complex issues to be addressed as scientists and clinicians move forward. The formation of the Biorepository Coordinating Committee was part of the seminal infrastructure that would proceed to identify an urgent need for standardization and oversight of repositories. The committee recognized that clinicians were continually collecting biospecimens, but that procedures across NCI-funded institutions remained unstandardized and unregulated.

Figure 7-5. Milestones in Regulatory and Infrastructure Development for Biobanking

---

2002—National Cancer Institute (NCI) begins an internal and external review of biospecimen practices.

2003—NCI publishes *National Biospecimen Network Blueprint.*
NCI forms Biorepository Coordinating Committee (BCC).

2004—BCC evaluates existing best practices.

2005—NCI establishes Office of Biorepositories and Biospecimen Research (OBBR).

2006—Biospecimen Research Network formed.
NCI publishes the *First-Generation Guidelines for NCI-Supported Biorepositories.*

2007—OBBR hosts forums attended by clinicians, scientists, cancer research advocates, and the public.

2008—OBBR forms national biobank resource.

2009—OBBR establishes the Cancer Human Biobank (caHUB).

2010—NCI receives $1.3 billion through the American Recovery and Reinvestment Act, $70 million of which will be devoted to caHUB.

2011—NCI hosts Biospecimen Research Network Symposium: Advancing Cancer Research Through Science.
NCI caHUB and the Critical Path Institute (a 501(c)(3) organization) establish a collaborative agreement to perform biospecimen research.
NCI Center to Reduce Cancer Health Disparities established Community Networks Program (CNP). Minnesota begins storing biospecimens for potential use in biobanking or other proteomic research, in collaboration with the Centers for Disease Control and Prevention's Arctic Investigations Program.
OBBR hosts Workshop on Biospecimen Reference Sets and Drug-Diagnostic Co-development.

Public support is key to infrastructure development. This support requires broad understanding of the state of the science and consensus on goals and objectives. This was accomplished through a series of workshops and forums in 2007. OBBR became the instrumental link among the funding agencies, clinicians, and scientists. This role took on greater import when, in 2008, OBBR formed a national biobank resource following the National Biospecimen Network Blueprint, which garnered approval and clearance from the U.S. Office of Budget and Management. In 2009, under the direction of Dr. Carolyn Compton, OBBR established the United States' first national biobank, which was called "a safe house for tissue samples, tumor cells, DNA and . . . blood—that would be used for research into new treatments for diseases" (Park, 2009, para. 2). This biobank, the Cancer Human Biobank (caHUB), was funded in 2010 through the American Recovery and Reinvestment Act. During the following two years, OBBR engaged the public and private sectors in discussing evolving issues and identifying mechanisms to integrate biospecimen reference sets with drug and diagnostic developments.

The efforts of the OBBR have been largely successful in establishing guidelines and organizing public support. However, the successes apply to a limited cohort of institutions and organizations involved in biospecimen collection and cancer research, as the network represents only a portion of all functioning repositories.

Implications for Future Health Policy

The problems surrounding biospecimen standard operating procedures have a large public health impact. Several weaknesses have been identified in biosampling practices and policy that are obstacles to best practice and ultimately will have health policy implications. They include (a) sampling and analyses are often done noncollaboratively, (b) researchers have difficulty acquiring high-quality and high-quantity samples, and (c) researchers limit their scope of work due to shortages in biospecimens.

Future health policy relies on researchers' access to adequate samples. Principle issues include the need to ensure that biorepositories continue to apply best practices and that all those in existence are included in the network. NCI's extramural research programs and nongovernmental biomedical research organizations rely on networks for shared biospecimens and are significantly affected by the variability of human biospecimens. Large-scale genomic and proteomic studies, such as the Cancer Genome Atlas project (http://cancergenome.nih.gov), require a sufficient number of quality-controlled biospecimens. Not all existing biobanks are part of the network. Unfortunately, no current funding opportunities are available for adding biobanks and medical institutions that are interested but not yet part of the caHUB network. According to NCI (n.d.), all contractual awards for establishment of the caHUB infrastructure have been made. Expanding the network will be essential to the development of quality, effective, and broadly applicable cancer diagnostics and treatments.

Obstacles to Cancer Research

Cancer is a complex, heterogeneous disease; therefore, research will rely on access to a large, complex, and heterogeneous biobank of samples. For most cancers, gene and environmental interactions hold the key to diagnosis, treatment, and prevention. A significant limiting factor to the translation of basic science studies to improved patient outcomes is the lack of "access to large, appropriate and well-annotated cohorts of human tissue" (Watson et al., 2010, p. 646). A researcher will need approximately 2,000–5,000 samples for genetic main-effects studies, and 2,000–20,000 samples for lifestyle main-effects studies (Caporaso, 2001). When gene-lifestyle interaction is studied (a main category of cancer research), 20,000–50,000 samples are needed (Burton et al., 2009). Enormous, diverse samples are therefore essential to cancer research that aims to uncover the important interactions among genes, lifestyle, environment, and disease, and to convert these to diagnostics and therapeutics.

Specific Challenges in Biobanking

Three challenges created by the process of biobanking must be overcome as researchers work to develop resilient and enduring governance of the process: the heterogeneity of biobanks, the uncertainty of purpose, and the temporality (Fullerton, Anderson, Guzauskas, Freeman, & Fryer-Edwards, 2010). First, biobanks are diverse in nature and may be established for general collection or for specific cancers. This creates a challenge to the development and adoption of standardized policies and procedures. Not all policies are broadly applicable to all situations. Second, many biobanks have a clearly defined purpose, but some do not. This creates a challenge if the aim is to design policies that are sufficiently flexible to allow adaptation to emerging interests and technologies that also respect the rights of donors. Lastly, Laurie (2011) asserted that timing issues arise because of scientific and natural restraints. Time is needed to generate sufficient data, and biobanks are set up as long-term initiatives (Laurie, 2011). Thus, policy and governance must balance the competing elements of immediate and long-term needs. An additional challenge is the trend toward virtual networking, which might enable single biobanks to communicate with multiple entities in real time. Naturally, the need will arise to establish "e-governance" of biobanks with policies that respond to the virtual medical research community

(Kaye, 2011). In this environment, new regulatory issues will continually emerge.

According to Kolata (2013), research is steadily eroding scientists' faith that the anonymity of DNA can be maintained. Even fragments of genetic information can compromise privacy. Identification of donors will always be a risk, and policies cannot prevent such risks. As a result, George Church, a geneticist at Harvard University, shared in a *New York Times* interview that "people who provide genetic information should be informed that a loss of privacy is likely, rather than unlikely, and agree to provide DNA with that understanding" (Kolata, 2013). In the same report, David Altshuler of the Broad Institute of Harvard and the Massachusetts Institute of Technology stated, "the amount of genetic data [available in biobanks] that has been gathered so far is miniscule compared with what will be coming in the next few years" (Kolata, 2013, para. 17). These privacy issues will increase as biobanks grow in number and usage. Policies can only guide actions.

Key Players

In the absence of adequate funding, the number of biosamples for cancer research will continue to be limited. The public, composed of patients, clinicians, and advocates for scientific infrastructure development, plays a key role. Legislators respond to unified and strong requests for action and financial support.

Future Health Policies

In addition to biobanking guidelines, health policies must anticipate future problems and respond to existing ones. First, with regard to sampling and analyses that are often done noncollaboratively, policies might be developed to guide the research in identifying and securing viable collaborations. Legislators may work with OBBR to extend their networking services to facilitate the formation of alliances among researchers with similar or related studies and to create incentives for the process with financial benefits provided to the collaborative enterprise.

Second, when researchers limit their scope of work because of shortages in biospecimens, policies are urgently needed to direct and oversee the expansion of approved repositories in the network. Along with this, advocates might lobby for substantial increases in funding opportunities made available to new repositories. Lobbying activities are not appropriate for government agencies, such as NCI, but they are appropriate for advocacy organizations, such as the Oncology Nursing Society, American Cancer Society, and others. Through lobbying efforts, these organizations can support and promote consumer engagement and capacity building, and can contribute to developing procedures to protect, promote, and defend the public's rights to affordable, safe, and quality health care that evolves from the use of biospecimens.

Third, given the advancements in clinical genetics and genome-based therapeutics, the quality of the product is directly related to the quality of the data sources and analysis of genomics, proteomics, and metabolomics across samples. Future policies will need to guide the approach to molecular analysis of tissue samples and cell lines to ensure that biodata are precise, complete, and reliable.

Lastly, in the interests of transparency and the public's right to know, policies are needed to specifically guide how the public is informed of the sources, collection, and quality control of biospecimens used by private and public agencies in the development of diagnostics and drug therapies. Such a policy may have a great impact on healthcare consumers and patients with cancer. They may serve to ensure that the most ethical procedures are followed and that the most scientifically valid data are collected and verified.

The Future of Biobanking—An Exemplar for Practice

The GTEx Project is an excellent example of researchers' ability to explore the mysteries of cancer when they have access to biobanks. This program's goal is to establish a resource database and tissue bank in which to study the relationship between genetic variation and gene expression in reference (nondiseased) human tissue. Sponsored by NIH, the project has more than 4,500 samples of healthy human tissue from about 175 donors. It has developed 150 standard operating procedures to ensure that all tissue samples are collected, processed, and stored in exactly the same way. GTEx partners with organizations involved in tissue and organ donations in several cities. Biospecimen source sites include LifeNet Health (Virginia Beach, Virginia), Gift of Life Donor Program (Philadelphia, Pennsylvania), Drexel University College of Medicine (Philadelphia, Pennsylvania), Albert Einstein College of Medicine (Bronx, New York), Virginia Commonwealth University (Richmond, Virginia), Roswell Park Cancer Institute (Buffalo, New York), and others. Biorepository operations and pathology review are conducted by the Van Andel Institute in Grand Rapids, Michigan. The Broad Institute in Cambridge, Massachusetts, serves as the laboratory, data analysis, and coordinating center. By comparing genetic variants to normal genes, the project aims to explain how variants might affect gene regulation in different tissues in the disease process. GTEx uses a web-based data processing application that allows project members to communicate in real time and monitor the progress of specimen processing and data collection. Pathologists review images of all tissue samples to assess the quality of the biospecimens and add comments to the dataset. Dr. Sherilyn Sawyer co-led the development of the GTEx biobank and described in the *NCI Bulletin* the process for collecting samples and increasing capacity (Winstead, 2012). According to NHGRI (2012a), the GTEx Project will more than triple its pool of donors by 2015.

Conclusion

Policy on biospecimen collection must ensure inclusiveness of all biorepositories and standardization of the collection, storage, and use of human biospecimens. Such policies are essential to conducting the highest quality molecular research for the purpose of advancing genomic therapeutics. The most significant challenges for translational research are in ensuring that all biobanks conduct the business of biosampling using identical criteria and standards for consenting donors, labeling and storing samples, and handling and transferring samples to investigators. The key challenges when this is not done are that biospecimens will vary and analytical outcomes will not be accurate, reliable, or reproducible. Policies must exist to certify that accurate clinical information is linked to specimens. This will ensure that scientists know about the patients and understand the biologic context of samples. Finally, there must be uniform standards on what scientists may do with specimens and data. This includes policies regarding patient consent and how scientists will address emerging ethical, legal, and social issues. Such policies should be adopted by all biobanks, regardless of proprietor or location. The ultimate results will be improved patient care, improved treatment outcomes, and public engagement in an important and evolving scientific discussion.

References

Appel Consulting. (2011, September 10). Biobanking Global Summit Sept 20–21, London UK (organiser Appel Consulting). Retrieved from http://www.prlog.org/11640986-biobanking-global-summit-sept-20-21-london-uk-organiser-appel-consulting.html

Burton, P.R., Hansell, A.L., Fortier, I., Manolio, T.A., Khoury, M.J., Little, J., & Elliott, P. (2009). Size matters: Just how big is BIG? Quantifying realistic sample size requirements for human genome epidemiology. *International Journal of Epidemiology, 38,* 263–273. doi:10.1093/ije/dyn147

Caporaso, N.E. (2001). Why have we failed to find the low penetrance genetic constituents of common cancers? *Cancer Epidemiology, Biomarkers and Prevention, 11,* 1544–1549. Retrieved from http://cebp.aacrjournals.org/content/11/12/1544.long

Caulfield, T., Einsiedel, E., Merz, J.F., & Nicol, D. (2006). Trust, patents, and public perceptions: The governance of controversial biotechnology research. *Nature Biotechnology, 24,* 1352–1354.

Daviss, B. (2005). Growing pains for metabolomics. *Scientist.* Retrieved from http://www.the-scientist.com/?articles.view/articleNo/16400/title/Growing-Pains-for-Metabolomics

De Cecco, L., Musella, V., Veneroni, S., Cappelletti, V., Bongarzone, I., Callari, M., ... Daidone, M.G. (2009). Impact of biospecimens handling on biomarker research in breast cancer. *BMC Cancer, 9,* 409. doi:10.1186/1471-2407-9-409

Druker, B.J. (2002). Perspectives on the development of a molecularly targeted agent. *Cancer Cell, 1,* 31–36. doi:10.1016/S1535-6108(02)00025-9

Eiseman, E., Bloom, G., Brower, J., Clancy, N., & Olmsted, S.S. (2003). *Case studies of existing human tissue repositories: "Best practices" for a biospecimen resource for the genomic and proteomic era* (Document No. MG-120-NDC/NCI). Santa Monica, CA: RAND Corporation.

Eiseman, E., & Haga, S.B. (2009). *Handbook of human tissue sources: A national resource of human tissue samples* (Document No. MR-954-OSTP). Santa Monica, CA: RAND Corporation.

Engel, K.B., & Moore, H.M. (2011). Effects of preanalytical variables on the detection of proteins by immunohistochemistry in formalin-fixed, paraffin-embedded tissue. *Archives of Pathology and Laboratory Medicine, 135,* 536–543. Retrieved from http://www.archivesofpathology.org/doi/full/10.1043/2010-0702-RAIR.1

Fearon, E.R. (1997). Human cancer syndromes: Clues to the origin and nature of cancer. *Science, 278,* 1043–1050. doi:10.1126/science.278.5340.1043

Friede, A., Grossman, R., Hunt, R., Li, R.M., & Stern, S. (Eds.). (2003). *National Biospecimen Network blueprint.* Retrieved from http://biospecimens.cancer.gov/global/pdfs/FINAL_NBN_Blueprint.pdf

Fullerton, S.M., Anderson, N.R., Guzauskas, G., Freeman, D., & Fryer-Edwards, K. (2010). Meeting the governance challenges of next-generation biorepository research [Commentary]. *Science Translational Medicine, 2,* 15cm3. doi:10.1126/scitranslmed.3000361

Gertz, R. (2008). Withdrawing from participating in a biobank—A comparative study. *European Journal of Health Law, 15,* 381–389. doi:10.1163/157180908X338269

Gottweis, H., & Zatloukal, K. (2007). Biobank governance: Trends and perspectives. *Pathology, 74,* 206–211. doi:10.1159/000104446

Greenman, C., Stephens, P., Smith, R., Dalgliesh, G.L., Hunter, C., Bignell, G., ... Stratton, M.R. (2007). Patterns of somatic mutation in human cancer genomes. *Nature, 446,* 153–158.

Guttmacher, A.E., & Collins, F.S. (2002). Genomic medicine—A primer. *New England Journal of Medicine, 347,* 1512–1520. doi:10.1056/NEJMra012240

Hakimian, R., & Korn, D. (2004). Ownership and use of tissue specimens for research. *JAMA, 292,* 2500–2505. doi:10.1001/jama.292.20.2500

Hansson, M.G., Dillner, J., Bartram, C.R., Carlson, J.A., & Helgesson, G. (2006). Should donors be allowed to give broad consent to future biobank research? *Lancet Oncology, 7,* 266–269. doi:10.1016/S1470-2045(06)70618-0

Hartl, D.L., & Jones, E.W. (2011). *Genetics: Analysis of genes and genomes* (8th ed.). Burlington, MA: Jones & Bartlett Learning.

Hawkins, A.K., & O'Doherty, K.C. (2011). "Who owns your poop?": Insights regarding the intersection of human microbiome research and the ELSI aspects of biobanking and related studies. *BMC Medical Genomics, 4,* 72. doi:10.1186/1755-8794-4-72

Horlick-Jones, T., Rowe, G., & Walls, J. (2007). Citizen engagement processes as information systems: The role of knowledge and the concept of translation quality. *Public Understanding of Science, 16,* 259–278. doi:10.1177/0963662506074792

Jeffers, B.R. (2001). Human biological materials in research: Ethical issues and the role of stewardship in minimizing research risks. *Advances in Nursing Science, 24*(2), 32–46.

Kaye, J. (2011). From single biobanks to international networks: Developing e-governance. *Human Genetics, 130,* 377–382. doi:10.1007/s00439-011-1063-0

Khoury, T., Sait, S., Hwang, J., Chandrasekhar, R., Wilding, G., Tan, D., & Kulkarni, S. (2009). Delay to formalin fixation effect on breast biomarkers. *Modern Pathology, 22,* 1457–1467. doi:10.1038/modpathol.2009.117

Kinzler, K.W., & Vogelstein, B. (2002). Introduction. In B. Vogelstein & K.W. Kinzler (Eds.), *The genetic basis of human cancer* (2nd ed., pp. 3–6). New York, NY: McGraw-Hill.

Kolata, G. (2013, June 16). Poking holes in genetic privacy. *New York Times.* Retrieved from http://www.nytimes.com/2013/06/18/science/poking-holes-in-the-privacy-of-dna.html?pagewanted=all&_r=0

Laurie, G. (2011). Reflexive governance in biobanking: On the value of policy led approaches and the need to recognise the limits of law. *Human Genetics, 130,* 347–356. doi:10.1007/s00439-011-1066-x

Lockhart, D.J., & Winzeler, E.A. (2000). Genomics, gene expression and DNA arrays. *Nature, 405,* 827–836.

Mardis, E.R. (2008). The impact of next-generation sequencing technology on genetics. *Trends in Genetics, 24,* 133–141. doi:10.1016/j.tig.2007.12.007

Master, Z., Nelson, E., Murdoch, B., & Caulfield, T. (2012). Biobanks, consent and claims of consensus. *Nature Methods, 9,* 885–888.

McDonald, S.A., Velasco, E., & Ilasi, N.T. (2010). Business process flow diagrams in tissue bank informatics system design, and identification and communication of best practices: The pharmaceutical industry experience. *Biopreservation and Biobanking, 8,* 203–209. doi:10.1089/bio.2010.0020

McDonald, S.A., Watson, M.A., Rossi, J., Becker, C.M., Jaques, D.P., & Pfeifer, J.D. (2011). A new paradigm for biospecimen banking in the personalized medicine era. *American Journal of Clinical Pathology, 136,* 679–684. doi:10.1309/AJCP7DWCQ1SWJTWU

Mongoven, A.M., & Solomon, S. (2012). Biobanking: Shifting the analogy from consent to surrogacy. *Genetics in Medicine, 14,* 183–188. doi:10.1038/gim.2011.49

Moore, H.M. (2012). The NCI Biospecimen Research Network. *Biotechnic and Histochemistry, 87,* 18–23. doi:10.3109/10520295.2011.591833

Murphy, J., Scott, J., Kaufman, D., Geller, G., LeRoy, L., & Hudson, K. (2009). Public perspectives on informed consent for biobanking. *American Journal of Public Health, 99,* 2128–2134. Retrieved from http://www.ncbi.nlm.nih.gov/pmc/articles/PMC2775766/

National Cancer Institute. (n.d.). About caHUB. Retrieved from http://cahub.cancer.gov/about/Default.asp?p=5

National Cancer Institute. (2010, June 16). *White paper entitled "labeling of biological specimens."* Retrieved from http://ncifrederick.cancer.gov/repository/cr/docs/WhitePaper.pdf

National Cancer Institute. (2012). *How you can help medical research: Donating your blood, tissue, and other samples* (Publication No. 12-7933). Retrieved from http://biospecimens.cancer.gov/global/pdfs/MedicalResearchPatientBrochure-508.pdf

National Cancer Institute. (2013a). Biospecimen Research Network. Retrieved from http://biospecimens.cancer.gov/researchnetwork/default.asp

National Cancer Institute. (2013b). NCI best practices for biospecimen resources. Retrieved from http://biospecimens.cancer.gov/bestpractices

National Cancer Institute. (2013c). Patient corner: What are biospecimens and biorepositories? Retrieved from http://biospecimens.cancer.gov/patientcorner

National Cancer Institute. (2013d). Resources for public use: Standard operating procedures for biospecimen collection. Fresh frozen tissue protocol. Retrieved from http://epi.grants.cancer.gov/CFR/biospecimen_fresh_tissue.html

National Cancer Institute Center for Cancer Research. (2013). *Laboratory of Pathology policy manual* [Electronic version]. Retrieved from http://home.ccr.cancer.gov/lop/intranet/PolicyManual/default.asp

National Human Genome Research Institute. (n.d.). Career profiles: Molecular geneticist. Retrieved from http://www.genome.gov/GenomicCareers/career.cfm?id=28

National Human Genome Research Institute. (2011a). A brief guide to genomics: DNA, genes and genomes. Retrieved from https://www.genome.gov/18016863

National Human Genome Research Institute. (2011b). DNA sequencing. Retrieved from https://www.genome.gov/10001177

National Human Genome Research Institute. (2012a). Building a biobank to explore mysteries of the genome: The GTEx Project could help researchers learn about diseases such as cancer. Retrieved from http://www.genome.gov/pfv.cfm?pageID=27550100

National Human Genome Research Institute. (2012b). Genetic mapping. Retrieved from https://www.genome.gov/10000715

National Human Genome Research Institute. (2013a). Division of Policy, Communications, and Education. Retrieved from http://www.genome.gov/10001084

National Human Genome Research Institute. (2013b). Research Funding Divisions. Retrieved from http://www.genome.gov/27552836

National Human Genome Research Institute. (2014). Cancer Genetics and Comparative Genomics Branch. Retrieved from http://www.genome.gov/10000012

National Institutes of Health. (2000, July 17). NIH working definition of bioinformatics and computational biology. Retrieved from http://www.bisti.nih.gov/docs/CompuBioDef.pdf

National Institutes of Health. (2012, September 14). Request for information (RFI) regarding potential uses of stored biospecimens from the Common Fund GTEx Project (Notice No. NOT-RM-12-028). Retrieved from http://grants.nih.gov/grants/guide/notice-files/NOT-RM-12-028.html

National Institutes of Health Office of Technology Transfer. (n.d.). Forms and model agreements. Retrieved from http://www.ott.nih.gov/forms-model-agreements

Okasha, S. (2012, July). Population genetics. In E.N. Zalta (Ed.), *The Stanford encyclopedia of philosophy* (Fall 2012 ed.). Retrieved from http://plato.stanford.edu/archives/fall2012/entries/population-genetics

Pagon, R.A. (2004). Molecular genetic testing for inherited disorders. *Expert Review of Molecular Diagnostics, 4*, 135–140. doi:10.1586/14737159.4.2.135

Park, A. (2009). 10 ideas changing the world right now: Biobanks. *Time Magazine*. Retrieved from http://content.time.com/time/specials/packages/article/0,28804,1884779_1884782_1884766,00.html

Peters, K.F., & Hadley, D.W. (1997). Programmed instruction: The Human Genome Project. *Cancer Nursing, 20*, 62–71. doi:10.1097/00002820-199702000-00008

Preti, G. (2005). Metabolomics comes of age? [Letter]. *Scientist, 19*(11), 8. Retrieved from http://www.the-scientist.com/?articles.view/articleNo/16506/title/Metabolomics-comes-of-age-

Pullman, D., Etchegary, H., Gallagher, K., Hodgkinson, K., Keough, M., Morgan, D., & Street, C. (2012). Personal privacy, public benefits, and biobanks: A conjoint analysis of policy priorities and public perceptions. *Genetics in Medicine, 14*, 229–235. doi:10.1038/gim.0b013e31822e578f

Rai, A.J., Gelfand, C.A., Haywood, B.C., Warunek, D.J., Yi, J., Schuchard, M.D., ... Chan, D.W. (2005). HUPO Plasma Proteome Project specimen collection and handling: Towards the standardization of parameters for plasma proteome samples. *Proteomics, 5*, 3262–3277. doi:10.1002/pmic.200401245

Recombinant DNA technology. (2014). In *Encyclopaedia Britannica*. Retrieved from http://www.britannica.com/EBchecked/topic/493667/recombinant-DNA-technology

Rial-Sebbag, E., & Cambon-Thomsen, A. (2012). The emergence of biobanks in the legal landscape: Towards a new model of governance. *Journal of Law and Society, 39*, 113–130. doi:10.1111/j.1467-6478.2012.00573.x

Risch, N.J. (2000). Searching for genetic determinants in the new millennium. *Nature, 405*, 847–856.

Rowe, G., & Frewer, L.J. (2005). A typology of public engagement mechanisms. *Science, Technology, and Human Values, 30*, 251–290.

Salter, B., & Jones, J. (2005). Biobanks and bioethics: The politics of legitimation. *Journal of European Public Policy, 12*, 710–732. doi:10.1080/13501760500160623

Simon, C.M., L'Heureux, J., Murray, J.C., Winokur, P., Weiner, G., Newbury, E., ... Zimmerman, B. (2011). Active choice but not too active: Public perspectives on biobank consent models. *Genetics in Medicine, 13*, 821–831. Retrieved from http://www.ncbi.nlm.nih.gov/pmc/articles/PMC3658114

Skloot, R. (2010). *The immortal life of Henrietta Lacks.* New York, NY: Crown Publishers.

Stanford University. (1995). Master agreement regarding use of the Uniform Biological Material Transfer Agreement (UBMTA). Retrieved from http://www.stanford.edu/group/ICO/researchAdmins/documents/ubmta_000.pdf

Sulmasy, D.P., & Snyder, L. (2010). Substituted interests and best judgments: An integrated model of surrogate decision making [Commentary]. *JAMA, 304*, 1946–1947. doi:10.1001/jama.2010.1595

Tutton, R. (2007). Constructing participation in genetic databases: Citizenship, governance, and ambivalence. *Science, Technology, and Human Values, 32*, 172–195. doi:10.1177/0162243906296853

Vaught, J., & Lockhart, N.C. (2012). The evolution of biobanking best practices. *Clinica Chimica Acta, 413*, 1569–1575. doi:10.1016/j.cca.2012.04.030

Vaught, J., Rogers, J., Carolin, T., & Compton, C. (2011). Biobankonomics: Developing a sustainable business model approach for the formation of a human tissue biobank. *Journal of the National Cancer Institute Monographs, 2011*(42), 24–31. doi:10.1093/jncimonographs/lgr009

Vaught, J.B. (2006). Blood collection, shipment, processing, and storage. *Cancer Epidemiology, Biomarkers and Prevention, 15*, 1582–1584. doi:10.1158/1055-9965.EPI-06-0630

von Elm, E., Altman, D.G., Egger, M., Pocock, S.J., Gøtzsche, P.C., & Vandenbroucke, J.P. (2008). The Strengthening the Reporting of Observational Studies in Epidemiology (STROBE) statement: Guidelines for reporting observational studies. *Journal of Clinical Epidemiology, 61*, 344–349. doi:10.1016/j.jclinepi.2007.11.008

Watson, R.W.G., Kay, E.W., & Smith, D. (2010). Integrating biobanks: Addressing the practical and ethical issues to deliver a valuable tool for cancer research. *Nature Reviews Cancer, 10*, 646–651.

Weedn, V.W. (1996). Forensic DNA tests. *Clinics in Laboratory Medicine, 16*, 187–196.

Williams, P.H., Schepp, K., McGrath, B., & Mitchell, P. (2010). The stewardship model: Current viability for genetic biobank practice development. *Advances in Nursing Science, 33*(1), E41–E49. doi:10.1097/ANS.0b013e3181cd8367

Winstead, E.R. (2012, February 18). Building a biobank to explore mysteries of the genome. *NCI Cancer Bulletin, 9*(18). Retrieved from http://www.cancer.gov/ncicancerbulletin/091812/page6

Wolff, A.C., Hammond, M.E.H., Schwartz, J.N., Hagerty, K.L., Allred, D.C., Cote, R.J., … Hayes, D.F. (2007). American Society of Clinical Oncology/College of American Pathologists guideline recommendations for human epidermal growth factor receptor 2 testing in breast cancer. *Archives of Pathology and Laboratory Medicine, 131*, 18–43. Retrieved from http://www.archivesofpathology.org/doi/full/10.1043/1543-2165(2007)131[18:ASOCCO]2.0.CO;2

World Health Organization. (2002). *Genomics and world health: Report of the Advisory Committee on Health Research.* Retrieved from http://www.who.int/rpc/genomics_report.pdf

Yassin, R., Lockhart, N., González del Riego, M., Pitt, K., Thomas, J.W., Weiss, L., & Compton, C. (2010). Custodianship as an ethical framework for biospecimen-based research. *Cancer Epidemiology, Biomarkers and Prevention, 19*, 1012–1015. doi:10.1158/1055-9965.EPI-10-0029

CHAPTER 8

Policy Considerations in Cancer Pain Management

Robert Twillman, PhD, FAPM

Introduction

Although healthcare providers frequently encounter, and are frustrated by, policies that affect their ability to deliver optimal cancer care, few have more than a rudimentary understanding of how and why policy is made, and even fewer are aware of the extent to which they can play a role in policy making. In fact, healthcare providers, with their detailed technical knowledge and vital clinical experience, represent some of the most effective potential advocates for good pain management policy, alongside people with pain. To realize that potential, providers need to understand basic information about types of policies and how they are made, as well as the issues underlying the most important policy debates of the day. This chapter will cover both of these educational needs with the intent of producing a better-educated group of healthcare providers who can be more effective spokespeople in the effort to promulgate good pain management policy.

What Is a Policy?

For this discussion, *policy* refers to the formal means used by legislative and regulatory bodies to control the practice of pain management. In general, such policy is permissive rather than prescriptive—it allows a healthcare provider to do what is necessary to provide good, effective care, but it does not dictate specific practices except where safety is the primary consideration. In part, this is because pain management, like much of the practice of medicine, is too complex and individualized to permit policy makers to dictate good practice with any degree of success.

While this lack of prescriptive policy permits the necessary degrees of freedom to provide good pain care, it also means that it is possible for a governmental jurisdiction to have good pain policy but poor pain care. Another way of thinking of this is that good pain policy is necessary, but not sufficient, for the existence of good pain care. Once good policy is in place, it becomes necessary to address practice improvement through means such as continuing education, development of practice guidelines, and outcomes research. Outcomes research also can provide information suggesting necessary revisions to policy to further promote good practice.

It also is important to recognize that policy development occurs at different levels of government. Federal policy is developed by the U.S. Congress; the federal executive branch, including cabinet departments and agencies within them; and the federal court system. The Supremacy Clause of the U.S. Constitution (U.S. Const. art. VI, cl. 2) dictates that federal policy trumps state and local policy, so that state and local policy can only be more restrictive than federal policy, not less so. An example of this is found in federal and state controlled substance acts. As of mid-2014, the federal Controlled Substances Act lists hydrocodone-containing combination medications in Schedule III (U.S. Drug Enforcement Administration [DEA], 2014a), while the New York State Controlled Substances Act listed them in Schedule II as of February 2013 (New York State Controlled Substances Act, 2013). This greater restriction is allowable, but New York would not be permitted to move these medications to Schedules IV or V or to make them noncontrolled, because the authority of the federal legislation is greater. It is also important to recognize that the Constitution delegates certain powers to the federal government but leaves all "unenumerated" powers to state governments. Because the power to regulate medical practice is not listed as a federal power, this function is left to states, meaning that state policy often has far greater impact on pain management and other forms of medical practice.

Understanding the three general types of policy and how they are made is the first key in advocating for effective pain policy. Knowing this information enables advocates to target the appropriate policy makers and provides some idea about which groups will be the most effective allies in that effort. It also has implications for the degree of difficulty to expect in making a change, the potential for negative unintended consequences, and the extent to which advocating for a change will involve primarily education, primarily persuasion, or a mix of both.

Statutes and ordinances, generically known as *laws,* are policies that are passed by federal, state, or local legislative bodies, either with the approval of the chief executive or by overriding his or her objections. When most people think about policy advocacy, it is legislative advocacy that comes to mind. From the time a legislator begins to consider introducing a bill and up until the time a bill officially becomes a statute, advocates have opportunities to influence the content and the survival of this type of policy. Even after a bill becomes law, opportunities may exist for advocates to modify its impact, either through challenges in the judicial branch or by influencing the development of rules and regulations by the responsible executive branch agency. In pain management, perhaps the most influential statutes are federal and state controlled substances acts. These laws designate which medications are classified into which controlled substance schedules, define the requirements for lawful use of these substances, and grant certain law enforcement agencies the authority to enforce these requirements.

Legislative advocacy often involves both education and persuasion, although in many cases, it is education that is most needed. Although some legislators do specialize in certain content areas, most of them do not, and they may not understand either the contents or the implications of a bill related to pain care. Legislators may go from a committee meeting about the need to legislate clean air standards, to a floor debate about whether to build a bridge in a certain location, to a meeting with a pain policy advocate about a bill regulating prescribing patterns. At times, legislators can feel a bit like they are trying to drink from a gushing fire hose, with an overwhelming amount and variety of information coming at them. For state legislators in particular (who may have minimal or no staffers, compared to federal legislators), it may be necessary for pain management advocates to start with very basic education about how effective pain care is delivered and about the effect the proposed legislation would have on the ability to deliver that care.

A second type of policy is known as *rules or regulations*. These policy instruments are developed by executive branch agencies as a means of carrying out mandates contained in laws (USA.gov, 2014). Often, a law will expressly grant authority to the relevant regulatory body or bodies to make necessary rules, as those agencies are thought to be better equipped to understand the details necessary to properly regulate that area of practice. Regulatory bodies, which may include cabinet-level departments, agencies of those departments, or professional licensing boards (which sometimes operate outside the department structure), typically are required to follow a set process for proposing, considering, revising, and adopting rules or regulations. Because rules and regulations are directly linked to laws, they have the force of law and can be enforced as such. Examples of federal rules and regulations include requirements for health insurance arising from the Patient Protection and Affordable Care Act, such as requirements for essential health benefits, development of accountable care organizations, and others. State rules and regulations include policies outlining the composition of Medicaid formularies, including preferred drug lists, and the specific continuing education requirements necessary to renew a professional license.

Regulatory advocacy often involves far less of the educational aspect found in legislative advocacy. The people responsible for making pain management rules and regulations, because they oversee at least some aspect of medical practice, often have extensive training or experience in health care. For advocates, regulatory advocacy often involves more persuasion, as the key is to convince regulators that the advocate's proposal vis-à-vis the rules and regulations is the best way to proceed. Policy experts generally prefer regulatory advocacy to legislative advocacy as a means of seeking needed changes because the legislative process is often driven by political motivations and lacks the intimate knowledge of what constitutes good practice. The regulatory process is typically more predictable, with the discussion focusing on the finer points of providing good pain care. The needs for education and for persuasion to influence rules and regulations are relatively balanced.

The final type of policy to consider is *guidelines*. Unlike statutes and regulations, guidelines are not considered to have the force of law. Instead, guidelines reflect less-formal rules and issues for consideration when regulatory bodies evaluate the behavior of healthcare providers. For instance, most state medical licensing boards have adopted at least some portion, or some revised version, of the Federation of State Medical Boards' *Model Policy for the Use of Controlled Substances for the Treatment of Pain* (Federation of State Medical Boards, 2004). These guidelines list, with a moderate degree of specificity, the boards' expectations for physicians' behavior in their treatment of pain. Most state boards' guidelines assert that, should a complaint be lodged with the board regarding a physician's treatment of pain, it is the content of these guidelines that will serve as the standard against which the board will judge the physician's behavior. In a sense, guidelines like these typically serve to express the board's sense of what constitutes an adequate standard of practice in this area. This information applies as well to other licensed professions involved in prescribing, administering, and dispensing controlled substances, including nurses, physician assistants, pharmacists, dentists, and others.

Guideline development also presents an opportunity for healthcare practitioner advocacy. Because of the specificity of guidelines, coupled with the diverse composition of licensing boards, expert practitioners often are consulted to assist in their drafting. Guidelines are considered by boards in open public meetings, presenting opportunities for advocates to weigh in with their opinions and to suggest alternatives. Given the expert level of knowledge among the bodies creating the rules, persuasion often trumps education as an advocacy technique.

Policy Specific to Cancer Pain Management

By the late 1980s and early 1990s, unrelieved cancer pain was gaining recognition as a significant healthcare issue, and efforts began, both on the education front and on the policy front, to remedy this. While educators focused on a variety of healthcare providers, policy makers set about ensuring that people with cancer and their healthcare providers had access to and the ability to freely use opioid analgesics. In 1994, the Agency for Healthcare Policy and Research issued clinical practice guidelines for cancer pain management (Jacox, Carr, & Payne, 1994), and policy makers set about passing legislation such as Intractable Pain Treatment Acts, ensuring that all people with chronic pain had access to necessary treatments, including opioid analgesics (Gilson, Joranson, & Maurer, 2007).

For the rest of the 20th century and into the first decade of the 21st, these policies continued to proliferate with little opposition. However, with sharp increases in opioid use and the simultaneous increase in evidence of misuse of these medications, leading to increased overdose deaths involving them, policy makers came under pressure to rein in opioid prescribing through a variety of policies that will be discussed here later. However, in many cases, people with cancer-related pain and those receiving hospice or palliative care services have been specifically exempted from such policies. While patients, their significant others, and healthcare providers are all undoubtedly grateful for these exclusions, a number of questions have been raised about the logic of such policy exclusions.

The most detailed public discussion of this issue occurred in 2012 and 2013 when a group of physicians and other concerned citizens petitioned the U.S. Food and Drug Administration (FDA) to change the label indications for opioid analgesics to limit their dose and duration of use. In so doing, however, the petition called for such restrictions only for noncancer pain, a distinction that was the subject of considerable discussion in both submitted comments and a public hearing (U.S. FDA, 2013b).

The petitioners asserted that people with chronic noncancer pain are both unlikely to benefit from extended use of opioid analgesics and more likely to develop harmful complications, including addiction. Requesting limitations only for noncancer pain, however, would seem to indicate that there was not a similar concern for people with cancer, and implies that there is something qualitatively different between pain associated with cancer and pain associated with other conditions. The logic involved in such a distinction seems strained, at best. Consider the following points.

1. Noncancer pain is too diverse in its response to opioids for a single indication to be appropriate for all types of pain in that class. Some noncancer pain conditions respond well to opioids (e.g., rheumatoid arthritis and osteoarthritis), whereas others (e.g., fibromyalgia and migraine) do not.

2. "Cancer pain" is ill-defined. Does it include only pain in individuals with evidence of active disease? Does it include only pain caused by the cancer itself? What about pain caused by cancer treatments—is that also cancer pain, or something else?

3. The same root causes for pain can exist in people with and without cancer. For example, the petition's request seems to suggest that it would be appropriate to use opioids to treat pain related to a vertebral compression fracture secondary to multiple myeloma, but not to treat pain related to the same fracture secondary to osteoporosis. This distinction defies logic.

4. No evidence has shown that the human nociceptive system or opiate receptors act differently based on the presence or absence of a malignancy.

In the end, FDA decided not to grant the petition's request to limit opioid treatment in cases of noncancer pain, but some in the pain management policy community remain concerned about potential future developments in this area (Bridge-Cook, 2013). Many more individuals diagnosed with cancer are becoming long-term survivors, thanks to the availability of increasingly effective (and increasingly toxic) treatment regimens. Many of these long-term survivors also become people with chronic pain, as they experience long-lasting (perhaps lifelong) painful sequelae of treatment, such as chemotherapy-related peripheral neuropathies. If "cancer pain" is deemed to include this type of pain, then some policies would bar third-party payers and others from limiting use of opioids and other medications in treating it—potentially exposing those payers to years of increased costs. The concern is then that these payers would press the position that such pain is not cancer pain, but is instead chronic noncancer pain, for which they can limit payment for treatment.

A second question in this area concerns the original intent of policies limiting exposure to opioids—the prevention of adverse effects, including addiction. The only logical basis for excluding people with cancer from such policies would appear to be the notion that people with cancer either do not develop these adverse effects, or that it is inconsequential if they do. Many would argue that this also is fallacious logic. First, people with cancer might be more susceptible to addiction than those without it, as some addictions (notably, to nicotine and alcohol) are actually risk factors for development of cancer. Second, if the risk these policies seek to control is one of overdose death, then exclusion of people with cancer would seem to indicate that policy makers are unconcerned about such deaths in people with cancer.

As can be the case in policy, these logical pitfalls suggest that policy makers may have responded to emotional appeals without full consideration of the issue and the potential consequences of their decisions. Although this is starkly clear in respect to policies excluding people with cancer from limitations in opioid therapy, it also appears in other ways throughout the pain management policy opus. The rest of this chapter will focus on current debates in the pain management policy environment. Many of these debates are overtly about using opioids to treat noncancer pain, but they may have unintended consequences for the treatment of pain in people with cancer, and thus are relevant to individuals providing pain management to people with cancer.

Controlled Substances Policy

Of all the content areas related to pain management policy, none has been as active, or as contentious, as controlled substances policy, especially as it involves opioid pain relievers. Many battles have been fought over the past century in the United States over the regulation of these vital medications, battles that continue largely unabated today. At the core of this policy debate are two public health issues: treatment of pain with opioids, and prescription drug misuse, abuse, and diversion.

The first significant national policy related to opioids was the Harrison Narcotics Tax Act of 1914 (Harrison Narcotics Tax Act, 1914). After several decades of debate about the ramifications of the international drug trade (principally involving Great Britain, India, and China), the Harrison Act was Congress's attempt to meet its obligations under the Hague Convention of 1912, which regulated the international opium trade. It also was intended to address the problems of cocaine and opium addiction in the United States by better regulating the trade in narcotics within the country. The bill provided that patent medicines containing low concentrations of opioids could be sold over the counter, with the manufacturers being exempt from registration and taxation. Higher-concentration products, however, were subjected to a tax, and everyone involved in the manufacture, importation, prescribing, and dispensing of these products was required to register with the government. The bill specifically stated that physicians had a right to supply these drugs in the course of professional practice, which would appear, on its face, to be an unambiguously good thing.

The unintended consequence of the Harrison Act, as is often the case in the policy arena, did not become apparent until after the law was passed. The contemporaneous cultural view of addiction was that it was not a disease but a moral weakness—a view that continues to affect policy efforts today to some extent. Therefore, a physician who provided opioids to someone with an addiction was not treating a disease but was supporting an immoral habit, making that physician subject to arrest and imprisonment. Naturally, this interpretation of the law exerted a profound chilling effect on physicians' prescribing behavior and caused many people with opioid addictions to seek the drugs on the black market. Much like the effects of the 18th Amendment's ban on alcohol, this unintended aspect of the Harrison Act seems to have exacerbated, and some would say created, a law enforcement problem that was practically nonexistent prior to passage of the law (Brecher & Editors of *Consumer Reports* Magazine, 1972).

The Harrison Act remained the primary federal opioid policy for half a century, albeit with a few modifications to tighten its provisions, such as an outright ban on the importation of heroin, added in 1924, and the creation of the Federal Bureau of Narcotics in 1930 as an agency of the Department of the Treasury. By the late 1960s, however, Congress had decided it was time for a complete overhaul of federal policies related to drug abuse. The instrument that accomplished this overhaul was the Comprehensive Drug Abuse Prevention and Control Act of 1970, of which Title II was the Controlled Substances Act (CSA).

Among the most visible legacies of the CSA is the system of "schedules" for controlled substances based on their medical utility and potential for abuse. Table 8-1 shows a summary of this classification scheme. It is subjective in nature, as it requires that regulators make judgments about a drug's abuse potential and propensity to cause physical and psychological dependence relative to other scheduled drugs. One controversial regulatory issue has been the appropriate placement of hydrocodone-containing combination products. These medications initially were placed into Schedule III by the CSA, but some argued that they should more properly be placed into Schedule II. In late 2013, FDA recommended this rescheduling to DEA (Woodcock, 2013), and DEA concurred, officially rescheduling these medications effective October 6, 2014 (U.S. DEA, 2014b).

As part of a reorganization plan for the executive branch, President Johnson proposed Reorganization Plan No. 1 in 1968. This plan included a pro-

Table 8-1. Federal Schedules of Controlled Substances

Schedule	Accepted Medical Use?	Abuse Potential	Physical/ Psychological Dependency Risk	Examples
I	No	High	High	Heroin, marijuana
II	Yes	High	Severe	Morphine, oxycodone, methadone, hydrocodone
III	Yes	Less than Schedules I and II	Low-to-moderate physical; high psychological	Codeine combinations, buprenorphine
IV	Yes	Less than Schedule III	Limited	Carisoprodol, tramadol, benzodiazepines, barbiturates
V	Yes	Less than Schedule IV	Limited	Pregabalin, cough preparations, antidiarrheals

Note. Based on information from U.S. Drug Enforcement Administration, 2014a.

posal to merge the existing Bureau of Narcotics (part of the Treasury Department) with the Bureau of Drug Abuse Control (in the Department of Health, Education, and Welfare) to create a new Bureau of Narcotics and Dangerous Drugs (BNDD), which was to be placed under the Department of Justice. This plan was approved, but BNDD's existence as an independent agency was to be short-lived.

In 1973, President Nixon proposed Reorganization Plan No. 2, resulting in an executive order creating the DEA. Under this reorganization, BNDD was merged with the Office of Drug Abuse Law Enforcement and the Office of National Narcotics Intelligence, both of which had been created just one year earlier. The new DEA was placed in the Department of Justice, where it remains to this day.

DEA's mission is wide ranging, with both domestic and international responsibilities. In terms of its relevance to pain management, DEA is responsible for enforcing the CSA's provisions regarding the manufacture, distribution, and dispensing of controlled substances. One notable aspect of DEA's official charge is the requirement, consistent with both international treaties and language in the CSA, that it continue to ensure that the availability of controlled substances for "useful and legitimate medical and scientific purposes will not be unduly restricted" (21 U.S.C. § 801a). This dual responsibility—to control and prevent access to drugs for purposes of abuse while also ensuring adequate supplies of them for legitimate medical use—is commonly known as the Principle of Balance (World Health Organization, 2011), which underlies much of pain management policy, at least as it relates to controlled substances.

At its core, the Principle of Balance embodies recognition of two coexisting (and perhaps competing) public health concerns, namely, the need to adequately care for people with pain and the need to prevent drug abuse and addiction (World Health Organization, 2011). Threading the policy needle in such a way as to address both of these issues has historically been challenging and continues to be so. One aspect of drug abuse control efforts, in particular, has complicated policy making: an imbalanced focus on controlling the supply of drugs of abuse rather than the demand for them.

Early in his administration's "War on Drugs," President Nixon made it clear that he believed as much as two-thirds of budget dollars dedicated to that effort should be directed toward providing treatment to people with drug abuse and addiction problems, with one-third spent on reducing the supply of drugs (Nixon, 1971). However, greater emphasis on supply-side efforts was more appealing to voters, and thus the die was cast. The result has been a 40-year emphasis on controlling supplies of drugs, focused largely on eliminating illicit drugs entirely.

When the drugs being targeted are illicit and have no legitimate medical use, the goal of completely eliminating their supplies is reasonable. However, when the drugs in question are used extensively to treat medical conditions such as pain, eliminating them is not only not a goal, but is inconsistent with federal law (including the CSA) and international treaties to which the United States is party (International Narcotics Control Board, n.d.). With the rise in prescription drug abuse during the late 1990s and into the 2000s, this conundrum moved to the forefront of policy making, as government has sought an elusive balance between the recognized undertreatment of pain and the surge in abuse of these vital medications. DEA has recognized these inherent difficulties and in 2001 issued a statement endorsed by 21 leading healthcare organizations, in which it officially recognized a statement of the Principle of Balance (U.S. DEA, 2001).

Prescription Opioid Misuse and Abuse

The current environment midway through the second decade of the 21st century is one of increasing tension between those who view prescription drug abuse and related overdose deaths as an epidemic (Centers for Disease Control and Prevention [CDC], 2011) and those who see chronic pain as having pandemic proportions, requiring a "cultural transformation" (Institute of Medicine, 2011) in the delivery of pain care. Because some of the same medications that relieve chronic pain and give people a greater quality of life can, for others, reduce quality and even quantity of life, much of the current policy environment involves a tug-of-war between forces representing these two "sides." Understanding the current policy environment requires at least a passing knowledge of some of the statistics underlying concerns about prescription drug abuse.

The National Survey on Drug Use and Health (NSDUH) is an annual survey conducted by the Substance Abuse and Mental Health Services Administration (SAMHSA), the Department of Health and Human Services agency responsible for overseeing substance abuse and mental health treatment in the United States. Since 2002, the NSDUH has included questions about nonmedical use of opioid pain relievers. *Nonmedical use* is defined as the use of medications by someone for whom they are not prescribed, or taking them just for the experience or feeling they cause (SAMHSA, 2003) (e.g., getting "high" or sedating oneself to escape unpleasant experiences). The distinction between these two types of nonmedical use can be substantial and meaningful, yet the NSDUH does not provide a breakdown of how many respondents endorse each motivation. Taking someone else's medication might be done to achieve pain relief, however illegal and dangerous that behavior might be. Those taking it only for the experience or feeling, however, are engaging in a form of drug abuse or addiction (SAMHSA, 2003).

Since SAMHSA began including this set of questions in the NSDUH, the percentage of respondents reporting nonmedical use within the past month or year has been essentially unchanged, albeit at a level that many find unacceptable (see Figure 8-1). The NSDUH also contains questions allowing researchers to ascertain the number of individuals who qualify for diagnoses of opioid abuse or opioid dependence according to the *Diagnostic and Statistical Manual* (American Psychiatric Association, 2000). Those numbers, also shown in Figure 8-1, have been remarkably stable as well. Thus, there is little evidence that the prevalence of prescription opioid abuse is increasing, although that is not to say that it had not increased before SAMHSA added this question set (SAMHSA, 2003).

Also instructive are data collected from NSDUH respondents indicating the source of the prescription opioids used the last time the respondent engaged in nonmedical use (see Figure 8-2). Most of the respondents (53%) were given those medications for free by a friend or relative; another 14.6% reported buying or stealing them from a friend or relative (SAMHSA, 2014). Taken together, these numbers suggest that nearly 70% of misused prescription opioids come from friends, relatives, and home medicine cabinets. Advocates for controlling prescription drug abuse frequently assert that this is an indication of an excess supply of medications, which they attribute to overprescribing by healthcare providers. While these data suggest that overprescribing may be partly to blame, it is also necessary to point out that had these medications been stored securely, and had people not made the risky, unfortunate (and felonious) decision to share medications with some-

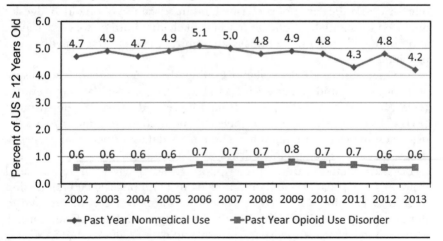

Figure 8-1. Percentage of Americans With Past-Year Nonmedical Use of Prescription Opioid Analgesics and With Opioid Use Disorders

Note. Based on information from Substance Abuse and Mental Health Services Administration, 2013b.

Figure 8-2. Sources of Medications Used for Nonmedical Purposes, National Survey on Drug Use and Health, 2012–2013

Source of Pain Relievers for Most Recent Nonmedical Use, Users 12 Years or Older

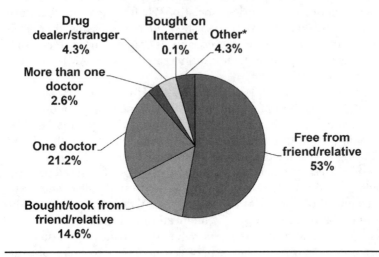

Drug dealer/stranger 4.3%

Bought on Internet 0.1%

Other* 4.3%

More than one doctor 2.6%

One doctor 21.2%

Bought/took from friend/relative 14.6%

Free from friend/relative 53%

* "Other" includes "Wrote fake prescription," "Stole from doctor's office/clinic/hospital/pharmacy," and "Some other way."

Note. From *Results From the 2013 National Survey on Drug Use and Health: Summary of National Findings,* by Substance Abuse and Mental Health Services Administration, September 2014. Retrieved from http://www.samhsa.gov/data/population-data-nsduh/reports?tab=32.

one for whom they are not prescribed, nonmedical use of opioid analgesics might be substantially reduced. It seems likely that both factors are at play, and optimal management of this issue requires interventions aimed at both problems.

Another source of data demonstrating the magnitude of the misuse and abuse of opioid analgesics is SAMHSA's Drug Abuse Warning Network (DAWN) (SAMHSA, 2013a). Data from drug-related emergency department (ED) visits in 48 urban areas are collected and used to generate DAWN's statistical estimates of national rates. The DAWN data set tracks many types of drugs, including licit and illicit drugs, as well as alcohol.

ED visits related to use of prescription opioid analgesics have increased from 49.4 per 100,000 population in 2004 to 117.5 per 100,000 population in 2011, suggesting a marked increase in serious adverse events related to the use of these medications, although the rate has leveled off substantially in the most recent three years' of available data (2009–2011) (SAMHSA, 2013a). These rates include all causes of opioid exposure, both intentional and unintentional. Nonetheless, opioid analgesics are associated with more ED visits than any other class of prescription drugs, although they are closely followed by benzodiazepines (114.8/100,000 in 2011), and they far outstrip rates for any illicit drugs and for alcohol.

In November 2011, CDC released data detailing the involvement of prescription opioids in overdose deaths (CDC, 2011). This report, using death certificate data, showed that 36,450 drug overdose deaths occurred in 2008, of which 27,153 had at least one specific drug named as the cause of death. Of those 27,153 deaths, 14,800 involved at least one prescription opioid analgesic. This number has increased to 16,600 for 2010, the most recent year available at this time (Office of National Drug Control Policy, 2013a). The report combines data from a number of sources to show that the morbidity associated with prescription opioid analgesics is even more dramatic than the mortality, as for every one death, there are 10 treatment admissions for abuse, 32 ED visits for misuse or abuse, 130 people who abuse or are dependent on prescription opioids, and 825 nonmedical users (Office of National Drug Control Policy, 2013a).

A 2011 CDC *Morbidity and Mortality Weekly Report* also showed that prescription opioid sales and admissions to substance abuse treatment related to prescription opioids both increased in parallel with prescription opioid-related overdose deaths (see Figure 8-3). CDC suggested that this apparent correlation between sales and overdose deaths indicates that efforts to rein in opioid prescribing may be an effective means of preventing overdose deaths (CDC, 2011).

When considering these data, it is necessary to remember that overdose deaths involving prescription opioids usually result from a combination of multiple drugs, and may, in most cases, occur in individuals who are using a medication not prescribed for them. Hall et al. (2008) studied overdose deaths in West Virginia and found that decedents in 79% of opioid-related deaths tested positive for other drugs, and 56% of those decedents did not have an active prescription for an opioid. More recent data from the Florida Medical Examiners Commission revealed that, in the first half of 2013, drug overdose decedents in Florida were found to have multiple drugs in their bodies 93.5% of the time (Florida Department of Law Enforcement, 2013). Thus, while prescription opioids are associated with a large number of overdose deaths, in seeking remedies, it is important to recognize the multifactorial nature of these deaths and the significant extent to which the people involved are obtaining their drugs outside the healthcare system.

Clearly, there are plenty of indications that misuse and abuse of prescription opioid analgesics are associated with substantial morbidity and mortality and that the status quo is unacceptable. Many policy initiatives have been undertaken to address this problem and have increased in number and magnitude over the past few years, as government agencies and non-

Figure 8-3. Rates* of Opioid Pain Reliever (OPR) Overdose Death, Treatment Admissions, and Kilograms of OPR Sold—United States, 1999–2010

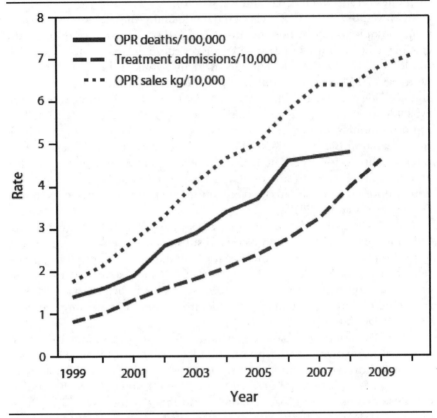

* Age-adjusted rates per 100,000 population for OPR deaths, crude rates per 10,000 population for OPR abuse treatment admissions, and crude rates per 10,000 population for kilograms of OPR sold.

Note. From "Vital Signs: Overdoses of Prescription Opioid Pain Relievers—United States, 1999–2008," by Centers for Disease Control and Prevention, 2011, *Morbidity and Mortality Weekly Report, 60,* p. 1491. Retrieved from http://www.cdc.gov/mmwr/preview/mmwrhtml/mm6043a4.htm?s_cid=mm6043a4_w.

governmental organizations (Association of State and Territorial Health Officers, 2013; National Governors Association Center for Best Practices, n.d.; Office of National Drug Control Policy, 2013b) have sounded the alarm. What makes this such a challenging area for policy makers, however, is the need to maintain access to opioid analgesics in order to provide adequate care for people with pain, who far outnumber those being harmed by opioids. Unlike illicit drugs, where complete elimination of the drug supply can be a goal, the Principle of Balance dictates that policy efforts cannot simply focus on eliminating the problematic drug, because opioid analgesics have a legitimate medical use.

Proposed Policy Solutions

A number of governmental and nongovernmental agencies have proposed comprehensive plans to address the pain management and prescription drug abuse conundrum (Association of State and Territorial Health Officers, 2013; National Governors Association Center for Best Practices, n.d.; Office of National Drug Control Policy, 2013b). Specific recommendations that could affect the ability of healthcare professionals to treat pain are found in most, if not all, comprehensive plans proposed by these agencies. At the core of these recommendations are efforts to control prescribing that may be excessive and/or ineffective, as well as methods of checking to ensure that patients are adhering to the regimens prescribed by their healthcare providers. Following is a review of five of the most common of these recommendations.

Prescribing Guidelines

Several states (e.g., Washington, Ohio, Florida) have passed legislation in recent years designed to decrease excess prescribing by instituting guidelines for prescriber behavior (see National Alliance for Model State Drug Laws, 2012, for a summary of all such state laws). Some of these laws (notably, in Florida and Ohio) have been in response to widely publicized problems with "pill mills," rogue medical practices that prescribe and dispense (from their own in-house pharmacy) thousands of doses of controlled substances with no medical justification. In other cases, concerns about the use of high doses of opioids in treating pain that is not associated with cancer have led to these actions.

In general, prescribing guidelines prompted by this legislation specify that providers must examine patients and their records thoroughly; clearly and completely document their findings; develop a written treatment plan; schedule regular follow-up visits; and make use of prescription monitoring programs (PMPs), drug testing, and patient-provider agreements (see following sections for discussion of these three items). Additionally, some require providers to seek consultation with other providers under certain circumstances. Typically, these policies will state that when a patient reaches a certain dose or duration in the course of his or her opioid treatment, the prescriber must reassess the patient and the treatment plan and/or seek advice from a third party through a required consultation with a pain management expert.

While the requirement that providers reassess patients' progress at certain points is eminently reasonable, multiple anecdotal reports and one published study (Franklin, Fulton-Kehoe, Turner, Sullivan, & Wickizer, 2013) suggest that one unintended consequence of such requirements is a restriction of access to care. Many primary care providers report that they are confused by the complex nature of the rules, and rather than risk accidentally violating them and exposing themselves to sanction, some choose instead to stop prescribing opioids (or at least Schedule II opioids) altogether. Others seem to be using these rules as a sort of scapegoat, citing their stringent nature as an excuse for ridding their practices of people with chronic pain—who they do not feel adequately equipped to treat and who require an inordinate amount of time from practitioners with very busy practices. This is a classic example of a policy with good intent and sound requirements, yet imbalanced results from an outcome perspective.

Prescription Monitoring Programs

PMPs are state-run databases that collect, store, and disseminate information about controlled substances prescriptions. At this writing, 49 states, the District of Columbia, and the territory of Guam have passed legislation to implement PMPs, leaving only Missouri and the other U.S. territories without them (National Alliance for Model State Drug Laws, 2014). Initially conceived and designed to enable law enforcement agencies to detect and intervene with so-called "doctor shoppers" (individuals who visit multiple prescribers, take prescriptions to multiple pharmacies, and use multiple payment methods to accumulate large amounts of medications for purposes of abuse and/or diversion while avoiding detection), these programs are touted by virtually every authority as a key policy in addressing prescription drug abuse.

While it is true that universal use of PMPs could virtually eliminate doctor shopping, PMPs are also a valuable patient care tool for healthcare providers. Using PMP data, providers can (a) feel more secure in prescribing for patients whose PMP profiles indicate behavior consistent with adherence to a good pain management regimen, (b) detect and diagnose individuals whose PMP results suggest substance use disorders and refer them for appropriate treatment, and (c) avoid potentially deadly drug-drug interactions by learning about all controlled substances currently prescribed to the patient, even if the patient cannot remember or does not disclose them. In fact, it is these healthcare uses of PMPs that predominate; in Kansas, data from the fourth quarter of 2012 revealed that 99.97% of requests for reports on patients came from healthcare providers (C. Morris, personal communication, January 23, 2013), a number that is consistent with anecdotal reports from other states.

Much of the challenge with PMPs results from lack of use. In most states, fewer than one-third of all eligible prescribers and dispensers use the databases on a regular basis (Kentucky All Schedule Prescription Electronic Reporting Program Evaluation Team, 2010). Many providers complain that obtaining reports is time consuming and outside their normal work flow, especially if they are using electronic health records that do not pull in PMP data automatically. Rather than subject themselves to what could be an hour or more of additional work each day, many providers choose to query only patients who raise suspicions about their behavior. Some states (notably, Kentucky, Ohio, and Tennessee) have addressed this by establishing rules requiring prescribers to obtain a PMP report before writing an initial prescription for controlled substances and then periodically thereafter (National Alliance for Model State Drug Laws, 2013). The impact of these policies is still unknown, as they have been in place for only a short time. However, there is concern that such requirements could have a chilling effect, as prescribers choose to eliminate what amounts to an unfunded mandate by ceasing to prescribe opioids.

Several initiatives with PMPs could make them more useful and effective, including development of validated, easy-to-use "ratings" that can help providers know at a glance the extent to which a given patient's profile suggests problematic behavior; expansion of the use of multidisciplinary advisory committees composed of PMP stakeholders who can advise programs on enhancements and general functional issues; shortening of the time allowed between filling a prescription and reporting it to the PMP to no longer than 24 hours; and enhanced use of validated data mining techniques to better flag providers and patients who are extreme outliers so that the appropriate authorities can investigate the reasons for their behavior.

Routine Drug Testing

Urine drug testing (UDT) has become a big business, with some laboratory companies becoming very successful in providing this service. Increasingly, both policy makers and healthcare providers are coming to view routine use of UDT as both desirable and necessary when using opioids to manage pain. Several states have mandated UDT in laws and rules. For instance, Georgia now requires patient monitoring that may include UDT every 90 days for patients who are using opioids on a long-term basis (Georgia Composite Medical Board, 2012). Other states have less stringent requirements, with many specifying a test at the initiation of opioid therapy and repeat testing on at least an annual basis, with the frequency determined by the provider's assessment of the patient's substance abuse risk. Note that people with cancer are not specifically excluded from these rules, unless they are judged to be terminally ill. Most other state requirements for UDT do not specifically exclude people with cancer.

UDT conducted in this setting has two purposes: (a) to ensure that patients are not using illicit drugs or medications not prescribed by their healthcare providers, and (b) to ensure that prescribed medications are present in a patient's body, implying at least some level of adherence to their regimen. While early office-based UDT used a qualitative methodology, indicating only the presence or absence of a substance, newer laboratory-based testing using gas chromatography–mass spectrometry (GC-MS) can provide quantitative results. Given the relatively high rate of false-negative results from office-based testing, the more definitive GC-MS testing is often used as confirmation before providers act on office-based test results. Finally, companies performing laboratory-based testing now supply more detailed results to providers, using proprietary algorithms to indicate whether patients are taking their medications as prescribed and providing an analysis of metabolites to suggest whether they have been doing so for some time prior to the latest office visit (Heit & Gourlay, 2014a).

The principal issue with UDT is reimbursement. Whereas office-based tests are inexpensive, laboratory tests can sometimes run as high as $500 or more (Cheves, 2012). Many third-party payers are reluctant to pay for this testing, to such an extent that even some Medicaid intermediaries have refused to pay for it in states where it is required by law. Patients can be billed exorbitant amounts for testing that they ordinarily would not need because their risk of substance abuse is negligible, and when they are unable to pay, their providers may find themselves responsible for these charges. At some point, patients may be forced to choose among carrying significant debt, paying out of pocket while neglecting other financial needs, or stopping opioid therapy to avoid additional charges. There is a growing need for outcomes research to demonstrate to third-party payers that use of routine UDT is financially beneficial to them; should that not be proven, reassessment of these policies is in order.

Patient-Provider Agreements

Another feature found in nearly every policy proposal regarding pain management and prescription drug abuse is a required patient-provider agreement (PPA). PPAs, also known as opioid treatment agreements or opioid contracts, are generally formal agreements in which terms are set for a patient's opioid therapy. Typically, PPAs will contain provisions that limit patients to one prescriber and one designated pharmacy or pharmacy chain, specify that early refills are not permitted, designate the frequency with which UDTs are conducted, and typically specify consequences for violation of the terms. Other provisions may also be included, and in some cases, PPAs also list the responsibilities of the clinician in providing care to the patient (Payne et al., 2010).

Although PPAs are proposed as good policy, very little outcome research exists to support their efficacy in preventing substance misuse, abuse, and diversion (Payne et al., 2010). Many patient advocates view the terms of many PPAs as demeaning and punitive to patients, especially when the only listed consequence for a violation of the agreement is termination of the patient's treatment. Some providers believe that requiring a PPA implies to patients that they are not trusted, and that providers feel the need to protect themselves by requiring the PPA.

More recently, the trend in PPAs has been to emphasize that they should serve primarily as an extension of an informed consent discussion with the patient (i.e., that the PPA be used to ensure that such discussions cover all the necessary topics and that patients understand the risks and benefits of opioid treatment). A model PPA currently under development by the FDA's Safe Use Initiative follows this trend (U.S. FDA, 2014). Additionally, proponents of expanded risk assessment and informed consent for opioid treatment now recommend that the consequences of violating a PPA be couched in terms of a reevaluation of the conditions under which treatment will be provided, as they have observed that some patients are much more adherent to their regimens if given more structure in their treatment (Heit & Gourlay, 2014b).

Policy makers considering requirements for PPAs should be aware of the lack of research regarding their efficacy and should consider supporting research to determine how helpful they are. Additionally, they should exercise caution in specifying the terms of a PPA, allowing some leeway for providers to exercise professional judgment in crafting agreements and individualizing them for patients on the basis of a risk assessment.

Tamper-Deterrent Formulations of Opioids

Many people who abuse prescription opioid analgesics do so by altering their form, typically crushing, cutting, or melting tablets and capsules so as to create a powdered or liquid form that can be inhaled or injected. Although this behavior is atypical among those who are relative novices to prescription drug abuse, those who are more experienced are more likely to engage in it than to simply swallow an intact dosage unit (McCabe, Cranford, Boyd, & Teter, 2007). When the medication being crushed contains a high dose of opioid (e.g., 80 mg of oxycodone), the results can be deadly, as patients consume a very high dose very rapidly. To deter patients from altering the manufactured products in these ways, drug makers have begun developing formulations that make tampering with them more difficult.

The tamper-deterrent formulations (TDFs) that have reached the market to date have taken two forms (Moorman-Li et al., 2012). One is a tablet that has been manufactured in such a way that it cannot be crushed into a powder or otherwise acted upon in ways that permit extraction of the opioid. The second is a capsule containing beads, each of which has a naltrexone core surrounded by an opioid. When this intact capsule is swallowed, it releases the beads into the digestive system, where the naltrexone remains sequestered and does not enter the bloodstream, while the opioid does, providing analgesia. On the other hand, if this product is crushed, the naltrexone is released and mixed with the opioid, so that it antagonizes the mu-opiate receptor and prevents development of both euphoria and respiratory depression.

FDA (which refers to this class of products as "abuse-deterrent" despite the fact that none of its features deter someone from abusing the products by swallowing them intact) is finalizing rules about what is required for pharmaceutical manufacturers to market their products as such, as well as taking other steps to assess and promote use of these technologies (U.S. FDA, 2013a). Additionally, Congress is considering legislation (Stop Tampering of Prescription Pills Act of 2013, H.R. 486) to encourage the further development of TDFs, viewing them as a key measure in combating overdose deaths related to prescription opioids.

For policy makers, the primary concern with TDFs has been the possibility that third-party payers will require pharmacies to substitute non-TDF generic products if they are available, as a means of saving money. To counter that possibility, legislation has been introduced in several states to prohibit such automatic substitution if the prescriber indicates that he or she specifically intends for the patient to have a TDF. Clinicians should decide whether a TDF is required based on complete assessment of the patient's risk of substance abuse, as well as the risk of someone in the patient's social milieu engaging in the same behavior. Patients at low risk, who report that no one in their social circles could reasonably be expected to acquire the medication for abuse or diversion, may be able to safely use the less expensive generic non-TDF products. These concerns remain to be resolved through the policymaking process.

Other Policy Issues Related to Pain Management

In addition to the issues discussed previously, all of which seek to balance concerns about prescription drug abuse and legitimate use of opioid analgesics, a number of other policy issues impact pain treatment. Some of these will be reviewed briefly.

Fail-First/Step Therapy Protocols

Some third-party payers have established policies, referred to as fail-first/step therapy protocols, that require patients to first try inexpensive generic medications, and find that they are ineffective or cause intolerable side effects, before progressing to more expensive brand-name medications. In some cases, these policies can be extensive and require considerable time to implement—one company is known to have required five steps before agreeing to pay for medications with official FDA indications for treating fibromyalgia (Coventry Health Care, 2009). Such policies may cause patients considerable delays in obtaining adequate pain relief while simultaneously exposing them to unnecessary risks. For providers, these protocols complicate treatment and require that they approve the use of medications that they may be reasonably certain will not work. Some states have addressed these protocols by limiting them to one or two steps before the requested medication must be supplied. (For a summary of existing laws, regulations, and current legislation, see Global Healthy Living Foundation, n.d.)

Specialty Tier Pricing

Most third-party payers with coverage for prescription medications use a tiered strategy, enabling them to reimburse for various medications at different rates and to require different co-pays from patients for each tier. Faced with the availability of very expensive new medications, some payers have begun instituting "specialty tier" pricing, wherein a patient does not pay a co-pay but instead is required to pay a certain percentage of the cost of the medication—a cost that can run into thousands of dollars per month. Patients have protested this development, and policy makers have shown some interest and have considered offering legislation to prohibit such practices (National Patient Advocate Foundation, 2013).

Prior Authorization

Third-party payers also may use a prior authorization process to control costs. Faced with a request for an expensive medication, the payer may require that the prescriber submit a request for approval before the prescription can be filled, with the request focused on justifying the use of the requested medication instead of less expensive alternatives. This process, as it has been practiced, is cumbersome, slow, and frustrating, sometimes requiring weeks to complete. Studies of medical practices have shown that completing all the required prior authorization requests can be extraordinarily costly in terms of provider and clerical staff time, and the frustrating nature of the process can lead some providers and patients to just give up and either use a less desirable medication or to use nothing at all (American Medical Association, 2011). States have begun addressing this by passing legislation requiring that all prior authorization requests use a single concise form that is available electronically. Payers are given a short period of time, often two to three days, to respond to the prior authorization request, and failure to do so is determined to constitute approval of the request. To date, such legislation has passed in at least 14 states and is in the implementation process.

Reimbursement for Nonpharmacologic Interventions

For many people with chronic pain, the most effective treatment regimens involve a considerable "dose" of nonpharmacologic interventions, such as physical and occupational therapy, psychotherapy, massage, acupuncture, chiropractic, and numerous other complementary and alternative therapies. Over the past decade or more, third-party payers have gravitated toward selectively reimbursing for invasive anesthetic procedures and prescribing, and away from nonpharmacologic therapies. The result, some believe, is an overemphasis on prescribing and procedures, resulting in poorer pain control and a proliferation of opioid analgesics that can be abused or diverted. In seeking to address the prescription drug abuse problem, some policy makers have begun considering ways to increase reimbursement for nonpharmacologic therapies with the hope of improving patients' pain care while reducing prescription drug abuse and diversion. Such policy changes seem logical, but until they are implemented and studied, it is difficult to say with certainty how much good they will do.

Medical Marijuana

Faced with popular opinion and a smattering of scientific evidence of its effectiveness in treating some types of pain (Martín-Sánchez, Furukawa, Taylor, & Martin, 2009), some state legislatures have passed legislation allowing patients to possess and use marijuana as a medical treatment, provided that those patients' healthcare providers have approved the practice. Such "medical marijuana" laws fly in the face of the federal government's classification of marijuana as a Schedule I drug, indicating that the federal government does not believe there is a legitimate medical use for it. Two states (Washington and Colorado) have taken this policy a step further, legalizing the possession and use of small amounts of marijuana. The Obama administration has issued a directive to U.S. Attorneys, saying that prosecution of patients and their medical marijuana suppliers is not a priority, unless there is clearly an inordinate profit motive on the part of suppliers or an inordinately large supply of marijuana involved, or if it involves harms to public safety and health or other law enforcement issues (e.g., distribution to minors, violence and use of firearms, drugged driving, trafficking of other illegal drugs or illegal activity, use of federal or public property) (U.S. Department of Justice Office of the Deputy Attorney General, 2013). In this area, the evidence for marijuana's effectiveness in providing pain relief is insufficient to convince FDA that it should be rescheduled, although there is a groundswell of support for doing so (Drug Policy Alliance, 2013).

Conclusion

As the nation struggles to deal with two major public health crises—undertreatment of pain, especially chronic pain; and the abuse, misuse, diversion, and overdose deaths related to the medications used to treat pain—policy solutions are frequently offered by well-meaning legislators and regulators. Unfortunately, in many cases, the solutions offered are overly simplistic, especially considering the extraordinarily complex nature of both of these public health problems. Often, the result of these simple policy solutions is a restriction of access to controlled substances for people who use them legitimately and benefit from them greatly. The magnitude of these negative unintended consequences is only beginning to be fully understood.

Throughout the late 1990s, 2000s, and even into the early 2010s, many policies related to the use of controlled substances to treat pain exempted people with cancer, and often people receiving hospice care as well. While this proved to be beneficial to those individuals and their healthcare providers, it ignored some inconvenient facts—namely, that having cancer or being at the end of life does not cure addiction or lessen one's risk of adverse effects (including accidental overdose) or of abusing controlled substances. Also, the high doses often required in those situations make these people inviting targets for someone seeking to obtain medications illicitly. Further, as more people with cancer become long-term survivors, often with persistent pain resulting from their cancer treatment, more of them will require long-term treatment with opioids and other pain medications, driving up the risks of adverse effects and costs for insurers.

Given those concerns, it seems reasonable to wonder if or when policy makers and payers will begin to see long-term cancer survivors as having noncancer pain as opposed to cancer pain, thereby subjecting them to restrictions they previously avoided. This issue is being closely watched by advocates for people with cancer, some of whom note that the noncancer versus cancer pain bifurcation is a distinction without a difference, as highlighted earlier. Those advocates support policies that promote adequate access to controlled substances for all people who need them, regardless of the diagnosis that led to the pain condition. Advocating for separate policies on the basis of a cancer diagnosis is illogical in this arena, as the human nervous system does not treat pain differently if it arises from cancer or from other causes and human opioid receptors do not function differently in the presence of a neoplasm. Clearly, this important issue bears watching.

This review of key issues in pain management policy, while extensive, is by no means exhaustive. It illustrates the need for concerned healthcare providers and people with pain to speak out insistently and regularly to ensure that policy continues to develop in a positive direction—one that ensures the ability of healthcare professionals to provide optimal pain care for all people with pain, regardless of its cause. No one understands the complexity of the problems and the magnitude of the unintended negative consequences more than those caring for people with pain. Failure of healthcare providers in particular to be involved in advocating for good policy could mean that those providers lose the ability to care for their patients. And that would be a tragedy for all of society.

References

American Medical Association. (2011). *Standardization of prior authorization process for medical services* (White paper). Retrieved from http://www.ama-assn.org

American Psychiatric Association. (2000). *Diagnostic and statistical manual of mental disorders* (4th ed., text rev.). Arlington, VA: American Psychiatric Publishing.

Association of State and Territorial Health Officials. (2013). ASTHO President's Challenge 2014: 15 by 15: Reduce Prescription Drug Abuse and Deaths 15% by 2015. Retrieved from http://www.astho.org/Rx/2014-Presidents-Challenge-Fact-Sheet

Brecher, E.M., & Editors of *Consumer Reports* Magazine. (1972). Chapter 8. The Harrison Narcotic Act (1914). In *The Consumers Union report on licit and illicit drugs.* Retrieved from http://www.druglibrary.org/schaffer/library/studies/cu/cu8.html

Bridge-Cook, P. (2013). Understanding FDA's views on opioid painkillers: The PROP petition. Retrieved from http://www.hormonesmatter.com/fda-views-opioid-painkillers-prop-petition

Centers for Disease Control and Prevention. (2011). Vital signs: Overdoses of prescription opioid pain relievers—United States, 1999–2008. *Morbidity and Mortality Weekly Report, 60,* 1487–1492. Retrieved from http://www.cdc.gov/mmwr/preview/mmwrhtml/mm6043a4.htm?s_cid=mm6043a4_w

Cheves, J. (2012, September 27). Urine tests required by new drug law can cost patients hundreds of dollars. *Lexington Herald-Leader.* Retrieved from http://www.kentucky.com/2012/09/27/2352733/drug-tests-required-by-new-law.html

Comprehensive Drug Abuse Prevention and Control Act of 1970, Pub. L. No. 91-513. Retrieved from http://www.gpo.gov/fdsys/pkg/STATUTE-84/pdf/STATUTE-84-Pg1236.pdf

Controlled Substances Act of 1970, 21 U.S.C. § 801 et seq.

Coventry Health Care. (2009). Fibromyalgia prior authorization form. Retrieved from http://altius.coventryhealthcare.com/web/groups/public/@cvty_regional_chcut/documents/document/c054190.pdf

Drug Policy Alliance. (2013, May). Removing marijuana from the Controlled Substances Act. Retrieved from http://www.drugpolicy.org/sites/default/files/DPA_Fact%20sheet_Marijuana%20Reclassification_May%202013.pdf

Federation of State Medical Boards. (2004, May). Model policy for the use of controlled substances for the treatment of pain. Retrieved from http://library.fsmb.org/pdf/2004_grpol_Controlled_Substances.pdf

Florida Department of Law Enforcement. (2013). *Drugs identified in deceased persons by Florida medical examiners: Interim report.* Retrieved from http://myfloridalegal.com/webfiles.nsf/WF/JMEE-9KKLMN/$file/DrugsIdentifiedInterimReport.pdf

Franklin, G.M., Fulton-Kehoe, D., Turner, J.A., Sullivan, M.D., & Wickizer, T.M. (2013). Changes in opioid prescribing for chronic pain in Washington State. *Journal of the American Board of Family Medicine, 26,* 394–400. doi:10.3122/jabfm.2013.04.120274

Georgia Composite Medical Board. (2012). Rule 360-3-.02: Unprofessional conduct defined. Retrieved from https://medicalboard.georgia.gov/sites/medicalboard.georgia.gov/files/Pain-Management-Rules.pdf

Gilson, A.M., Joranson, D.E., & Maurer, M.A. (2007). Improving state pain policies: Recent progress and continuing opportunities. *CA: A Cancer Journal for Clinicians, 57,* 341–353. doi:10.3322/CA.57.6.341

Global Healthy Living Foundation. (n.d.). Fail First Hurts: Fail First updates. Retrieved from http://failfirsthurts.org/fail-first-updates

Hall, A.J., Logan, J.E., Toblin, R.L., Kaplan, J.A., Kraner, J.C., Bixler, D., ... Paulozzi, L.J. (2008). Patterns of abuse among unintentional pharmaceutical overdose fatalities. *JAMA, 300,* 2613–2620. doi:10.1001/jama.2008.802

Harrison Narcotics Tax Act, 38 Stat. 785, Ch. 1 (1914). Retrieved from http://www.druglibrary .org/schaffer/history/e1910/harrisonact.htm

Heit, H.A., & Gourlay, D.L. (2014a). Philosophy of urine drug testing in pain management. Retrieved from http://www.prescriberesponsibly.com/articles/urine-drug-testing

Heit, H.A., & Gourlay, D.L. (2014b). What a prescriber should know before writing the first prescription. Retrieved from http://www.prescriberesponsibly.com/articles/before-prescribing -opioids

Institute of Medicine. (2011). *Relieving pain in America: A blueprint for transforming prevention, care, education, and research.* Washington, DC: National Academies Press.

International Narcotics Control Board. (n.d.). Single Convention on Narcotic Drugs, 1961. Retrieved from https://www.incb.org/incb/en/narcotic-drugs/1961_Convention.html

Jacox, A., Carr, D.B., & Payne, R. (1994, March). *Management of cancer pain* (Clinical Practice Guideline No. 9. AHCPR Publication No. 94-0592). Retrieved from http://www.ncbi.nlm .nih.gov/books/NBK52307

Kentucky All Schedule Prescription Electronic Reporting Program Evaluation Team. (2010, June). *Review of prescription drug monitoring programs in the United States.* Retrieved from http://chfs.ky.gov/NR/rdonlyres/85989824-1030-4AA6-91E1-7F9E3EF68827/0/KASPE REvaluationPDMPStatusFinalReport6242010.pdf

Martín-Sánchez, E., Furukawa, T.A., Taylor, J., & Martin, J.L.R. (2009). Systematic review and meta-analysis of cannabis treatment for chronic pain. *Pain Medicine, 10,* 1353–1368. doi:10.1111/j.1526-4637.2009.00703.x

McCabe, S.E., Cranford, J.A., Boyd, C.J., & Teter, C.J. (2007). Motives, diversion and routes of administration associated with nonmedical use of prescription opioids. *Addictive Behaviors, 32,* 562–575. doi:10.1016/j.addbeh.2006.05.022

Moorman-Li, R., Motycka, C.A., Inge, L.D., Congdon, J.M., Hobson, S., & Pokropski, B. (2012). A review of abuse-deterrent opioids for chronic nonmalignant pain. *Pharmacy and Therapeutics, 37,* 412–418. Retrieved from http://www.ncbi.nlm.nih.gov/pmc/articles/PMC3411218

National Alliance for Model State Drug Laws. (2012, June). *State statutes and regulations relative to chronic pain and pain management: Emphasis on pain management clinics. Brief summary of federal provisions.* Retrieved from http://www.namsdl.org/library/7C4DC653-1C23-D4F9-7411227356D4CFE3

National Alliance for Model State Drug Laws. (2013). *States that require prescribers and/or dispensers to access PMP database in certain circumstances.* Retrieved from http://www.namsdl.org/ library/14F3F3DF-1C23-D4F9-74143B7F8C041665/

National Alliance for Model State Drug Laws. (2014). Status of state prescription drug monitoring programs (PDMPs). Retrieved from http://www.namsdl.org/library/16666FCC-65BE -F4BB-A2BBAD44E1BC7031

National Governors Association Center for Best Practices. (n.d.). Prescription Drug Abuse Project. Retrieved from http://www.nga.org/cms/Rx

National Patient Advocate Foundation. (2013, May). *White paper: Specialty tiers.* Retrieved from http://www.npaf.org/files/5%207%2013%20Specialty%20Tiers%20White%20Paper%20 Final_0.pdf

New York State Controlled Substances Act, New York State Public Health Law, Article 33, Title 1, § 3306 (2013). Retrieved from http://www.health.ny.gov/regulations/public_health _law/article/33/docs/33.pdf

Nixon, R. (1971, June 17). Special message to the Congress on drug abuse prevention and control. *American Presidency Project.* Retrieved from http://www.presidency.ucsb.edu/ws/?pid=3048

Office of National Drug Control Policy. (2013a, August 28). Fact sheet: Preventing, treating, and surviving overdose. Retrieved from http://www.whitehouse.gov/sites/default/files/ondcp/prevention/overdose_fact_sheet.pdf

Office of National Drug Control Policy. (2013b). *National drug control strategy: 2013.* Retrieved from http://www.whitehouse.gov//sites/default/files/ondcp/policy-and-research/ndcs_2013.pdf

Payne, R., Anderson, E., Arnold, R., Duensing, L., Gilson, A., Green, C., … Christopher, M. (2010). A rose by any other name: Pain contracts/agreements. *American Journal of Bioethics, 10*(11), 5–12. doi:10.1080/15265161.2010.519425

Reorganization Plan No. 1 of 1968. (1968). 33 F.R. 5611, 82 Stat. 1367, as amended Pub. L. 90–623, § 7(c), Oct. 22, 1968, 82 Stat. 1316. Retrieved from http://uscode.house.gov/view.xhtml?req=granuleid:USC-prelim-title5a-node83-leaf170&num=0&edition=prelim

Reorganization Plan No. 2 of 1973. (1973). 33 F.R. 5611, 82 Stat. 1367, § 3, eff. July 1, 1973, 38 F.R. 15932, 87 Stat. 1091. Retrieved from http://www.gpo.gov/fdsys/pkg/USCODE-2011-title5/pdf/USCODE-2011-title5-app-reorganiz-other-dup96.pdf

Stop Tampering of Prescription Pills Act of 2013, H.R. 486, 113 Cong.

Substance Abuse and Mental Health Services Administration. (2003). *Results from the 2002 National Survey on Drug Use and Health: National findings* (HHS Publication No. SMA 03-3836, NHSDA Series H-22). Retrieved from http://www.samhsa.gov/data/nhsda/2k2nsduh/Results/2k2Results.htm

Substance Abuse and Mental Health Services Administration. (2013a). *Drug Abuse Warning Network, 2011: National estimates of drug-related emergency department visits* (HHS Publication No. SMA 13-4760, DAWN Series D-39). Retrieved from http://www.samhsa.gov/data/2k13/DAWN2k11ED/DAWN2k11ED.htm

Substance Abuse and Mental Health Services Administration. (2013b). National Survey on Drug Use and Health (NSDUH). Retrieved from http://www.samhsa.gov/data/population-data-nsduh

Substance Abuse and Mental Health Services Administration. (2014, September). *Results from the 2013 National Survey on Drug Use and Health: Summary of national findings.* Retrieved from http://www.samhsa.gov/data/population-data-nsduh/reports?tab=32

U.S. Const. art. VI, cl. 2.

U.S. Department of Justice Office of the Deputy Attorney General. (2013, August 29). Memorandum for all United States Attorneys. Retrieved from http://www.justice.gov/iso/opa/resources/3052013829132756857467.pdf

U.S. Drug Enforcement Administration. (2001, October 23). *Promoting pain relief and preventing abuse of pain medications: A critical balancing act.* Retrieved from http://www.deadiversion.usdoj.gov/pubs/advisories/painrelief.pdf

U.S. Drug Enforcement Administration. (2014a). Controlled substance schedules. Retrieved from http://www.deadiversion.usdoj.gov/schedules

U.S. Drug Enforcement Administration. (2014b). DEA to publish final rule rescheduling hydrocodone combination products [News release]. Retrieved from http://www.justice.gov/dea/divisions/hq/2014/hq082114.shtml

U.S. Food and Drug Administration. (2013a). FDA's efforts to address the misuse and abuse of opioids. Retrieved from http://www.fda.gov/Drugs/DrugSafety/InformationbyDrugClass/ucm337852.htm

U.S. Food and Drug Administration. (2013b). FDA/CDER response to physicians for responsible opioid prescribing—Partial petition approval and denial. Retrieved from http://www.regulations.gov/#!documentDetail;D=FDA-2012-P-0818-0793

U.S. Food and Drug Administration. (2014). Safe Use Initiative: Current projects. Retrieved from http://www.fda.gov/Drugs/DrugSafety/SafeUseInitiative/ucm188762.htm#opioidppa

USA.gov. (2014). Laws and regulations. Retrieved from http://www.usa.gov/Topics/Reference
-Shelf/Laws.shtml

Woodcock, J. (2013). Statement on proposed hydrocodone reclassification from Janet Woodcock, M.D., Director, Center for Drug Evaluation and Research. Retrieved from http://
www.fda.gov/drugs/drugsafety/ucm372089.htm

World Health Organization. (2011). *Ensuring balance in national policies on controlled substances: Guidance for availability and accessibility of controlled medicines.* Retrieved from http://
whqlibdoc.who.int/publications/2011/9789241564175_eng.pdf

CHAPTER 9

Eliminating Cancer Disparities Through Legislative Action

John Lunstroth, LLM, MPH, Lovell Jones, PhD, and Kimberly R. Enard, PhD, MBA, MSHA

Medicine is a social science, and politics is nothing more than medicine on a large scale.

—Rudolph Virchow

Social injustice is killing people on a grand scale.
—World Health Organization Commission
on Social Determinants of Health

Introduction

This chapter will focus on the role that policy plays in creating or determining cancer and in reducing the burden of cancer. It will describe the sources of policy; the language of policy; the history of health policy, introducing the concept of the "social determinants of health"; some ideas about how policy "determines" cancer; and various ways policy can be evaluated. The chapter will also illustrate the concepts discussed using the example of breast cancer and will provide tentative policy suggestions.

Sources of Health Policy on Cancer

Policy comes in two forms. "Hard" policy is law and the legal system. The central case of hard policy is legislation and judicial opinion. "Soft" policies are norms or guidelines issued by various authorities that are not laws. For example, when the Centers for Disease Control and Prevention (CDC) issues vaccine guidelines, it is setting policy, but the U.S. states and territories to whom the policy is addressed are not required to follow the policy recommendations. At the core of policy is the idea of an authority speaking in an authoritative role to advise or guide others who do not have either the authority or the knowledge required to make well-informed and prudent decisions in that particular area.

The most important health policy institutions unfortunately do not fit comfortably in the categories of "hard" or "soft" policy sources. Those are the large regulatory agencies such as the Environmental Protection Agency and the Food and Drug Administration (FDA). These agencies are created by law (hard policy), but because of their expertise in their field, they are given further authority to make regulations and enforce them with the state's police power.

The concept of *police power* is important in the discussion of policy development and enforcement. Max Weber (1864–1920), German sociologist, philosopher, and economist, famously defined the *state* as the entity that has a monopoly on the use of force, either through a police force, a military, or other means. The use of force is required, the theory says, to maintain order within the state and to maintain the state itself with regard to other states or actors. In modern federal states, there are numerous police forces to maintain internal order—local, state, and federal (e.g., the Department of Homeland Security). The military is used only toward other international states, not within the federal borders.

Public health is a catchall term that refers to the acts of the state to maintain the health of the population considered as groups, not as individuals. Physicians and other healthcare professionals provide health care to individuals, whereas states use means (laws, policies, regulatory agencies) that reach large numbers of individuals at once. Sometimes, the state's efforts to maintain, reestablish, or promote health are of such urgency or importance that the state mandates a health intervention, and that mandate is backed up by the police power of the state. If individuals or groups do not comply with the law or mandate, the state can then force them to act or refrain from acting through fines, taxes, quarantines, etc.

A state is organized legally by a constitution. The United States consists of fifty-one states (and some territories): there are the 50 states such as Texas, Arkansas, etc., each with its own constitution, and there is the federal state with its Constitution, which is distinguished by capitalizing the initial *c*. One of the things negotiated in the drafting of the Constitution was the distribution of police power between the federal state and the member states. This distribution is of fundamental importance to the public health community because it was that distribution of police power that has caused, and continues to cause, important policy issues. In essence, each state retained the police power for public health over its own citizens. An important example is that all health professionals are regulated at the state level through licensing and other schemes.

Each state has a three-part governing arrangement (the "three branches"). The legislature creates laws; the executive branch carries out the law; and the judiciary interprets the law in problems related to its execution. In each legislature there are committees that oversee and structure the health matters, or hard policy, within that state. If the state has an upper and lower house, each house will have a committee that deals with public health matters; if the state has only one house, it will have just one committee. In this system, the executive branch is where police power resides, and this branch can at its discretion delegate some of that power to subordinate or even semi-independent governmental bodies, such as a department of health or authority of some kind, respectively. Each state has a department of health that implements some of those policies, issues its own policies, and oversees the state health sector in general using the state's police power that is delegated to it. Considering about 18%, or some $3 trillion dollars, of the U.S. economy is spent in the health sector, these state legislatures are very important sources of health policy (Centers for Medicare and Medicaid Services [CMS], n.d.).

However, health policy is not only sourced at the state government level. Each major city has its own health policies, some of them, such as that of New York City, are of national importance. By far, however, the most important sources of health policy emanate from national or federal-level institutions.

At the federal level, apart from the legislature, three kinds of policy-setting institutions exist: federal agencies or departments; semiautonomous federal entities, such as the Institute of Medicine; and nonprofit groups. Several federal departments or agencies are very important for public health policy. The Department of Health and Human Services is massive and has under its jurisdiction 11 departments or administrations, some of which are among the most powerful governmental entities in the field of public health in the world, including FDA, the National Institutes of Health (NIH), CDC, and CMS. Because roughly half of every dollar spent in the health sector comes from the federal government and the Health and Human Services budget accounts for substantially all of that money, its policies are immensely influential (U.S. Department of Health and Human Services, 2014). FDA ensures the safety and efficacy of drugs, protects the safety of some of the food supply, and the safety of cosmetics. NIH spends roughly $30 billion every year researching health interventions through its 27 institutes and centers, and its decisions determine the direction of the life sciences in general (NIH Office of Budget, 2013). CDC monitors the health of the nation through an extensive statistical system; identifies, responds to, and coordinates responses to health problems; publishes the *Morbidity and Mortality Weekly Report*; and advises state health departments on numerous public health issues. CMS manages the health care of the very poor, the elderly, and the disabled in the nation's largest single-payer, government-sponsored healthcare system. All of these federal agencies and administrations not only exercise extraordinary influence in the United States, but their advice, efficiencies, and competencies are sought and imitated around the world.

Other cabinet-level departments that play a significant role in the nation's health include the Department of Agriculture (USDA), Department of Education, Department of Housing and Urban Development, Department of Labor, Department of Commerce, Department of Treasury, and Department of Defense (DOD). The Environmental Protection Agency is not a cabinet-level agency, but its administrator is often given cabinet rank. The role of USDA as overseer of the nation's food supply in protecting and promoting the public health is straightforward, but why the DOD plays a pivotal role is not as obvious. During national biologic emergencies, DOD can, by request or on its own, act by

- Providing disease surveillance and laboratory diagnostics
- Transporting response teams, vaccines, medical equipment, supplies, diagnostic devices, pharmaceuticals, and blood products
- Treating patients
- Evacuating the ill and injured
- Processing and tracking patients
- Providing base and installation support to federal, state, local, and tribal agencies
- Controlling movement into and out of areas, or across borders, with affected populations
- Supporting law enforcement
- Supporting quarantine enforcement
- Restoring damaged public utilities
- Providing mortuary services. (Kapp & Jansen, 2009, p. 7)

The link between commerce, economics, transportation, education, housing, and workplace and the public's health will be discussed. In short, the federal government, with its own police powers and those it delegates to the agencies, wields unparalleled power over the public health infrastructure and practices of the nation through its policies, and therefore its spending and other coercive powers. This influence occurs in an environment of multiple overlapping and uncoordinated public health authorities and goes to the heart of a comprehensive policy approach to any disease, or to health in general.

One more high-level source of policy must be acknowledged, the World Health Organization (WHO). WHO is an independent United Nations (UN) organ that is like the CDC of the international community. Although it is a UN organ, it is considered independent because it has its own member states that determine its policies. It has origins in 19th century trade treaties and has limited legislative powers that are binding on member governments, but functions largely in the same capacity as CDC, with whom it works closely (McCarthy, 2002).

For all of these departments and agencies, cancer is of the utmost importance and plays a significant role in their policy deliberations.

The other major source of cancer policy is from nonprofits or nongovernmental organizations (NGOs). Typically these organizations employ or consist of experts in a particular field, such as breast cancer, or are organized around a particular intervention, such as tobacco. The example discussed later in this chapter will focus on policy recommendations concerning breast cancer made primarily by NGOs (Gostin, 2008, 2010; Grad, 2005).

Causes of Health and Disease

Three kinds of causation generally are recognized when discussing health and disease: biochemical or biomedical; individual choice; and sociopolitical causes. The first category is the province of medical and other kinds of doctors and individual professional providers. They enter into doctor-patient relationships and treat according to their training, which almost exclusively sees the causes of disease as biochemical events. At the next level, individual choice, doctors and many others exhort people to take more control over their diet, exercise regimen, and a host of other decisions in order for them to take control of their health. The cause of disease in this model is the individuals themselves. At the next level, disease (or health) is understood to be caused by large-scale social, environmental, economic, cultural, and political causes. In the first kind of causation, the focus is on invisible causes within an organism, whereas in the third kind of causation, the focus is on large-scale causes that are measured at the population level, not the individual level. The third kind of causation is often signaled by the use of the word *disparities*.

Disparities is a descriptive term arising from the uncontroversial observation that, at the population level, if a scale is drawn between the rich and poor (to put it simply), then the closer one gets to the poor end of the gradient, the greater the incidence and prevalence of disease and death (and many other markers). There is a disparity, in other words, between those with more wealth and those with less. The word "disparity," while correct, does not indicate anything about causation. A doctor, for example, while being well aware of the gradient, might counsel a patient who lives on a high-traffic street in an apartment with roaches and mice and has chronic asthma to take prophylactic antibiotics along with a bronchodilator. Doctors are not trained to address the other causes of disease, which might include having parents who could not afford to send their children (the patients) to a decent school, get them regular medical care, feed them well, or, most importantly, live in a home that is not covered with lead paint, infested with roaches or mice, and in a neighborhood that is not in the plume from a chemical plant, highway, or other source of airborne pollutants. In other words, *disparities* is a depoliticized word that permits a discussion of the phenomenon of the gradient without making implications about its cause. *Inequities* is a more accurate term as it refers to the underlying problem with disparities, a sociopolitical injustice.

For the purposes of treatment or intervention, it is helpful to use names that convey causative information. The convention in public health is to use the word *determinant* to refer to causative classes or types (e.g., social determinants). An entire body of scholarship has arisen under the category of social determinants of health created by social epidemiologists looking at social inequities as the primary cause of disease across populations. In the past few years, as a greater part of the public health community embraced the idea of social determinants, other phrases have come into use: environmental determinants, individual determinants, biologic determinants, political determinants, and so on, including the word *disparities*.

The idea of policy determinants can be narrow or broad. This chapter takes a broad perspective, and because environmental, economic, social, biologic, and other determinants, including genetic and neurologic determinants, are caused or determined by policy decisions, the phrase *sociopolitical determinants* will be used to refer to the entire spectrum of causes of disease considered at the population level.

Mechanisms by Which Policy Influences Cancer Rates

Cancer is generally understood as a noncommunicable, chronic, and often fatal disease with obscure origins. Typically, cancer causation is discussed in terms of "intrinsic factors such as heredity, diet, and hormones, [and] scientific studies point to key extrinsic factors that contribute to the cancer's development: chemicals (e.g., smoking), radiation, and viruses or bacteria" (National Cancer Institute [NCI], 2009, slide 24). Those are proximate causes, each of which is or can be controlled by policy.

Diet can be controlled by agricultural and various economic and safety policies (Bakst, 2013). In turn, diet affects the expression of genes (Wanjek, 2012). Hormone levels can be influenced by a variety of external factors, including visual, tactile, olfactory, and auditory cues (Silver, 1992); exercise (Parr, 2009); diseases, drugs, and stress (Anawalt, Kirk, & Shulman, 2013); alcohol (Thiel, n.d.); and environmental chemicals (Environmental Working Group, 2013), all of which can be directly influenced through policies. Exposure to chemicals and radiation in general is controlled by policies mediated through the Environmental Protection Agency and other federal regulatory bodies. Exposures to harmful microorganisms are controlled by agricultural policy and through regulation of places such as hospitals (Alliance for the Prudent Use of Antibiotics, n.d.; CDC, 2013a).

The Social Determinants of Health

As the Industrial Revolution took off in the early 19th century, it quickly became apparent that a link existed among poverty, a subjugated, depressing lifestyle and working conditions, and disease (Rosen, 1993). Friedrich Engels, who would go on to work with Karl Marx, lived in Manchester, England, from 1842 to 1844, and from his experiences and observations wrote what can be described as the first work documenting and theorizing about the link between sociopolitical conditions and disease, *The Condition of the Working Class in England*, in 1845 (Navarro, 2009). Those sociopolitical conditions are now referred to as the *social determinants of health* (or *disease*), or, at NIH, *disparities*.

The social theory of disease developed until about the 1880s, with the onset of the Bacteriological Era, which dominated into the 1960s and still carries considerable power in the medical community (Kennedy, 2008). The bacteriological model of medicine emphasizes the power of the physician to use medicines and techniques developed in the laboratory to combat the individual case of disease with a magic bullet, such as an antibiotic. In this model, disease is the result of a bacteria or virus and can be eliminated by eradicating the bug. This kind of medicine, *biomedicine*, put medical doctors and the pharmaceutical companies at the center of delivering health to the people (Kennedy, 2008; Starr, 1982).

Meanwhile, the social determinants of health began to slowly reemerge in the 1940s under the rubric of "social medicine" (Galdston, 1949; Susser, 1966). Most notably, Thomas McKeown in a series of articles and books beginning in the 1950s launched a powerful argument known as the McKeown thesis (McKeown, 1976a, 1976b; McKeown & Brown, 1955; McKeown, Brown, & Record, 1972; McKeown & Record, 1962; McKeown, Record, & Turner, 1975). It is well summarized by historian James Colgrove:

> The physician and demographic historian Thomas McKeown put forth the view that the growth in population in the industrialized world from the late 1700s to the present was due not to life-saving advancements in the field of medicine or public health, but instead to improvements in overall standards of living, especially diet and nutritional status, resulting from better economic conditions. His historical analysis called into question the effectiveness of some of the most basic and widely applied techniques in the public health armamentarium, including sanitary reforms,

vaccination, and quarantine. The "McKeown thesis" sparked the inquiries and shaped the research hypotheses of many scholars and became the subject of an extended controversy. (Colgrove, 2002, p. 725)

McKeown's theory formed the backbone of Malthusian arguments about the food supply, economic development, population growth, and the allocation of medical resources (Colgrove, 2002). Although they were criticized through the 1980s and 1990s, they continue to forcefully reemerge (Floud, Fogel, Harris, & Hong, 2011). Simultaneous with McKeown's work, the first generation of social epidemiologists began to establish the theoretical and empirical tools with which to document the social determinants of health (Syme, 2005). Social epidemiology uses the tools of epidemiology to study the effects of sociopolitical independent variables on the health of populations and other groups (Susser, 1973).

Nancy Kreiger, Michael Marmot, Richard Wilkinson, and Lisa Berkman, the second generation of researchers prominent among those who developed the social determinants of health movement, began working in the 1970s (Syme, 2005). It was a time of incredible sociopolitical ferment, and what we now call "social justice" was in the air. The foundations of medical authority were being questioned on all fronts (Illich, 1976; Lalonde, 1974; Starr, 1982; Zola, 1972).

Although the social authority of physicians was challenged and the sociopolitical environment of biomedicine changed radically with the growth in influence of corporate medicine and the pharmaceutical industry, doctors remained, and still remain, at the heart of the health sector. However, in the 1990s, the social determinants of health movement took off, relatively speaking (Marmot, 2005). The sensitivity and receptivity to its perspectives were probably a result of the end of the Cold War, which loosened ideologic structures, permitted the growth of the human rights and development movements at the international level, and brought widespread technical scrutiny to the extent of global poverty and human security (or rather, insecurity).

It continues to be an unusual idea that health is determined largely by sociopolitical factors. However, after about 1995, there has been a veritable (and relative) explosion of work on the social determinants of health (Syme, 2005). WHO, CDC, and NIH have institutionalized these approaches to disease, but most importantly the WHO Commission on Social Determinants of Health published a groundbreaking report in 2008. The commission consisted of very prominent researchers in the field, such as Amartya Sen, Sir Michael Marmot, and others. The report considered substantially all of the empirical evidence for the social determinants of health and, as a compendium of data and analysis, is the starting point for research into the social determinants of health. The commission took

a holistic view of social determinants of health. The poor health of the poor, the social gradient in health within countries, and the marked health inequities between countries are caused by the unequal distribution of power, income, goods, and services, globally and nationally, the consequent unfairness in the immediate, visible circumstances of people's lives—their access to health care, schools, and education, their conditions of work and leisure, their homes, communities, towns, or cities—and their chances of leading a flourishing life. This unequal distribution of health-damaging experiences is not in any sense a "natural" phenomenon but is the result of a toxic combination of poor social policies and programmes, unfair economic arrangements, and bad politics. Together, the structural determinants and conditions of daily life constitute the social determinants of health and are responsible for a major part of health inequities between and within countries. . . . Deep inequities in the distribution of power and economic arrangements, globally, are of key relevance to health equity. . . . And of course climate change has profound implications for the global system—how it affects the way of life and health of individuals and the planet. (WHO Commission on Social Determinants of Health, 2008, p. 1)

The commission had three overarching recommendations, all of which are direct results of policy decisions regarding the human, political, and economic spheres.

• Improve daily living conditions. The commission determined that five subgoals more completely described this recommendation, which were
  – A more equitable start in life
  – A flourishing living or built environment
  – Fair employment and decent work
  – Social protection across the life course
  – Universal health care.
• Tackle the inequitable distribution of power, money, and resources. This meant
  – A coherent approach to health equity in all policies, systems, and programs
  – Fair financing
  – Market responsibility, especially by the private sector
  – Gender equity
  – Political empowerment through inclusion and voice
  – Good global governance.
• Measure and understand the problem, and assess the impact of action. This recommendation refers to the need to responsibly measure the impact of the various policy interventions.

In an earlier list, Wilkinson and Marmot (2003) similarly identified the social determinants in a more streamlined fashion, which were

- The social gradient (in general, the lower an individual's socioeconomic position, the worse their health—it runs from top to bottom of the socioeconomic spectrum)
- Stress
- Early life
- Social exclusion
- Work
- Unemployment
- Social support
- Addiction
- Food
- Transport.

From even a cursory reading of the foregoing list, it is evident why the Departments of Transportation, Labor, Housing, Commerce, and Treasury are important to health policy. Virchow's statement quoted at the beginning of this chapter, that "medicine is a social science, and politics is nothing more than medicine on a large scale," was prescient and is now substantiated by a significant body of empirical data. Virtually all policies have an impact on health, according to the social determinants of health approach to health and well-being. The more profoundly the policy affects the lifestyle and course of life of the people and/or the economy, the more profoundly it will affect their health.

Evaluating Health Policy

The making of policy is an ethical act in the political sphere and thus embodies some kind of justice, hopefully for good, but sometimes for bad. For example, economic policies associated with globalization are understood by many to be very good for transnational corporations, including those in the pharmaceutical sector, but those policies also create and maintain significant levels of poverty (Farmer, 2003). Poverty and disease are inextricably linked (Health Poverty Action, n.d.).

In general, the best policies benefit both the few (wealthy) and the many (poor), but many policies are either passed without careful consideration or, if they are considered, they are not systematically considered and are passed with a hope and a prayer. In response to the uncertainty in which many policies are passed, at least three different frameworks have been described that can be used in the policy deliberation process to ensure that policies are ethical and just: the cost-benefit approach, the capabilities approach, and the procedural approach.

The cost-benefit approach (CBA) is straightforward (Sunstein, 2004). To simplify, two columns are drawn, one with risks and one with benefits, and then they are compared. The stronger the benefits are compared to the risks, the better the policy appears to be. In a typical cost-benefit analysis, all risks and rewards are monetized, but in a policy analysis, human, environmental, and other risks and benefits must be considered. One of the controversial aspects of this approach comes into play when its proponents recommend that *all* risks and benefits be monetized, even those, such as quality of life, that seem to be degraded and meaningless when reduced to a dollar value.

The capabilities approach begins with an idea of what it means to have a just policy outcome. It is an outcome that improves the capacity of all participants to flourish both individually and as a sociopolitical group (Nussbaum, 1997, 2000, 2006; Ruger, 2008, 2010; Sen, 1999, 2009). This approach shares an important feature with the procedural approach in that all stakeholders are consulted. In the capabilities approach, the stakeholders prioritize the intended outcome and adjust the policies with that in mind, using the rules and tools (including a cost-benefit analysis) that make sense.

In the procedural approach, the stakeholders are not concerned with the outcome directly; rather they use a predetermined framework of rules and benchmarks to guide their policy decisions, understanding that justice will best be served if just procedures are followed (Daniels, 2006, 2008; Daniels et al., 2000). CBA is a kind of procedural approach, but not a strong one because it is created without the formal involvement of the stakeholders and the resulting political deliberations that must occur when they participate. Rather, CBA is an approach in which economic scientists (i.e., technocrats) produce the analysis.

An emerging trend in health policy analysis is the use of empirical methods to evaluate whether the policy or law achieved its ends (Mello & Parmet, 2013). It is referred to as *public health law research* (PHLR). PHLR is the scientific study of the relation of law and legal practices to population health. It consists of (Mello & Parmet, 2013)

- Policy-making studies, which seek to identify factors that influence the adoption of public health legal interventions
- Mapping studies, which employ systematic and rigorous methods of review and characterization to determine the current state of the law on an issue relevant to population health
- Implementation studies, which examine the gap, if any, between the "law on the books" and the law on the ground
- Intervention studies, which examine the effect of law on health outcomes or proximal factors
- Mechanism studies, which examine the means by which legal interventions influence health.

The following section will illustrate the use of one policy approach to address breast cancer disparities in the United States and will then follow with a discussion of the procedural approach outlined by Daniels et al. (2000) to frame related policy recommendations.

Cancer and the Social Determinants

The Case of Breast Cancer

Breast cancer is the most commonly diagnosed cancer among women of all races and Hispanic ethnicities in the United States, except for some skin cancers (CDC, 2014a). It also represents the leading cause of cancer death among Hispanic women and the second leading cause of cancer death among White, Black, Asian/Native Hawaiian/Pacific Islander, and American Indian/Alaska Native women (CDC, 2014a). In 2011, an estimated 220,097 women in the United States were diagnosed with breast cancer, and 40,931 women died from the disease in the same year (CDC, 2014a). In 2000, an estimated $7 billion was spent on the treatment of breast cancer in the United States (Brown, Lipscomb, & Snyder, 2001). In 2014, that number jumped to $19 billion according to NCI (n.d.).

When breast cancer is found in the early stages, the five-year survival rate is as high as 90%. The five-year survival rate for women with advanced (stage IV) breast cancer drops to 15% (American Cancer Society, 2013). The most effective method for early detection of breast cancer is mammography, which is associated with reductions of breast cancer mortality and is most effective when women undergo regular screenings (CDC, 2012; NCI, 2014). According to current U.S. Preventive Services Task Force guidelines, women should receive screening mammography every two years beginning at age 50 and continuing until age 74 (U.S. Preventive Services Task Force, 2013). Although recommended breast cancer screening guidelines have become somewhat controversial in recent years, studies demonstrate that timely mammography can reduce breast cancer mortality by approximately 20%–25% during a period of 10 years (CDC, 2008). For certain racial and ethnic minorities and women who are uninsured or covered by Medicaid, however, mammography screening rates are disproportionately low. These disparities in mammography screening between socially disadvantaged and socially advantaged women in the United States are associated with wide gaps in breast cancer outcomes (Hunt, Whitman, & Hurlbert, 2014; Peek & Han, 2004).

Targeting Breast Cancer Disparities Through Legislative Action

National Breast and Cervical Cancer Early Detection Program

In an effort to address disparities in cancer outcomes among low-income, uninsured, and underserved women, Congress authorized the National Breast and Cervical Cancer Early Detection Program (NBCCEDP) in 1990, a public health program to be administered by CDC to help socially disadvantaged women gain access to screening services for the early detection of breast and cervical cancers (Ryerson, Benard, & Major, 2004). To be eligible for breast screening services through NBCCEDP, women must be 40–64 years of age, uninsured or underinsured, with a household income at or below 250% of the federal poverty level (FPL) (CDC, 2014b). Approximately 9% of women in the United States are eligible for NBCCEDP breast cancer screening services (CDC, 2014b). NBCCEDP initiatives also focus on outreach efforts to serve women in high-priority populations, including older women, racial and ethnic minorities, foreign-born women, women with disabilities, lesbians, and women living in rural areas. Congress initially appropriated $30 million in 1991 to fund efforts by the first eight states to establish early detection programs and added a capacity building program in 1992 to fund an additional 18 states to develop the infrastructure necessary to deliver screening programs (Ryerson et al., 2004).

Despite the potential benefits of the NBCCEDP, a clear policy gap soon became apparent. Although program providers received reimbursement for most diagnostic procedures, including diagnostic mammography, breast ultrasound, fine-needle aspiration of the breast, and breast biopsies, the legislation prohibited use of federal program funds for any part of treatment, based on the rationale that payment for treatment services would rapidly deplete resources available for screening services (Lawson, Henson, Bobo, & Kaeser, 2000). Instead, NBCCEDP-sponsored programs were required to identify and secure resources for treatment from other sources. This strategy, however, was considered to be resource intensive and to diminish the effectiveness of screening activities, according to some stakeholders involved with program implementation (Lawson et al., 2000).

In 1999, CDC received increased congressional appropriations to expand case-management activities to assist women in overcoming financial, logistical, and other barriers to obtaining these services (Lawson et al., 2000). A year later, Congress expanded the scope of the program by passing the Breast and Cervical Cancer Prevention and Treatment Act, which granted states the option to offer women in the NBCCEDP access to treatment through Medicaid (Ryerson et al., 2004). In 2001, Congress clarified that this option also applied to American Indians/Alaska Natives eligible for health services provided by the Indian Health Service or by a tribal organization with passage of the Native American Breast and Cervical Cancer Treatment Technical Amendment Act (Ryerson et al., 2004). All 50 states and the District of Columbia approved the Medicaid option. NBCCEDP-sponsored programs are implemented through cooperative agreements with state and territorial health departments, tribes, and tribal organizations (grantees), with 60% of federal funds designated for provision of direct services to women and 40% designated to support program management, public and provider education, quality assurance, and surveillance and other evaluation activities (Ryerson et al., 2004). Direct services include clinical breast examinations, screening mammograms, diagnostic testing for women whose screening outcome is abnormal, surgical consultations, and referrals to treatment (CDC, 2014b). The NBCCEDP, however, is still considered a payer of last resort—

program funds are not permitted when other coverage is available through any state, private health insurance, or other government health benefits program such as Medicaid or Medicare. In addition, grantees must contribute $1 for every $3 of federal funds. Grantees contract with provider agencies, including federally qualified health centers and community health centers, to deliver screening and other services. From 2008 to 2013, nearly 1.1 million women received an NBCCEDP-funded mammogram, and nearly 18,000 breast cancers were diagnosed (CDC, 2013b).

Trends in Breast Cancer Screening and Mortality Post NBCCEDP Implementation

From 1990 to 2010, the crude percentage of women aged 40 or older who reported receiving a mammogram within the past two years increased from 51.4% to 61.7%. During this period, the greatest increase occurred among American Indian/Alaska Native women (from 43.2% in 1990 to 71.2% in 2010), followed by Black women (from 46.4% in 1990 to 67.9% in 2010), Hispanic women (from 45.2% in 1990 to 64.2% in 2010), and Asian women (from 46% in 1990 to 62.4% in 2010) (see Figure 9-1). The screening

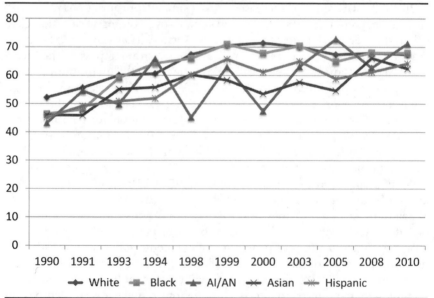

Figure 9-1. Crude Percentage of U.S. Women Aged 40+ Having a Mammogram Within the Past Two Years by Race/Ethnicity, 1990–2010 (Selected Years)

AI/AN—American Indian/Alaska Native

Note. Based on information from National Center for Health Statistics, 2013a.

rate in White women, who had the highest reported mammography rates in 1990, increased from 52.2% in 1990 to 67.4% in 2010. Mammography rates among low-income women also increased from 1990 to 2010, but rates were persistently higher for women with the highest incomes (see Figure 9-2). For example, for women with annual household incomes that were less than 100% of the FPL, mammography rates increased from 30.8% in 1990 to 51.4% in 2010, a net gain of 20.6%. Although mammography rate increases were more modest among women with household incomes that were 400% or more of the FPL (increase of 9.2% from 1990 to 2010), these women still reported mammography rates of 78.1% in 2010, nearly 27% higher than women in the lowest household income group. A similar trend was observed based on insurance status. From 1990 to 2010, mammography rates among women with Medicaid coverage increased from 51.9% to 61.4%, but were still much lower than privately insured women in 2010 (75.6%) (see Figure 9-3). Mammography rates were lowest and remained virtually unchanged among uninsured women (36% in 1990 and in 2010) (National Center for Health Statistics, 2013a).

Despite significant increases in mammography rates from 1990 to 2010, age-adjusted mortality rates remained relatively flat for all except White

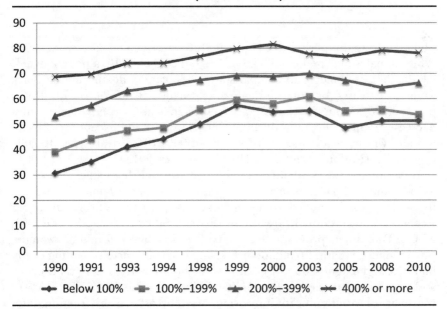

Figure 9-2. Crude Percentage of U.S. Women Aged 40+ Having a Mammogram Within the Past Two Years by Federal Poverty Level, 1990–2010 (Selected Years)

Note. Based on information from National Center for Health Statistics, 2013a.

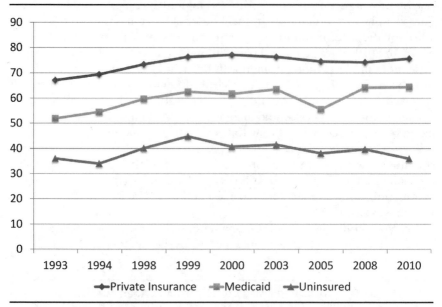

Figure 9-3. Crude Percentage of U.S. Women Aged 40+ Having a Mammogram Within the Past Two Years by Insurance Status, 1993–2010 (Selected Years)

Note. Based on information from National Center for Health Statistics, 2013a.

women during this period (see Figure 9-4). Breast cancer deaths per 100,000 White females declined from 35.9 in 1990 to 27.3 in 2010, a net change of 8.6 deaths per 100,000. In comparison, breast cancer deaths among Black women decreased by only 1.5 deaths per 100,000 (from 29 to 27.5 deaths per 100,000). Women of other races/ethnicities also experienced modest decreases in mortality rates during this period, with the exception of Asian women, whose death rates increased from 9.3 to 10.8 deaths per 100,000 population (National Center for Health Statistics, 2013a).

In summary, the NBCCEDP, established through legislative action, engaged multilevel partners in addressing the defined policy objective of helping socially disadvantaged women gain access to breast and cervical cancer screening and, eventually, treatment services. Since its inception in 1991, NBCCEDP-funded programs have served more than 4.6 million women, provided more than 11.6 million breast and cervical cancer screening examinations, and diagnosed more than 235,000 breast cancers, cervical cancers, and premalignant cervical lesions (CDC, 2014b). The NBCCEDP is clearly associated with significant improvements in breast cancer screening rates among racial and ethnic minority, low-income, and underinsured women.

The program, however, appears to have had little impact on overall breast cancer mortality for racial and ethnic groups other than White women.

Discussion and Future Directions

Although the NBCCEDP should be considered a major step forward in addressing cancer disparities, the program also represents an example of how legislative focus on a single metric defined by health system experts (in this case, mammography services) may not be sufficient to address the full spectrum of factors from the individual's sociopolitical environment that determine health.

However, as the benchmarks are applied, it becomes clear that in the same way a single-metric approach has unfortunate and incapacitating inefficiencies, focusing on a single disease suffers from the same problems. Rather, a comprehensive policy approach will produce widespread sociopolitical changes that have a general effect on improving population health. It is only after the general causes of illness patterns have been ameliorated

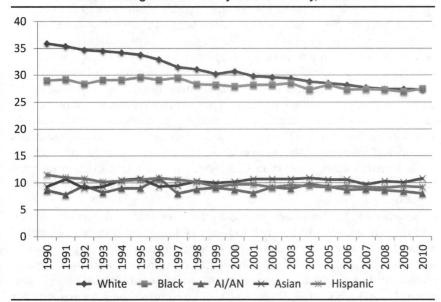

Figure 9-4. Age-Adjusted Mortality Rates for Malignant Neoplasm of the Breast Among U.S. Women by Race/Ethnicity, 1990–2010

— White — Black — AI/AN — Asian — Hispanic

AI/AN—American Indian/Alaska Native

Note. Based on information from National Center for Health Statistics, 2013a.

by the application of broad policies that remaining, if not residual, causes of disease (e.g., breast cancer) can be identified and appropriate interventions designed. Unfortunately, a full-bore policy approach is unlikely to be instituted in the United States because of the deep distrust in the American polity of the government, thus leaving health workers with an inherently inadequate set of tools for improving population health. The best that can be done, we think, is that health workers must never forget the primacy and fundamental importance of the policy approach. While designing and advocating for interventions, health workers must always place them in the broadest policy context possible using either the capabilities or the procedural frameworks.

Ultimately, policy goals are determined by the way the country sees itself in the context of its unique history. The United States, when compared to, for example, the United Kingdom and Germany, is more interested in providing liberty to its citizens then equality (Jasanoff, 2005). In both the United Kingdom and Germany, structures are in place at the highest levels of policy making that ensure, among other things, that citizens are not treated merely as consumers. When a population is made up primarily of consumers, then an important policy goal is the support of the private sector corporations that produce goods for the consumers to consume. Because corporations are driven by the profit motive, in such a system, the profit motive determines the lifestyles of the population, and the value of the population as citizens is degraded. This meta-ordering of policy goals in the United States is unavoidable and creates an ongoing tension between the "liberals" (who seek greater equality) and "conservatives" (who seek greater liberty) because it results in the institutionalization of some of the inequities and disparities that create disease.

We now will use the nine benchmarks developed by Daniels et al. (2000) to suggest policy approaches that will better address disparities in breast cancer and cancer disparities in general. Daniels' criteria were primarily designed for undeveloped countries, and it is for that reason we think they are salutary for the United States. The U.S. healthcare system is systematically problematic, and ad hoc fixes, while politically prudent, will not resolve its widespread inequities. Also, we are using Daniels' procedural approach because it makes more sense than CBA, which would justify existing inequalities, and it is more developed as a practical matter than any version of the capabilities approach.

Benchmark 1. The policy should be intersectoral. This benchmark establishes the general framework for approaching health disparities within a population. It calls for the creation of an appropriately stratified baseline assessment of the distribution of basic nutrition, decent housing, freedom from environmental causes, exposure to education and health literacy, and safety. It also calls for the development of an information infrastructure for ongoing monitoring of the changes in the baseline, and for the inclusion of local, regional, and national inputs, along with those of vulnerable groups.

An example of this is the National Health and Nutrition Examination Survey (NHANES). It is a program of the National Center for Health Statistics to assess the health and nutritional status of American adults and children through a combination of surveys and physical examinations (National Center for Health Statistics, 2013b). Nonetheless, NHANES is just a beginning, and there remains a need to enhance the collection of data on racial and ethnic minorities, such as expanding NCI's Surveillance, Epidemiology, and End Results Program to include underrepresented populations with differential cancer rates. The Patient Protection and Affordable Care Act of 2010 (ACA) goes a long way in addressing this through its mandates for new standards for collection of data related to race, ethnicity, sex, primary language, and disability status (Dorsey & Graham, 2011; Dorsey et al., 2014).

Benchmark 2. The policy should remove financial barriers to equitable access. A very basic package of health services and goods should be made available to the very poorest, and for those with more resources, policies should be in place to encourage better access. Policies should also make it easier to have adequate health insurance for those with the least income and to reduce corruption.

An example of this is the need to increase federal funding for government programs that provide greater access to cancer screening programs, such as the NBCCEDP. Unfortunately, with the ACA, the thought is that everyone will be covered and such safety net programs will not be needed. However, this is not the case with the large number of individuals who will not be covered by the ACA. This includes 30 million or more individuals who are not citizens or legal residents of the United States and individuals with low incomes who live in states that have elected to opt out of the Medicaid expansion (27 states and Washington, DC, as of December 2014) (Advisory Board Company, 2014; Congressional Budget Office, 2014; Nardin, Zallman, McCormick, Woolhandler, & Himmelstein, 2013).

Benchmark 3. The policy should remove nonfinancial barriers to access. This is another comprehensive sociopolitical group of interventions to reduce geographical maldistribution of health goods; minimize gender-related burdens that function through the family, restriction on access to transportation to providers, limitations on reproductive autonomy, and reduction in services available in poor communities (e.g., closures of family planning clinics or social service office locations); reduce cultural impediments to access and knowledge such as language and community stigmas related to disease and poverty; and reduce discrimination by race, religion, class, sexual orientation, disease, and other stigmas.

An example of this is the unfunded Patient Navigator Outreach and Chronic Disease Prevention Act of 2005, which helps patients—regardless of race, ethnicity, language, or geography—gain access to prevention, screening, and treatment. This act is inherently limited because it applies only to those with insurance, but it is a step in the right direction.

Benchmark 4. The policy should provide comprehensiveness of benefits across levels in the social gradient ("tiering"). The unequal distribution of benefits to different tiers is often based on factors addressed by Benchmarks 2 and 3, and this benchmark is intended to evaluate inequities in distribution more comprehensively, focusing on the idea that every human being has comparable health needs and should be treated the same.

NHANES would be the basis for this kind of evaluation and the design of appropriate responses. However, the fundamental basis for policy design in the United States is liberty, not equality. Thus, if everyone is equal as a consumer (of health care), then the fundamental characteristic of equality has been conferred by the policy, and the fact of deep disparities in the capacity to pay is of secondary concern. Rhetorically, this benchmark informs the periodic national discussions around health sector reform, but as the recent ACA demonstrates, people are still treated as consumers, not holders of some kind of right to health care.

Benchmark 5. The policy should provide for equitable financing. Funding, usually sourced from taxes, insurance premiums, and out-of-pocket payments, should result in a system in which people pay what they can afford, not what the provider can justify charging by market rationales.

The ACA takes steps to implement this policy goal, but because it is structured as reform to the health insurance market, it leaves deep market-driven forces in place that will continue to distort the entire health sector, such as the relatively unrestricted monopolies given to drugs and devices. The recent U.S. Supreme Court case of Myriad Genetics functions toward this policy goal in the court's finding that naturally occurring genes cannot be patented (*Association for Molecular Pathology v. Myriad Genetics,* 2013), casting doubt on the thousands of patents that purportedly cover as much as one-third of the human genome.

Benchmark 6. The policy should result in a system that is efficacious and efficient and provides a good quality of care. This and the following benchmark are focused on the best use of available resources, as the maldistribution of available resources results in inequitable distribution of health benefits. These two benchmarks address distributive justice. This benchmark recommends a principal focus on primary health care, rational use of evidence-based practice, and institutionalized quality improvement measures.

Benchmark 7. The policy should result in administrative efficiency. This standard focuses on ensuring the distribution of health benefits is structured with accountability and transparency measures to avoid excessive administrative overheads, cost shifting, fraud and abuse, and other inefficiencies.

An example here would be to fully implement and fund recommendations of the U.S. Department of Health and Human Services' Trans-HHS

Cancer Health Disparities Progress Review Group, which in 2004 listed 14 priority recommendations for Health and Human Services to take the lead in eliminating the unequal burden of cancer (NCI, 2004; Trans-HHS Cancer Health Disparities Progress Review Group, 2004). Although attempted, it still has not been fully implemented or funded.

Benchmark 8. The policy should result in democratic accountability and empowerment. Democratic accountability can be presumed if there is a significant component of each of the following factors.

- Explicit, public, detailed procedures for evaluating the services with public reports
- Explicit deliberative procedures for stakeholders to make decisions about distribution
- Comprehensive budgeting
- Fair legal and nonlegal grievance procedures
- Adequate privacy protection
- Institutions for enforcing compliance with laws and rules as needed
- Procedures and structures for strengthening civil society

As noted previously, because the private sector is privileged at the highest levels of policy making in the United States, and the highest levels of the health bureaucracy are filled with corporate executives, the possibility and reality of corruption pervades the entire health sector. It manifests in extensive fraud and abuse. It also manifests in widespread problems in the production of unbiased evidence-based knowledge about disease because most knowledge about drugs and devices is produced by the private sector and thus is saddled with quintessential conflicts of interest.

Benchmark 9. The policy should provide for patient and provider autonomy. The other benchmarks are aimed at ensuring that the structural features of the health delivery institutions are fair and ethical. This benchmark assigns value to the individuals whose decisions are most constrained by the other benchmarks and protects them from overly paternalistic structures that erode individual choice in unjust ways.

A beginning might be to formally recognize patient rights at the federal level. There have been numerous attempts to do this, but none have been successful (Law, 2013).

Conclusion

Premature death that is preventable or avoidable is the ultimate health inequity. Sustainable reductions in health inequities will not occur without comprehensive, multilevel strategies that consider the interactions between and among the multiple determinants of health. To achieve sustainable improvements in cancer and other health outcomes for vulnerable populations, health workers must move beyond legislative policies designed to influence specific screening practices or health behaviors to establish policies that will support the infrastructure needed to help individuals and communities flourish.

References

Advisory Board Company. (2014, December 17). Where the states stand on Medicaid expansion: 27 states, D.C. expanding Medicaid. Retrieved from http://www.advisory.com/daily-briefing/resources/primers/medicaidmap

Alliance for the Prudent Use of Antibiotics. (n.d.). Science of resistance: Antibiotics in agriculture. Retrieved from http://www.tufts.edu/med/apua/about_issue/antibiotic_agri.shtml

American Cancer Society. (2013, February 22). Survival rates for breast cancer. Retrieved from http://www.cancer.org/cancer/breastcancer/overviewguide/breast-cancer-overview-survival-rates

Anawalt, B.D., Kirk, S., & Shulman, D. (Eds.). (2013, May). The endocrine system: Factors that affect endocrine function. Retrieved from http://www.hormone.org/hormones-and-health/the-endocrine-system/factors-that-affect-endocrine-function

Association for Molecular Pathology v. Myriad Genetics, No. 12-398, slip op. (U.S. June 13, 2013).

Bakst, D. (2013, September 3). *Government control of your diet: Threats to "freedom to eat"* (Issue Brief No. 4033 on Health Care). Retrieved from http://www.heritage.org/research/reports/2013/09/obamacare-menu-labeling-requirement-government-control-of-your-diet

Brown, M., Lipscomb, J., & Snyder, C. (2001). The burden of illness of cancer: Economic cost and quality of life. *Annual Review of Public Health, 22,* 91–113. doi:10.1146/annurev.publhealth.22.1.91

Centers for Disease Control and Prevention. (2008, August). *Preventing chronic diseases: Investing wisely in health: Screening to prevent cancer deaths.* Retrieved from http://www.cdc.gov/nccdphp/publications/factsheets/prevention/pdf/cancer.pdf

Centers for Disease Control and Prevention. (2012, November 1). Breast cancer screening rates. Retrieved from http://www.cdc.gov/cancer/breast/statistics/screening.htm

Centers for Disease Control and Prevention. (2013a). *Antibiotic resistance threats in the United States, 2013.* Retrieved from http://www.cdc.gov/drugresistance/threat-report-2013/pdf/ar-threats-2013-508.pdf

Centers for Disease Control and Prevention. (2013b). National Breast and Cervical Cancer Early Detection Program (NBCCEDP): National aggregate; five-year summary: January 2008 to December 2012. Retrieved from http://www.cdc.gov/cancer/nbccedp/data/summaries/national_aggregate.htm

Centers for Disease Control and Prevention. (2014a, September 2). Breast cancer statistics. Retrieved from http://www.cdc.gov/cancer/breast/statistics

Centers for Disease Control and Prevention. (2014b). National Breast and Cervical Cancer Early Detection Program (NBCCEDP): About the program. Retrieved from http://www.cdc.gov/cancer/nbccedp/about.htm

Centers for Medicare and Medicaid Services. (n.d.). National health expenditure projections 2012–2022. Retrieved from http://www.cms.gov/Research-Statistics-Data-and-Systems/Statistics-Trends-and-Reports/NationalHealthExpendData/downloads/proj2012.pdf

Colgrove, J. (2002). The McKeown thesis: A historical controversy and its enduring influence. *American Journal of Public Health, 92,* 725–729. Retrieved from http://www.ncbi.nlm.nih.gov/pmc/articles/PMC1447153/pdf/0920725.pdf

Congressional Budget Office. (2014, April). Effects of the Affordable Care Act on health insurance coverage—Baseline projections. Retrieved from http://www.cbo.gov/publication/43900

Daniels, N. (2006). Toward ethical review of health system transformations. *American Journal of Public Health, 96*, 447–451. doi:10.2105/AJPH.2005.065706

Daniels, N. (2008). *Just health: Meeting health needs fairly*. Cambridge, United Kingdom: Cambridge University Press.

Daniels, N., Bryant, J., Castano, R.A., Dantes, O.G., Khan, K.S., & Pannarunothai, S. (2000). Benchmarks of fairness for health care reform: A policy tool for developing countries. *Bulletin of the World Health Organization, 78*, 740–750. Retrieved from http://www.ncbi.nlm.nih.gov/pmc/articles/PMC2560780/pdf/10916911.pdf

Dorsey, R., & Graham, G. (2011). New HHS data standards for race, ethnicity, sex, primary language, and disability status. *JAMA, 306*, 2378–2379. doi:10.1001/jama.2011.1789

Dorsey, R., Graham, G., Glied, S., Meyers, D., Clancy, C., & Koh, H. (2014). Implementing health reform: Improved data collection and the monitoring of health disparities. *Annual Review of Public Health, 35*, 123–138. doi:10.1146/annurev-publhealth-032013-182423

Environmental Working Group. (2013, October 28). Dirty dozen list of endocrine disruptors: 12 hormone-altering chemicals and how to avoid them. Retrieved from http://www.ewg.org/research/dirty-dozen-list-endocrine-disruptors

Farmer, P. (2003). *Pathologies of power: Health, human rights, and the new war on the poor*. Berkeley, CA: University of California Press.

Floud, R., Fogel, R.W., Harris, B., & Hong, S.C. (2011). *The changing body: Health, nutrition, and human development in the western world since 1700*. Cambridge, United Kingdom: Cambridge University Press.

Galdston, I. (Ed.). (1949). *Social medicine: Its derivations and objectives*. New York, NY: Commonwealth Fund.

Gostin, L.O. (2008). *Public health law: Power, duty, restraint* (2nd ed.). Berkeley, CA: University of California Press.

Gostin, L.O. (Ed.). (2010). *Public health law and ethics: A reader* (2nd ed.). Berkeley, CA: University of California Press.

Grad, F.P. (2005). *The public health law manual* (3rd ed.). Washington, DC: American Public Health Association.

Health Poverty Action. (n.d.). Key facts: Poverty and poor health. Retrieved from http://www.healthpovertyaction.org/policy-and-resources/the-cycle-of-poverty-and-poor-health/the-cycle-of-poverty-and-poor-health1

Hunt, P.R., Whitman, S., & Hurlbert, M.S. (2014). Increasing Black:White disparities in breast cancer mortality in the 50 largest cities in the United States. *Cancer Epidemiology, 38*, 118–123. doi:10.1016/j.canep.2013.09.009

Illich, I. (1976). *Limits to medicine: Medical nemesis: The expropriation of health*. London, England: Marion Boyars.

Jasanoff, S. (2005). *Designs on nature: Science and democracy in Europe and the United States*. Princeton, NJ: Princeton University Press.

Kapp, L., & Jansen, D.J. (2009). *The role of the Department of Defense during a flu pandemic* (Congressional Research Service report). Retrieved from http://fas.org/sgp/crs/natsec/R40619.pdf

Kennedy, M. (2008). The second era of bacteriology [Web log post]. Retrieved from http://abriefhistory.org/?p=306

Lalonde, M. (1974). *A new perspective on the health of Canadians*. Ottawa, Ontario, Canada: Government of Canada.

Law, S. (2013). Do we still need a federal patients' bill of rights? *Yale Journal of Health Policy, Law, and Ethics, 3*(1), Article 1. Retrieved from http://digitalcommons.law.yale.edu/yjhple/vol3/iss1/1

Lawson, H.W., Henson, R., Bobo, J.K., & Kaeser, M.K. (2000). Implementing recommendations for the early detection of breast and cervical cancer among low-income women. *MMWR Recommendations and Reports, 49*(RR02), 35–55. Retrieved from http://www.cdc.gov/mmwr/preview/mmwrhtml/rr4902a4.htm

Marmot, M. (2005). Historical perspective: The social determinants of disease—Some blossoms. *Epidemiologic Perspectives and Innovations, 2,* 4. Retrieved from http://www.ncbi.nlm.nih.gov/pmc/articles/PMC1180841

McCarthy, M. (2002). A brief history of the World Health Organization. *Lancet, 360,* 1111–1112. doi:10.1016/S0140-6736(02)11244-X

McKeown, T. (1976a). *The modern rise of population.* New York, NY: Academic Press.

McKeown, T. (1976b). *The role of medicine: Dream, mirage, or nemesis?* London, England: Nuffield Provincial Hospitals Trust.

McKeown, T., & Brown, R.G. (1955). Medical evidence related to English population changes in the eighteenth century. *Population Studies, 9,* 119–141. doi:10.1080/00324728.1955.10404688

McKeown, T., Brown, R.G., & Record, R.G. (1972). An interpretation of the modern rise of population in Europe. *Population Studies, 26,* 345–382. doi:10.1080/00324728.1972.10405908

McKeown, T., & Record, R.G. (1962). Reasons for the decline of mortality in England and Wales during the nineteenth century. *Population Studies, 16,* 94–122. doi:10.1080/0032472 8.1962.10414870

McKeown, T., Record, R.G., & Turner, R.D. (1975). An interpretation of the decline of mortality in England and Wales during the twentieth century. *Population Studies, 29,* 391–422. doi: 10.1080/00324728.1975.10412707

Mello, M.M., & Parmet, W.E. (2013). Public health law research: Editors' introduction. *Journal of Health Politics, Policy and Law, 38,* 629–643. doi:10.1215/03616878-2208558

Nardin, R., Zallman, L., McCormick, D., Woolhandler, S., & Himmelstein, D. (2013, June 6). The uninsured after implementation of the Affordable Care Act: A demographic and geographic analysis. *Health Affairs Blog.* Retrieved from http://healthaffairs.org/blog/2013/06/06/the-uninsured-after-implementation-of-the-affordable-care-act-a-demographic-and-geographic-analysis/

National Cancer Institute. (n.d.). Cancer prevalence and cost of care projections: Graph by cancer site and phase of care. Retrieved from http://costprojections.cancer.gov/graph.php

National Cancer Institute. (2004). Trans-HHS Cancer Health Disparities Progress Review Group: Fact sheet. Retrieved from https://web.archive.org/web/20111015041223/http://www.cancer.gov/newscenter/qa/2004/health-disparities-prgqa

National Cancer Institute. (2009, September). Understanding cancer series. Retrieved from http://www.cancer.gov/cancertopics/understandingcancer/cancer/AllPages

National Cancer Institute. (2014, March 25). Factsheet: Mammograms. Retrieved from http://www.cancer.gov/cancertopics/factsheet/detection/mammograms

National Center for Health Statistics. (2013a). *Health, United States, 2012: With special feature on emergency care.* Retrieved from http://www.cdc.gov/nchs/data/hus/hus12.pdf

National Center for Health Statistics. (2013b). *National Health and Nutrition Examination Survey,* 2013–2014. Retrieved from http://www.cdc.gov/nchs/data/nhanes/nhanes_13_14/2013-14_overview_brochure.pdf

National Institutes of Health Office of Budget. (2013). Overview of FY 2014 President's budget. Retrieved from http://officeofbudget.od.nih.gov/br.html

Navarro, V. (2009). History of the social determinants of health: Global histories, contemporary debates [Review]. *Bulletin of the History of Medicine, 83,* 620–622. doi:10.1353/bhm.0.0261

Nussbaum, M.C. (1997). Capabilities and human rights. *Fordham Law Review, 66,* 273–300. Retrieved from http://ir.lawnet.fordham.edu/flr/vol66/iss2/2

Nussbaum, M.C. (2000). *Women and human development: The capabilities approach* [The Seeley Lectures (No. 3)]. Cambridge, United Kingdom: Cambridge University Press. doi:10.1017/CBO9780511841286

Nussbaum, M.C. (2006). *Frontiers of justice: Disability, nationality, species membership.* Cambridge, MA: Belknap Press.

Parr, B.B. (2009). Hormonal responses to exercise [Presentation]. In S.K. Powers & E.T. Howley (Eds.), *Exercise physiology: Theory and application to fitness and performance* (7th ed.). New York, NY: McGraw-Hill.

Patient Navigator Outreach and Chronic Disease Prevention Act of 2005, Pub. L. 109-18, 119 Stat. 340.

Patient Protection and Affordable Care Act, Pub. L. 111-148, 124 Stat. 119 (2010).

Peek, M.E., & Han, J.H. (2004). Disparities in screening mammography: Current status, interventions and implications. *Journal of General Internal Medicine, 19,* 184–194. Retrieved from http://www.ncbi.nlm.nih.gov/pmc/articles/PMC1492136/pdf/jgi_30254.pdf

Rosen, G. (1993). *A history of public health.* Baltimore, MD: Johns Hopkins University Press.

Ruger, J.P. (2008). Normative foundations of global health law. *Georgetown Law Journal, 96,* 423–443. Retrieved from http://georgetownlawjournal.org/files/pdf/96-2/PrahRuger.PDF

Ruger, J.P. (2010). Health capability: Conceptualization and operationalization. *American Journal of Public Health, 100,* 41–49. Retrieved from http://www.ncbi.nlm.nih.gov/pmc/articles/PMC2791246/pdf/41.pdf

Ryerson, A.B., Benard, V.B., & Major, A.C. (2004). *National Breast and Cervical Cancer Early Detection Program: 1991–2002 national report.* Retrieved from http://www.cdc.gov/cancer/nbccedp/pdf/national_report.pdf

Sen, A. (1999). *Development as freedom.* New York, NY: Anchor Books.

Sen, A. (2009). *The idea of justice.* Cambridge, MA: Belknap Press.

Silver, R. (1992). Environmental factors influencing hormone secretion. In J.B. Becker, S.M. Breedlove, & D. Crews (Eds.), *Behavioral endocrinology* (pp. 401–422). Cambridge, MA: MIT Press.

Starr, P. (1982). *The social transformation of American medicine.* New York, NY: Basic Books.

Sunstein, C.R. (2004). *Risk and reason: Safety, law, and the environment.* Cambridge, United Kingdom: Cambridge University Press.

Susser, M. (1966). Teaching social medicine in the United States. *Milbank Memorial Fund Quarterly, 44,* 389–413. doi:10.2307/3348994

Susser, M. (1973). *Causal thinking in the health sciences: Concepts and strategies of epidemiology.* New York, NY: Oxford University Press.

Syme, S.L. (2005). Historical perspective: The social determinants of disease—Some roots of the movement. *Epidemiologic Perspectives and Innovations, 2,* 2. Retrieved from http://www.ncbi.nlm.nih.gov/pmc/articles/PMC1087863

Thiel, M.J. (n.d.). Factors affecting estrogen levels. Retrieved from http://www.melissathielmd.com/Documents/EduMeno/Factors%20Affecting%20Estrogen%20Levels.pdf

Trans-HHS Cancer Health Disparities Progress Review Group. (2004). *Making cancer health disparities history.* Retrieved from http://planning.cancer.gov/library/2004chdprg.pdf

U.S. Department of Health and Human Services. (2014). *Fiscal year 2014 budget in brief: Strengthening health and opportunity for all Americans.* Retrieved from http://www.hhs.gov/budget/fy2014/fy-2014-budget-in-brief.pdf

U.S. Preventive Services Task Force. (2013, September). Recommendation summary: Breast cancer: Screening. Retrieved from http://www.uspreventiveservicestaskforce.org/uspstf/uspsbrca.htm

Wanjek, C. (2012, July 27). Your diet affects your grandchildren's DNA, scientists say. Retrieved from http://www.livescience.com/21902-diet-epigenetics-grandchildren.html

Wilkinson, R., & Marmot, M. (Eds.). (2003). *The social determinants of health: The solid facts* (2nd ed.). Retrieved from http://www.euro.who.int/__data/assets/pdf_file/0005/98438/e81384.pdf

World Health Organization Commission on Social Determinants of Health. (2008). *Closing the gap in a generation: Health equity through action on the social determinants of health. Final report*

of the Commission on Social Determinants of Health. Retrieved from http://www.who.int/social
_determinants/thecommission/finalreport/en

Zola, I.K. (1972). Medicine as an institution of social control. *Sociological Review, 20,* 487–504.
doi:10.1111/j.1467-954X.1972.tb00220.x

CHAPTER **10**

Latinos and Cancer

Guadalupe Palos, DrPH, LMSW, RN

Introduction

Policies related to cancer and public health in the United States will be markedly influenced by the projected growth in its Latino population (Humes, Jones, & Ramirez, 2011; Taylor, Lopez, Martínez, & Velasco, 2012; U.S. Census Bureau, 2014). Significant changes in America's demographic composition, the accelerating advances in the science of cancer medicine, and legislative public health policies are rapidly transforming health care. These changes reflect the urgent need for oncology nurses, other providers, policy makers, researchers, survivors, and the general public to better understand their impact across the cancer continuum. Another factor that will have a profound influence on these changes is the fact that Latinos continue to experience a disproportionate burden of cancer risk, incidence, mortality, and poor outcomes (Byrd & Clayton, 2003; DuBard & Gizlice, 2008; Elk et al., 2012; Fenelon, 2013; Morales, Lara, Kington, Valdez, & Escarce, 2002; Smedley, Stith, & Nelson, 2003; Villa, Wallace, Bagdasaryan, & Aranda, 2012). Research shows that despite the tremendous advances made in cancer oncology, Latinos are less likely to have insurance, a regular source of care, and access to high-quality cancer care (DuBard & Gizlice; 2008; Morales et al., 2002; Vega, Rodriguez, & Gruskin, 2009). Factors intensifying Latinos' disparities are related to challenges in the collection and analysis of epidemiologic data, socioeconomic and sociocultural determinants, and health policies (see Figure 10-1). Ample evidence supports the challenges of data collection and analysis related to Latinos (Reuben, Milliken, & Paradis, 2011) and the contributions of patient, provider, and health system factors to the unequal burden of cancer in Latinos. To date, however, limited published evidence exists examining how U.S. public healthcare policies and political views advance or prevent disparities in the care of Latino patients with cancer and their families. Based on estimates from the U.S. Census Bu-

---

Figure 10-1. Factors Affecting Health Care and Cancer for U.S. Latinos

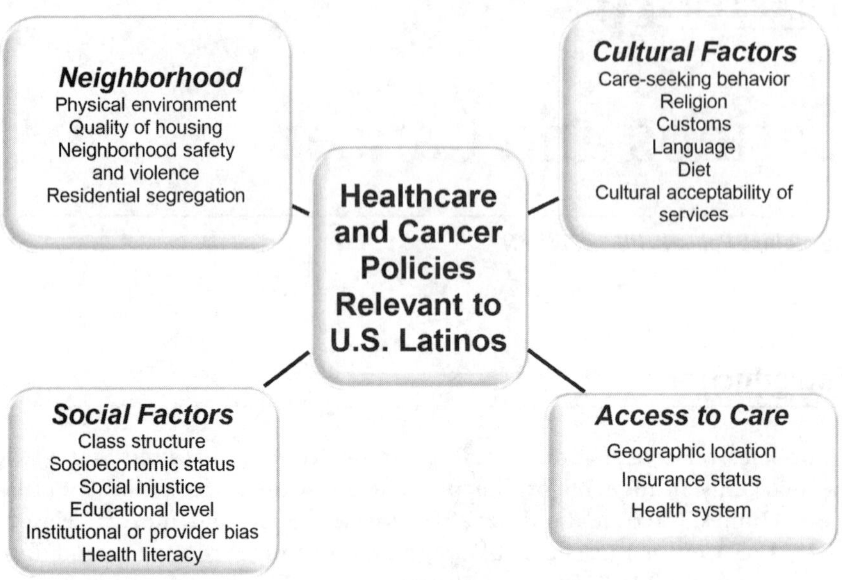

Neighborhood
Physical environment
Quality of housing
Neighborhood safety
and violence
Residential segregation

Cultural Factors
Care-seeking behavior
Religion
Customs
Language
Diet
Cultural acceptability of
services

**Healthcare
and Cancer
Policies
Relevant to
U.S. Latinos**

Social Factors
Class structure
Socioeconomic status
Social injustice
Educational level
Institutional or provider bias
Health literacy

Access to Care
Geographic location
Insurance status
Health system

---

reau, in 2013, 17% of the total population in America was of Hispanic origin (U.S. Census Bureau, 2014). Demographic trends indicate that by 2050, 30% of the U.S. population will be classified as being Latino/Hispanic (Motel & Patten, 2012). Interestingly, this population is the largest foreign-born ethnic group, with more than 50% of its population having non-U.S. nativity. The projected increase in America's Latino population, in addition to the inequalities in their cancer care, signify that oncology nurses need to better understand the role of health policy in the care of Latino patients with cancer.

Professional organizations such as the Oncology Nursing Society (ONS), American Nurses Association (ANA), American Society of Clinical Oncology (ASCO), and American Public Health Association (APHA) also recognize the significant impact that public health policies, both in and outside the cancer purview, have on Americans' health and risk for disparities in access. In 2009, ASCO published a policy statement outlining a plan to guarantee equal access to quality cancer care (Goss et al., 2009). Similarly, APHA (n.d.) has supported policies to reduce disparities in health care. In addition, the ANA House of Delegates reasserted that "health is a basic human right" (p. 1) and all people living in the United States should have access to that right (ANA, 2010). Two strategic resolutions, which also emerged from the assembly, posited that ANA (a) "speak for nurses collectively in shaping health care" in the United States, and (b) "address health policies that affect accessibility, quality, cost, and the violation of human rights" (ANA, 2010, pp. 6–7). ONS stated similar views in its health policy agenda for the 113th Congress, second session, which encouraged President Obama and Congress to ensure access to quality cancer prevention and care (ONS, 2014). In addition, the ONS agenda advocated for comprehensive health reform legislation that would ensure access to health insurance coverage and action to address health disparities and access challenges for at-risk and underserved populations. An example of such legislation is the Patient Protection and Affordable Care Act of 2010, known as the ACA, whose purpose is to provide adequate health care to a greater number of U.S. citizens. This healthcare reform act has contributed to unanticipated consequences on cancer care. For example, a recent study found that some individuals enrolled in Medicaid may not have access to preventive cancer care services such as mammograms or colonoscopies. The investigators suggest that this gap may occur because some states do not cover preventive services and the vague language of the ACA contributes to misunderstanding as to which services are covered by the Medicaid program (Wilensky & Gray, 2013). It is certain that all healthcare professionals will encounter change in their oncology care and practice as a result of current payment and healthcare reform. Therefore, consumers, healthcare professionals, and policy makers will benefit if they are proactive and learn how the nation's governmental bodies influence the implementation of health policies, particularly in regard to medically underserved groups such as Latinos.

This chapter will address how U.S. Latino patients with cancer and their families are affected by healthcare policies related to access to and delivery of high-quality cancer care. First, the diverse demographic, sociocultural, and socioeconomic determinants shown to contribute to cancer disparities among Latinos will be reviewed. Next, the chapter will discuss the challenges in collecting and analyzing epidemiologic data required to make appropriate policy recommendations for allocation of financial resources and delivery of program services. This chapter also will describe past, current, and future policies and legislative actions that affect cancer care for Latinos across the disease trajectory. Finally, the latter part of the chapter will discuss the implications of current healthcare reform on future oncology nursing practice, education, and research.

Self-Report of Latinos' Ethnicity and Race

As defined by the Office of Management and Budget (1997), the terms *Latino* and *Hispanic* will be used interchangeably throughout this chapter.

Debate exists as to which is the politically correct term to use. Four factors determine which term is preferred, including attitudes toward government labels, country of origin, generational status, and geographic location (Taylor et al., 2012). Although the U.S. Census Bureau has been using the term *Hispanic* for more than four decades and the term *Latino* for almost 15 years, a large majority of Latinos do not support the terms to describe their ethnicity. Similar attitudes have been identified regarding the terms *Chicano, Spanish, Latin,* or *Latin American*—many Latinos believe these terms often are inadequately defined, poorly understood, and often not used at all (Motel & Patten, 2012; Taylor et al., 2012).

The Pew Hispanic Center conducted a nationwide survey to identify Latinos' preferences for reporting their ethnicity and race (Motel & Patten, 2012). Interestingly, the researchers found that the majority (51%) preferred to use their family's country of origin to self-identify their ethnicity (e.g., Mexican American, Cuban, Dominican). Twenty-four percent preferred Latino or Hispanic; 21% preferred pan-ethnic terms such as American; and some did not know or care to use any self-descriptor (4%) (Taylor et al., 2012). The Pew survey also noted that generational differences affected one's personal preference for which term to use. This study found that first- and second-generation individuals used their country of origin to describe their ethnicity, whereas third- and later-generation Latinos chose the term *American.* The geographic diversity of Latinos contributes to preferences in how to describe their ethnicity (Hispanic vs. non-Hispanic), race (Black, White, mixed), and country of origin (more than 20 countries) (Humes et al., 2011; Motel & Patten, 2012). Other elements contributing to preferences on self-identifying include worldviews, cultural values, and degree of acculturation, incorporation, or enculturation. Table 10-1 summarizes definitions of these and other key concepts to explain how they are used in this chapter.

Demographic and Social Determinants of Latinos

Despite the current and projected increase in the U.S. Latino population, oncology nurses and other healthcare providers may not understand how the demographic heterogeneity of Latinos shapes cancer and public health policies. Policy makers recognize that the popularity of a target population or social group can influence the opportunity and type of governmental actions related to public policies (Oliver, 2006). In fact, Schneider and Ingram, political scientists, believe it is critical to understand the "cultural characterizations or popular images of the persons or groups whose behavior and well-being are affected by public policy" (Schneider & Ingram, 1993, p. 334). These researchers also point out that the social, cultural, and economic determinants of a specific group affect both the policy's intention and the overall policy agenda. The implications of this perspective on health policy relevant to Latinos' cancer care will be further discussed later in this chapter. To assist oncology nurses to better understand the social construction of this target popula-

Table 10-1. Definitions Related to Health and Cancer Policy and U.S. Latinos

Term	Definition
Ancestry	Refers to a person's ethnic roots, heritage, or the place of birth of the person's parents or ancestors before coming to the United States (U.S. Census Bureau, 2012)
Culture	Serves as the blueprint or tool kit for living life, solving problems, and informing decisions; provides meaning for being (Singer, 2012)
Ethnicity	A shared culture and way of life especially reflected in language, folkways, religious and institutional forms; material culture such as clothing and food; and cultural products such as music, literature, and art (Smedley et al., 2003)
First-generation/ foreign-born immigrant	Refers to foreign-born people or those outside the United States born to parents who are not U.S. citizens; terms used interchangeably (Taylor et al., 2012)
Hispanic or Latino	A person of Cuban, Mexican, Puerto Rican, South or Central American, or other Spanish culture or origin, regardless of race. The term "Spanish origin" can be used in addition to "Hispanic or Latino" (Office of Management and Budget, 1997).
Origin	Viewed as the heritage, nationality, or country of birth of the person or the person's ancestors before arriving in the United States (Humes et al., 2011)
Race	Refers to a social definition of race recognized in this country. It is not meant to define race biologically, anthropologically, or genetically. The Office of Management and Budget mandates five groups: White; Black or African American; American Indian or Alaska Native; Asian; and Native Hawaiian or other Pacific Islander (U.S. Census Bureau, 2013).
Second generation	Describes a person born in the United States, with at least one first-generation parent (Taylor et al., 2012)
Third or higher generation	Describes a person born in the United States and whose parents were both born in the United States (Taylor et al., 2012)
U.S. or native born	Describes a person born in the United States or a person born in another country but with at least one parent who is a U.S. citizen (Taylor et al., 2012)

tion—Latinos—the following section will discuss demographic, cultural, and social characteristics.

Demographic Profile of U.S. Latinos

Current population projections estimate by 2050, 30% of the U.S. population will be classified as Latinos, with 82% of that increase due to immigrants arriving after 2005 and the births of their U.S.-born descendants (Passel & Cohn, 2008). The vast diversity of the U.S. Latino population is due to the numerous subethnic groups originating from Mexico, Central America, South America, and the Caribbean Islands (Motel & Patten, 2012). In 2010, 92% of Latinos originated from 10 countries with wide differences among the groups in terms of demographic, cultural, economic, and health profiles. The countries of origin with the highest populations in the United States were Mexico, Puerto Rico, Cuba, and El Salvador. Not surprisingly, marked differences were noted in the social determinants in individuals from these four countries (Byrd & Clayton, 2003; Motel & Patten, 2012). For example, Puerto Ricans had the highest rates of English proficiency (82%), followed by Mexicans (64%), Cubans (58%), and Salvadorans (46%). Median age, poverty level, and insurance status also varied among the groups (Motel & Patten, 2012). For example, Mexican Americans were less educated and had a greater risk of living below the poverty level compared to Cubans. In addition, Central and South American groups were better educated and less likely to live in poverty. Determinants of the Puerto Rican population, although not an immigrant population, were similar to those of Mexican Americans (Motel & Patten, 2012).

In general, Latinos are primarily a young population, of immigrant background, live below the poverty level, and often have no to limited insurance coverage. According to the U.S. Census, unemployment among Latinos is more likely to be higher than in White, non-Hispanics but lower than in African Americans (Motel & Patten, 2012; U.S. Census Bureau, 2014). Latinos are employed in greater proportion in lower status occupations such as laborers, service workers, and production employees (Humes et al., 2011; Motel & Patten, 2012). Because of Latinos' wide geographic diversity in their countries of origin, this population has consistently reported different levels of ethnic and racial admixture across several U.S. Census reports. Consequently, Latinos are more likely to identify themselves as a mixed race or as being a White or Black Latino. This genomic and genetic diversity of Latinos also contributes to differences in skin color, cancer risk, and self-identification.

Latinos or Hispanics often are regarded as one ethnic group with similar demographic characteristics. These definitions do not make clear distinctions among the multiple subethnic groups of the Latino population. This perspective is evident in the lack of health indicators, epidemiologic data, and evidence-based research in subethnic Latino groups. This "one group fits all" approach restricts the reliability and availability of epidemiologic data and also often contributes to stereotyping, biases, and racism toward Latinos (Reuben et al., 2011). For instance, accurate morbidity and mortality data are lacking, which limits the ability to calculate reliable life expectancies for Latinos. Another factor contributing to the inability to accurately calculate life expectancies is the underreporting of Latino origin on death certificates (Reuben et al., 2011). Nurses can better advocate for relevant cancer policies if they understand the influence of demographic trends and nuances in the Latino population.

Cancer Epidemiology in Latinos

Evidence suggests that Latinos face a disproportionate burden of higher incidence and mortality rates for specific cancers (American Cancer Society, 2012; Vega et al., 2009). A combination of multiple, complex factors contributes to Latinos' epidemiologic trends, primarily associated with behavior (i.e., lower participation in cancer screening programs), environment (i.e., occupational exposures), migration patterns (i.e., different countries of origin), and generational level (i.e., first–third generation). Other factors include cultural attitudes toward cancer, late stage at diagnosis and treatment, and untimely follow-up for continuity of care.

Table 10-2 lists the top four cancers with higher incidence and mortality rates among Latino men and women. In general, Latinos have higher incidence rates than non-Hispanic Whites for cervical, gallbladder, gastric, and liver cancer. Cancers with high mortality rates in Latinos include gastric, cervical, gallbladder, liver, and thyroid cancer. Interestingly, death rates in Latinos exceeded those of non-Hispanic Whites by 50% for four cancers: acute lymphocytic leukemia, and cervical, gastric, and liver cancer (Ameri-

Table 10-2. Cancers With Highest Incidence and Mortality Among Latinos, 2012 Estimates

Indicator	Males	Females
Incidence (new cases)	Prostate Colon and rectum Lung and bronchus Kidney	Breast Thyroid Lung and bronchus Uterine corpus
Mortality (deaths)	Lung and bronchus Colon and rectum Liver and intrahepatic bile duct Prostate	Breast Lung and bronchus Colon and rectum Pancreas

Note. Based on information from American Cancer Society, 2012; ThisNation.com, n.d.

can Cancer Society, 2012; Haile et al., 2012). It is important to note that statistics are reported collectively for Latinos and do not address the wide heterogeneity in cancer rates for Latino subgroups. Some empirical evidence has suggested that Latinos have better health outcomes despite certain risk factors, which has been referred to as the *Latino Paradox* (Pinheiro et al., 2011). Embedded in this phenomenon is the belief that Latinos in the United States tend to have better health and mortality rates than the general population despite their poor socioeconomic status (Pinheiro et al., 2011). The factors contributing to better outcomes evolve from cultural and psychosocial characteristics embedded in the Latino/Hispanic cultural values (Gallo, Penedo, Espinosa de los Monteros, & Arguelles, 2009). The protective impact of these factors has been addressed in a few studies that focus on how psychosocial and cultural factors relate to risk and resiliency in Latinos. Preliminary findings from one study suggested that strong family integration and support can help foster resilience and contribute to better outcomes in Latinos with cancer (Penedo et al., 2007).

Preventive policies and programs most often focus on cancers of the cervix, colon, rectum, breast, and prostate. Yet, as noted by the high incidence and mortality rates of other cancers in Latinos such as gastric and gallbladder cancer and acute lymphocytic leukemia, oncology nurses may need to increase their own knowledge and awareness of these cancers when planning culturally competent nursing care, interventions, and policy recommendations.

Determinants Affecting Health Policy

Social Determinants and Health Policy for Latinos

The following social determinants have been found to influence health policy related to Latinos' health: cultural values, health status, healthcare utilization, and sociocultural factors (e.g., country of origin or ethnic identity, language preference, generational status). Acculturation is a major determinant affecting every dimension of their life and will be discussed in greater detail in the following sections. The level of acculturation achieved by a person of Latino heritage will have an impact across the spectrum of these dimensions. For example, a Latina from Ecuador who recently migrated to the United States may not be familiar with cervical cancer screening recommendations because Ecuador may not have had the governmental infrastructure to offer preventive cancer policies. Legal status also can influence her cancer care, particularly if the woman is an undocumented immigrant. Access to insurance for medical care or social services may be denied due to current policies, such as the Personal Responsibility and Work Opportunity Reconciliation Act of 1996.

These policies will have a profound effect on whether a person can afford or access the best cancer treatment and follow-up.

Latinos' Core Values and Cultural Factors

Although cultural factors significantly influence how people perceive and respond to health, little is known about how these elements are associated with barriers to care. The Institute of Medicine report *Unequal Treatment: Confronting Racial and Ethnic Disparities in Health Care* identified communication barriers, particularly language, as contributing to disparate care in non-English-speaking groups (Smedley et al., 2003). One study concluded that lack of a regular source of care was associated with limited English proficiency (Pérez-Stable, 2007). Evidence has shown that Spanish-speaking Latinos reported less satisfaction with provider communication, outpatient services, and overall care than English-speaking Latinos (Mead et al., 2008). DuBard and Gizlice (2008) concluded that Spanish-speaking Latinos reported poor health status, lower participation in preventive care, and less access to health care. Generational differences also affect access to care and health status (see Table 10-1). Studies have concluded that first-generation Latinos have a better health status compared to second- or third-generation Latinos. In fact, Latinos born in the United States who are more acculturated also report barriers such as limited knowledge of how to navigate the healthcare system and cultural fears or misconceptions of the disease (DuBard & Gizlice, 2008). By recognizing which factors can reduce unequal cancer care the most, policy makers can support cancer policy reform that is most likely to decrease these inequalities.

Although great heterogeneity exists among Latino subgroups, core values that are fundamental to worldviews, expectations, and coping methods are relevant to the entire cancer trajectory. These values include *confianza* (trust), *familismo* (family), respect (respecto), *simpatía* (being agreeable), *compadres* (kinship), *machismo* (manliness), and *marianismo* (feminine and unselfish) (Caballero, 2011; Palos, 1998). Understanding the role and importance of these values will help when advocating for policy changes, adherence to screening recommendations, and access to timely and quality treatment when government policies support these activities.

Health Status

Compelling evidence shows that the health of the Latino population has improved over the decades; however, health disparities still exist. Latinos have poorer health and higher rates of certain chronic conditions (e.g., diabetes), disability (decline in functional status), and other diseases requiring ongoing health surveillance. Over the past 30 years, health disparities research has concluded that adult Latinos have lower mortality rates compared to White non-

Hispanic adults (Fenelon, 2013). The relatively positive health outcomes support the Hispanic Paradox that the health status of U.S. Latinos is quite good compared to other ethnic or racial groups (Morales et al., 2002).

Healthcare Utilization

Numerous factors affect healthcare utilization by Latinos, including insurance status, income level, lack of a usual source of care, and cultural factors (Morales et al., 2002). Latinos of every income level have the greatest proportion of uninsured residents of all ethnic and racial groups (DuBard & Gizlice, 2008; Morales et al., 2002). Factors contributing to this disparity include no or limited employee benefits, citizenship status, and, most important, immigration reform policies that exclude immigrants from government programs (Morales et al., 2002). In addition, Latinos' low income level affects their ability to purchase private insurance. Ethnic and racial minorities are the least likely to have a regular healthcare provider. Evidence shows that Latinos are more than three times more likely than non-Hispanic Whites to not have a consistent provider. Other factors that influence healthcare utilization include limited English proficiency, perceived provider bias, and location of care (Ramirez et al., 2008; Saha, Fernandez, & Perez-Stable, 2007). Factors that impede healthcare utilization patterns will affect Latinos' cancer morbidity and mortality rates as well as their overall quality of life. Many of the barriers to healthcare utilization can be addressed through well-planned and insightful healthcare policies. One promising policy to provide equitable access and use of health care for Latinos and other citizens is the recently passed ACA, which will be discussed later in this chapter.

Acculturation and Related Determinants

According to recent literature, there is a strong debate on how acculturation is defined, measured, and used in social science (Thomson & Hoffman-Goetz, 2009). Acculturation has been identified as an important process and concept when working with Latino families. Acculturation is often referred to as *cultural assimilation* and indicates a person changing his or her cultural worldviews to be like others in dominant society (Thomson & Hoffman-Goetz, 2009).

On the other hand, immigrants may go through an opposite process beginning with enculturation, incorporation, and full integration into their new or dominant society. Latinos often choose to keep their language, ethnic values, behavior, and views toward health and cancer (Palos, 1998). This process is regarded as *enculturation* or *integration,* which preserves one's own cultural heritage worldview while blending aspects of the nontraditional society to achieve a better quality of life (Thomson & Hoffman-Goetz, 2009). An example of this process can be seen with the growing number of ethnic enclaves, including those of Latinos, throughout the United States. Interestingly, growing research suggests that communal communities may have a protective factor in moderating distress in Latinos (Aranda, Ray, Snih, Ottenbacher, & Markides, 2011; Fuentes & Aranda, 2012). However, immigrants can also become separated or marginalized from their culture of origin and their new society.

Acculturation has been studied as a unidimensional, bidimensional, and multidimensional construct. Accordingly, different instruments are used to measure acculturation—too many to discuss in this chapter. Thomson and Hoffman-Goetz's (2009) systematic review is an excellent reference to obtain further details on acculturation and measurement tools.

Health Policies and U.S. Latinos

Patients and families are considered the heart of cancer medicine, yet there is an increasing disconnect between public policies, national politics, and the implications for cancer nurses, patients, and their loved ones. In recent years, considerable debate has taken place on how to best provide and finance public health care and, equally important, for whom it should be provided. Thomas Oliver, a noted political sociologist, argued that "politics is central in determining how citizens and policy makers recognize and define problems with existing social conditions and policies, and in facilitating certain kinds of public health interventions but not others, and in generating a variety of challenges" (Oliver, 2006, p. 196). Legislators have voiced negative attitudes that can affect the health policy process for Latinos, for example, "I will do anything short of shooting immigrants" (stated by Representative Mo Brooks [R-AL], as cited in Hinojosa, 2011). The influence of such perspectives reflects the importance for nurses to understand and recognize that public health policies in the United States often inadvertently contribute to Latinos' unequal burden of cancer.

Many past, current, and future policies related to health and cancer policies have been supported through legislative action, public health initiatives, and requirements for data collection on race and ethnicity. Detailed discussion of all policies affecting Latinos is beyond the purview of this chapter. In this section, three major U.S. policies (the Decennial Census Improvement Act, Public Law 94-31, and the ACA) affecting Latinos' health, as well as collection and analysis of national health data, will be reviewed.

U.S. Census

The first U.S. Census was taken in 1790 to describe the characteristics of the U.S. population for accurately apportioning congressional districts. The census was not intended to use for epidemiologic or health purposes. However, data from the racial categories was used to create laws to define groups who may not have had equitable access to resources or freedom. Figure 10-2 lists other critical uses of census data with the potential to affect health policy making and outcomes (ThisNation.com, n.d.). In 1991, the Decennial Census Improvement Act was passed to collect the most accurate population count and description. However, because of growing criticism and suggestions to change the data collection methods and categories, Statistical Policy Directive No. 15, Race and Ethnic Standards for Federal Statistics and Administrative Reporting, was revised. The most recent change was implemented in 1997 by the Office of Management and Budget and is known as the "Revisions to the Standards for the Classification of Federal Data on Race and Ethnicity."

With this change, the Office of Management and Budget developed a more precise definition for the Hispanic/Latino category. The current form allows people to identify their ethnicity as Hispanic or Latino and then select one or more race categories. It also provides data indicating that not all Latinos are Spanish-speaking. For instance, four South American countries are regarded as non-Spanish-speaking territories, including Brazil, French Guiana, Guyana, and Suriname. Current census categories do not capture certain groups, such as Brazilians, other non-Spanish-speaking groups, or those of Middle Eastern descent (Reuben et al., 2011).

Designation of Hispanic Versus Latino Categories

Significant confusion and debate exists regarding which term to use when identifying or reporting Latino or Hispanic ethnicity. The term *Hispanic* originated from the 1976 Public Law 94-31, which was revised in the 1997 Office of Management and Budget Statistical Policy Directive No. 15 to include *Latino* in the definition. Currently, in the United States, Hispanic or Latino is defined as "a person of Cuban, Mexican, Puerto Rican, South or Central American, or other Spanish culture or origin, regardless of race" (Office of

---

Figure 10-2. How the Census Affects Cancer and Health Policies

- Provides national health and social statistics to federal, state, and local agencies to develop policies
- Uses data from economic indicators that become the foundation for forming economic policies
- Supplies data to guide allocation of federal funds for federally financed activities and programs
- Furnishes data to guide allocation of federal funds for state and local educational programs

---

Note. Based on information from ThisNation.com, n.d.

Management and Budget, 1997). The Office of Management and Budget considers Hispanic to be an ethnic group. However, Hispanics represent a variety of ancestries within each racial or ethnic group. This broad diversity contributes to the debate among Latinos/Hispanics on how to self-report their own ethnicity or race. Crucial elements to consider in this discussion include the person's country of origin, generation, and level of acculturation.

Patient Protection and Affordable Care Act

The ACA was passed in 2010 to provide comprehensive health reform. The primary purpose of the law is to provide accessible and affordable preventive care—including family planning and related services—to a greater number of Americans. To date, some provisions of the law have taken effect; however, several other provisions will be implemented over the next few years (Patient Protection and Affordable Care Act, 2010).

Despite national initiatives to educate Americans about the ACA, many still are unaware of the new law or do not understand its guidelines and provisions. In a recent study supported by the Robert Wood Johnson Foundation Center for Health Policy at the University of New Mexico, the authors concluded that the nation's federal government must increase educational and outreach efforts to inform Latinos about the new healthcare law and how the ACA will affect rising healthcare costs. Survey results showed that only 12% of 800 respondents were "very informed" about the law, compared to 52% who reported being "not at all informed" or "not that informed." The survey also reported that 45% of Latino adults did not have permanent or regular access to care (Barreto & Sanchez, 2013).

Despite the results of this study, the ACA has promising outcomes for Latinos, particularly those who do not have insurance or are underinsured. Benefits associated with the ACA include free preventive health care, lower costs for coverage, and coverage for preexisting conditions (Centers for Medicare and Medicaid Services, n.d.). At this time, it is still too early to determine if this public health policy will make a difference in the outcomes of Latinos diagnosed with cancer.

Collection and Analysis of Epidemiologic Data

The growth and diversity of U.S. Latinos will greatly affect future cancer outcomes (American Cancer Society, 2012; Haile et al., 2012; Reuben et al., 2011). Despite the significant increase and visibility of the Latino population, limitations exist in collecting, analyzing, and reporting cancer data for Latinos. First, the state of the science on how cancer develops, progresses, and is managed has been primarily studied in homogenous groups of White non-Hispanic populations. Clearly, the same science does not reflect the socioeconomic, demographic, and cultural characteristics of U.S. Latinos. Second, the cancer surveillance data available on Latinos are limited in their use, primarily because of inadequate data collection methods regarding race and ethnicity for national data sets such as those provided by the National Cancer Institute's Surveillance, Epidemiology, and End Results Program or other cancer registries. The primary factors complicating collection are self-reporting, misclassification, and lack of standardization in methods used to collect data on race and ethnicity (Haile et al., 2012; Vega et al., 2009). Third, the majority of available federal, state, or municipal data sets (i.e., vital statistics such as births or deaths) do not address the variability within Latino groups. For example, there is a dearth of data on incidence, survival, and death rates by Latino subgroups such as South American, Puerto Rican, or Mexican American. In fact, data sets on Latinos were not available until the early 1990s (Haile et al., 2012; Reuben et al., 2011). Other barriers contributing to the limited availability of data include nonadherence of national data sets to federal standards for collection of ethnicity and race, lack of understanding of the purpose and role for standardizing data collection methods and categories, and other provider- and system-related factors. Given the wide variation among Latinos groups, oncology nurses, policy makers, administrators, and researchers need to be mindful of these limitations and identify other sources that may have data sets reflecting these groups' diversity.

Implications for Oncology Providers

Cancer policies that increase costs and decrease eligibility, benefits, and services to Latinos will have a significant impact on cancer morbidity, survival, and mortality rates. The following exemplar illustrates the positive benefits of shaping cancer policy to improve outcomes.

Cervical Cancer in Latinas and Cancer Policy: An Exemplar

Cancer research shows that Latinas experience an inordinate burden of cervical cancer rates compared to women of other ethnic and racial groups (American Cancer Society, 2012). This trend is particularly disheartening because cervical cancer is one of the most preventable cancers. Factors contributing to this disparity include lack of a regular provider or source of care; no or limited awareness of cervical cancer symptoms; lower income, employed in an occupation that does not offer insurance benefits, or unemployed; and being uncomfortable with navigating a healthcare system not prepared to meet their needs (i.e., absence of policies that provide translation services or mandate provider and organizational cultural competency) (Saraiya, Watson, & Benard, 2012). The confluence of these factors contributes to lower participation in preventive services or delays in seeking treatment. In 1990, Congress sought to improve access to preventive services for cervical cancer by passing the Breast and Cervical Cancer Mortality Prevention Act (Benard et al., 2012). The purpose of the act was to provide screening and diagnostic services to low-income women. In 2000, Congress passed a similar bill, the Breast and Cervical Cancer Prevention and Treatment Act, which went one step further by providing a full range of services to meet the needs of women from all ethnic and racial populations, including the 12 American Indian tribes (Benard et al., 2012).

Regrettably, these landmark congressional acts were unable to meet the needs of women who were rarely or never screened, including Latinas (Benard et al., 2012). This gap was attributed to the need for policies that would provide additional resources to conduct special outreach efforts and to establish programs in communities specifically targeting Latinas. The outcome of these policy initiatives demonstrated the need to change the current U.S. disease-focused system to a stronger public health system that focuses on preventive services. Future cancer policies must be passed that include strategies to decrease the excessive burden of cervical cancer in Latinas.

Conclusion

According to the recently released Oncology Nursing Society *Statement on the Scope and Standards of Oncology Nursing Practice*, oncology nurses have the professional knowledge and expertise to serve "as a liaison to institutional, local, state, and national legislative bodies . . . regarding issues related to oncology nursing and oncology, with the ultimate goal of improving oncology patient outcomes" (Brant & Wickham, 2013, p. 57).

In the preceding exemplar, healthcare clinicians, researchers, and educators can make a significant contribution by outlining recommendations to federal policy makers for future policies that will increase Latinas' access to and use of preventive screening programs for cervical cancer. An example of a recommendation would be to strengthen the public health system by providing funding to increase the diversity and cultural competency of the oncology workforce.

Oncology providers must have or develop the skills and abilities to advocate for cancer policies that will provide equitable cancer care across all racial and ethnic groups. To support future changes, oncology providers as a collective group can advocate for public policies that respect the cultural values of Latinos and other ethnically and racially diverse populations.

References

American Cancer Society. (2012). *Cancer facts and figures for Hispanics/Latinos 2012–2014*. Retrieved from http://www.cancer.org/research/cancerfactsfigures/cancerfactsfiguresforhispanicslatinos

American Nurses Association. (2010). Nursing beyond borders: Access to health care for documented and undocumented immigrants living in the US. *ANA Issue Brief*. Retrieved from http://www.nursingworld.org/MainMenuCategories/Policy-Advocacy/Positions-and-Resolutions/Issue-Briefs/Access-to-care-for-immigrants.pdf

American Public Health Association. (n.d.). Ensuring the right to health and health care. Retrieved from http://www.apha.org/advocacy/priorities/issues/access

Aranda, M.P., Ray, L.A., Snih, S.A., Ottenbacher, K.J., & Markides, K.S. (2011). The protective effect of neighborhood composition on increasing frailty among older Mexican Americans: A barrio advantage? *Journal of Aging and Health, 23*, 1189–1217. doi:10.1177/0898264311421961

Barreto, M., & Sanchez, G. (2013). New National Latino Health Care Survey results. Retrieved from http://www.latinodecisions.com/blog/2013/05/01/new-national-latino-health-care-survey-results

Benard, V.B., Howe, W., Royalty, J., Helsel, W., Kammerer, W., & Richardson, L.C. (2012). Timeliness of cervical cancer diagnosis and initiation of treatment in the National Breast and Cervical Cancer Early Detection Program. *Journal of Women's Health, 21*, 776–782. doi:10.1089/jwh.2011.3224

Brant, J.M., & Wickham, R. (Eds.). (2013). *Statement on the scope and standards of oncology nursing practice: Generalist and advanced practice*. Pittsburgh, PA: Oncology Nursing Society.

Byrd, M.W., & Clayton, L.A. (2003). Racial and ethnic disparities in healthcare: A background and history. In B.D. Smedley, A.Y. Stith, & A.R. Nelson (Eds.), *Unequal treatment: Confronting racial and ethnic disparities in health care* (pp. 455–527). Washington, DC: National Academies Press.

Caballero, A.E. (2011). Understanding the Hispanic/Latino patient. *American Journal of Medicine, 124*(Suppl. 10), S10–S15. doi:10.1016/j.amjmed.2011.07.018

Centers for Medicare and Medicaid Services. (n.d.). A one-page guide to the Health Insurance Marketplace. Retrieved from https://www.healthcare.gov/get-covered-a-1-page-guide-to-the-health-insurance-marketplace

Decennial Census Improvement Act of 1991, Pub. L. No. 102-135, 105 Stat. 635.

DuBard, C.A., & Gizlice, Z. (2008). Language spoken and differences in health status, access to care, and receipt of preventive services among US Hispanics. *American Journal of Public Health, 98*, 2021–2028. doi:10.2105/AJPH.2007.119008

Elk, R., Morris, A., Onega, T.L., Ganschow, P., Hershmann, D., Brawley, O.W., & Cykert, S. (2012). Disparities in cancer treatment: Factors that impact health equity in breast, colon, and lung cancer. In R. Elk & H. Landrine (Eds.), *Cancer disparities: Causes and evidence-based solutions* (pp. 89–120). New York, NY: Springer.

Fenelon, A. (2013). Revisiting the Hispanic mortality advantage in the United States: The role of smoking. *Social Science and Medicine, 82*, 1–9. doi:10.1016/j.socscimed.2012.12.028

Fuentes, D., & Aranda, M.P. (2012). Depression interventions among racial and ethnic minority older adults: A systematic review across 20 years. *American Journal of Geriatric Psychiatry, 20*, 915–931. doi:10.1097/JGP.0b013e31825d091a

Gallo, L.C., Penedo, F.J., Espinosa de los Monteros, K., & Arguelles, W. (2009). Resiliency in the face of disadvantage: Do Hispanic cultural characteristics protect health outcomes? *Journal of Personality, 77*, 1707–1746. doi:10.1111/j.1467-6494.2009.00598.x

Goss, E., Lopez, A.M., Brown, C.L., Wollins, D.S., Brawley, O.W., & Raghavan, D. (2009). American Society of Clinical Oncology policy statement: Disparities in cancer care. *Journal of Clinical Oncology, 27*, 2881–2885. doi:10.1200/JCO.2008.21.1680

Haile, R.W., John, E.M., Levine, A.J., Cortessis, V.K., Unger, J.B., Gonzales, M., … Boffetta, P. (2012). A review of cancer in U.S. Hispanic populations. *Cancer Prevention Research, 5,* 150–163. doi:10.1158/1940-6207.CAPR-11-0447

Hinojosa, R. (2011, October 4). Democrats are fighting for jobs for America's Hispanics and their families. *Editorial and Blogs.* Retrieved from http://chc-hinojosa.house.gov/112th-congress-democratic-vs-republican-record-issues-key-hispanics

Humes, K.R., Jones, N.A., & Ramirez, R.R. (2011, March). *Overview of race and Hispanic origin: 2010.* Retrieved from http://www.census.gov/prod/cen2010/briefs/c2010br-02.pdf

Mead, H., Cartwright-Smith, L., Jones, K., Ramos, C., Woods, K., & Siegel, B. (2008). *Racial and ethnic disparities in U.S. health care: A chartbook.* Retrieved from http://www.commonwealthfund.org/publications/chartbooks/2008/mar/racial-and-ethnic-disparities-in-u-s–health-care–a-chartbook

Morales, L.S., Lara, M., Kington, R.S., Valdez, R.O., & Escarce, J.J. (2002). Socioeconomic, cultural, and behavioral factors affecting Hispanic health outcomes. *Journal of Health Care for the Poor and Underserved, 13,* 477–503. doi:10.1353/hpu.2010.0630

Motel, S., & Patten, E. (2012). *The 10 largest Hispanic origin groups: Characteristics, rankings, top counties.* Retrieved from http://www.pewhispanic.org/2012/06/27/the-10-largest-hispanic-origin-groups-characteristics-rankings-top-counties

Office of Management and Budget. (1997). *Revisions to the standards for the classification of federal data on race and ethnicity* (62 F.R. 36874–36946). *Federal Register* Notice, October 30, 1997. Retrieved from http://www.whitehouse.gov/omb/fedreg_1997standards

Oliver, T.R. (2006). The politics of public health policy. *Annual Review of Public Health, 27,* 195–233. doi:10.1146/annurev.publhealth.25.101802.123126

Oncology Nursing Society. (2014, January). *Health policy agenda, 113th Congress, 2nd session.* Pittsburgh, PA: Author.

Palos, G.R. (1998). Culture and pain assessment in Hispanic patients. In R. Payne, R.B. Patt, & C.S. Hill Jr. (Eds.), *Assessment and treatment of cancer pain* (pp. 35–51). Seattle, WA: IASP Press.

Passel, J.S., & Cohn, D. (2008). *U.S. population projections: 2005–2050.* Retrieved from http://www.pewhispanic.org/2008/02/11/us-population-projections-2005-2050

Patient Protection and Affordable Care Act, Pub. L. 111-148, 124 Stat. 119 (2010).

Penedo, F.J., Traeger, L., Dahn, J., Molton, I., Gonzalez, J.S., Schneiderman, N., & Antoni, M.H. (2007). Cognitive behavioral stress management intervention improves quality of life in Spanish monolingual Hispanic men treated for localized prostate cancer: Results of a randomized controlled trial. *International Journal of Behavioral Medicine, 14,* 164–172. doi:10.1007/BF03000188

Pérez-Stable, E.J. (2007). Language access and Latino health care disparities. *Medical Care, 45,* 1009–1011. doi:10.1097/MLR.0b013e31815b9440

Personal Responsibility and Work Opportunity Reconciliation Act of 1996, Pub. L. 104-193, 110 Stat. 2105.

Pinheiro, P.S., Williams, M., Miller, E.A., Easterday, S., Moonie, S., & Trapido, E.J. (2011). Cancer survival among Latinos and the Hispanic Paradox. *Cancer Causes and Control, 22,* 553–561. doi:10.1007/s10552-011-9727-6

Ramirez, A.G., Wildes, K., Talavera, G., Nápoles-Springer, A., Gallion, K., & Pérez-Stable, E.J. (2008). Clinical trials attitudes and practices of Latino physicians. *Contemporary Clinical Trials, 29,* 482–492. doi:10.1016/j.cct.2007.11.001

Reuben, S.H., Milliken, E.L., & Paradis, L.J. (2011). *President's Cancer Panel: 2009–2010 annual report. America's demographic and cultural transformation: Implications for cancer.* Retrieved from http://deainfo.nci.nih.gov/advisory/pcp/annualReports/pcp09-10rpt/pcp09-10rpt.pdf

Saha, S., Fernandez, A., & Perez-Stable, E. (2007). Reducing language barriers and racial/ethnic disparities in health care: An investment in our future. *Journal of General Internal Medicine, 22*(Suppl. 2), 371–372. doi:10.1007/s11606-007-0372-4

Saraiya, M., Watson, M., & Benard, V.B. (2012). Cervical cancer screening measures need to evolve to continue to tell the story. *Journal of Women's Health, 21,* 1128–1129. doi:10.1089/jwh.2012.3994

Schneider, A., & Ingram, H. (1993). Social construction of target populations: Implications for politics and policy. *American Political Science Review, 87,* 334–347. doi:10.2307/2939044

Singer, M.K. (2012). Applying the concept of culture to reduce health disparities through health behavior research. *Preventive Medicine, 55,* 356–361. doi:10.1016/j.ypmed.2012.02.011

Smedley, B.D., Stith, A.Y., & Nelson, A.R. (Eds.). (2003). *Unequal treatment: Confronting racial and ethnic disparities in health care.* Washington, DC: National Academies Press.

Taylor, P., Lopez, M.H., Martínez, J., & Velasco, G. (2012). *When labels don't fit: Hispanics and their views of identity.* Washington, DC: Pew Hispanic Center.

ThisNation.com. (n.d.). What is the purpose of the Census? What is the data used for? Retrieved from http://www.thisnation.com/question/022.html

Thomson, M.D., & Hoffman-Goetz, L. (2009). Defining and measuring acculturation: A systematic review of public health studies with Hispanic populations in the United States. *Social Science and Medicine, 69,* 983–991. doi:10.1016/j.socscimed.2009.05.011

U.S. Census Bureau. (2012). People and households: Ancestry. Retrieved from http://www.census.gov/population/ancestry

U.S. Census Bureau. (2013). Population: Race: About. Retrieved from http://www.census.gov/topics/population/race/about.html

U.S. Census Bureau. (2014). Hispanic Heritage Month 2014: Sept. 15–Oct. 15. Retrieved from http://www.census.gov/newsroom/facts-for-features/2014/cb14-ff22.html

Vega, W.A., Rodriguez, M.A., & Gruskin, E. (2009). Health disparities in the Latino population. *Epidemiologic Reviews, 31,* 99–112. doi:10.1093/epirev/mxp008

Villa, V.M., Wallace, S.P., Bagdasaryan, S., & Aranda, M.P. (2012). Hispanic Baby Boomers: Health inequities likely to persist in old age. *Gerontologist, 52,* 166–176. doi:10.1093/geront/gns002

Wilensky, S.E., & Gray, E.A. (2013). Existing Medicaid beneficiaries left off the Affordable Care Act's prevention bandwagon. *Health Affairs, 32,* 1188–1195. doi:10.1377/hlthaff.2013.0224

CHAPTER 11

American Indians and Alaska Natives and Cancer

Emily A. Haozous, PhD, RN, and Valerie Eschiti, PhD, RN, AHN-BC, CHTP, CTN-A

Introduction

Cancer health policy for American Indians (AIs) and Alaska Natives (ANs) is a complicated story with historic, cultural, and geographic factors. This chapter will provide context for the issues and will briefly outline the most salient points of this complex policy landscape. It is our intent to introduce this story here, and we invite interested readers to begin a journey of discovery that spans more than 500 years of health policy by following the citations provided at the end of the chapter. The readers may then continue the story as it relates to the AI/AN population or community closest to them.

AI/ANs represent more than 560 federally recognized tribes, 229 of which are located in Alaska (National Congress of American Indians [NCAI], 2013a), and hundreds more federally unrecognized tribes. The distribution of federally designated reservation land is predominantly in the western states, as shown in Figure 11-1. Although AI/ANs are discussed collectively in this chapter, each tribe is a social, cultural, and governmental unit unto itself with unique qualities too numerous to list here. AI/ANs have more individual qualities than shared, yet there are some similar and shared experiences that we will provide in the course of giving context to AI/AN health policy. This chapter will distinguish between AIs and ANs when necessary and will describe special circumstances that affect those living in Alaska.

Understanding AI/AN health policy requires an understanding of the history of health for AI/ANs in this country, as AI/AN health and cancer outcomes are directly related to the healthcare delivery system that has provided care for the nation's indigenous population for more than 150 years. This chapter will briefly detail the history of the Indian Health Service (IHS)

Figure 11-1. American Indian Reservations

American Indian Reservations

MAP KEY
■ Federal American Indian Reservations
• State American Indian Reservations

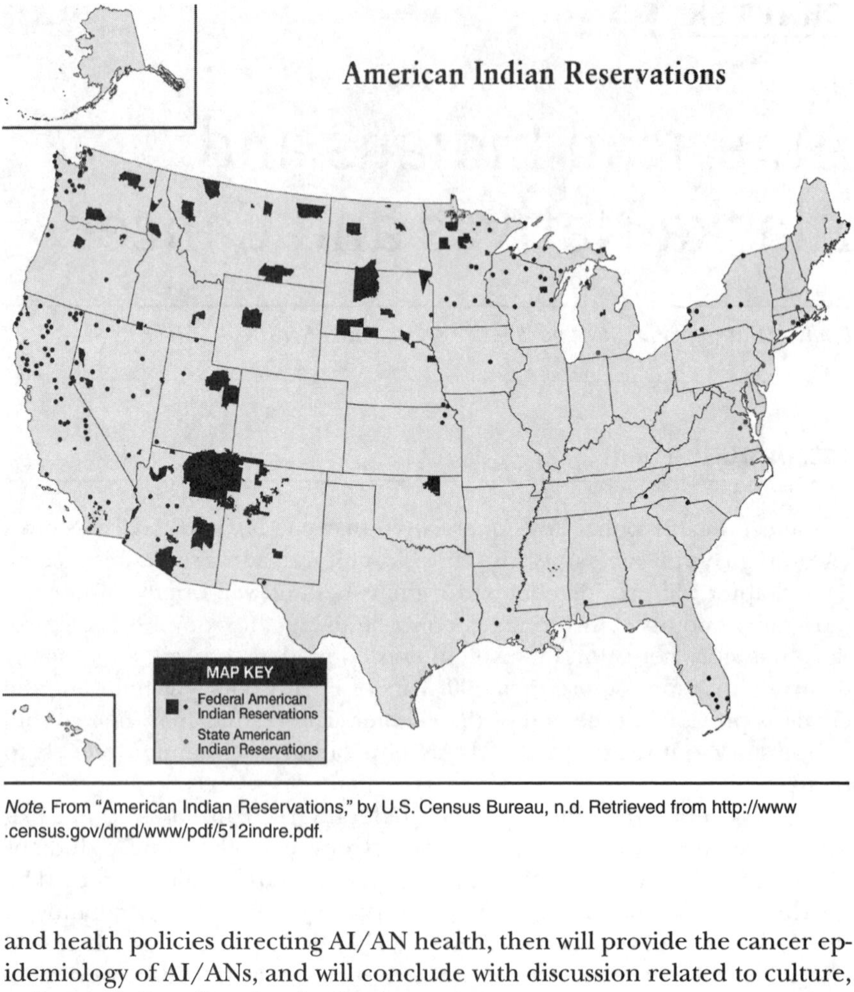

Note. From "American Indian Reservations," by U.S. Census Bureau, n.d. Retrieved from http://www .census.gov/dmd/www/pdf/512indre.pdf.

and health policies directing AI/AN health, then will provide the cancer epidemiology of AI/ANs, and will conclude with discussion related to culture, policy, and directions for the future.

Indian Health Service and Treaty Obligation

Indian Health Service

IHS provides health care for many AI/ANs. Federal responsibility for AI/AN health is not an altruistic gesture stemming from a desire to care for the nation's indigenous populations, but rather is based on treaty obligations established at the start of the reservation era (Schneider, 2005). In the late 18th and throughout the 19th century, the United States was a growing nation. Federal policies were created to manage and remove AI/AN groups from their historic homelands to reservations and allotments through a series of treaty agreements and executive orders to allow room for growth and westward expansion and to create access to natural resources (Shelton, 2001).

Historically, IHS grew out of a need to protect U.S. soldiers and neighboring settlers from the infectious disease epidemics that were running rampant through AI/AN communities (Shelton, 2001). As AI/AN removal and relocation populations grew, federally funded health care for AI/ANs followed suit, and military physicians cared for AI/ANs as part of the treaty agreements between the United States and AI/AN nations and as a public health measure to control infectious disease in and around reservation and allotment lands (Shelton, 2001; Warne, Kaur, & Perdue, 2012).

The Bureau of Indian Affairs managed health care for AI/ANs until 1954, when it was recognized that a distinct agency was needed to shoulder the treaty-bound responsibility for AI/AN health in the United States. In 1954, IHS was created as an agency of the Department of Health, Education, and Welfare (now the Department of Health and Human Services) through the Transfer Act (Indian Health Facilities Act of 1954) (Shelton, 2001). (For a list of the more than 370 treaties listed by state, see www.cr.nps.gov/nagpra/onlinedb/land_cessions/index.htm.)

Federal funding for AI/AN health has historically been low priority, and responsibility for AI/AN health has been juggled from agency to agency since the inception of the Bureau of Indian Affairs. Philosophies directing IHS policies have closely paralleled other federal policies concerning AI/ANs. U.S. government policies have progressed from a program geared toward AI/AN eradication to an assimilationist program to policies of sovereignty and self-determination (Thierry, Brenneman, Rhoades, & Chilton, 2009).

In the early 1970s, the Nixon administration rejected previous strategies of termination and then assimilation through the development of policies focused on AI self-determination. This focus eventually led to the passing of the Indian Self-Determination and Education Act (Public Law [P.L.] 93-638) in 1975 and the Indian Health Care Improvement Act (P.L. 94-437) in 1976 (Thierry et al., 2009).

Although well intentioned, these laws in fact intensified tribal competition for limited federal dollars. The policies surrounding self-determination further weakened AI/AN health care by decentralizing the individual funds, creating smaller healthcare units with fewer resources with which to provide care for recipients (Warne et al., 2012). Instead of large IHS-funded hospitals providing a variety of services, the trend has moved to smaller, tribal-run clinics that can only provide basic primary care.

638 Compacting of Tribes—At What Cost?

With the Indian Self-Determination and Education Act came the opportunity for AI/AN tribes to withdraw from the IHS system and create their own health clinics, called "638 Compacting," named after the law. This trend has gained popularity, and in recent years, AI/AN tribes have been seeking greater autonomy over tribal health by contracting with independent healthcare services, eschewing traditional IHS services. While this move has allowed tribes to determine their own priorities for health, it has further splintered the IHS system by withdrawing monies that would have otherwise funded the larger IHS system of hospitals and clinics (Thierry et al., 2009).

Decentralization has allowed tribes to prioritize healthcare issues, which has had a positive result in health status for those served. In particular, primary care has benefited from these changes. However, existing IHS facilities have seen resources dissipate and are no longer able to provide comprehensive care. Small tribal clinics have taken the major share of financial resources, while larger urban hospitals and clinics struggle to provide basic care for the population of AI/ANs living in urban areas. Specialty care has become increasingly complex over time, making decentralized health care the best model for rural primary care, but impractical for highly technical and expensive specialty care.

Patients with cancer are disproportionately affected by decentralization, as tribal clinics are ill equipped to manage tasks associated with a cancer diagnosis and treatment. Where the larger, centralized IHS hospitals used to have resources and staffing to perform uncomplicated surgeries and some infusions, and had equipment for monitoring and diagnosis of disease, these tasks now most frequently must be referred to providers outside the IHS system. This requires patients to rely more on a system called Contract Health Service/Purchased-Referred Care (CHS) funding and places patients who are living outside their IHS service unit area at a particular disadvantage. The CHS system will be described later in the chapter (Warne et al., 2012).

With the passage of the Patient Protection and Affordable Care Act (ACA), AI/ANs are being encouraged to enroll in private insurance to provide them with health insurance coverage and to supplement IHS coverage provided by tribal health (638) clinics when available. As observed by AI/AN health policy activists, the ACA provides an important opportunity for AI/AN communities to bring additional funding to their community clinics through available resources, such as Medicare and subsidized private insurance (McKosato, 2013).

Indian Health Service Funding

IHS has been historically underfunded. Despite steady increases in funding in recent years, per capita spending on health services for IHS is still significantly less than what is spent on health for the general U.S. population (Thierry et al., 2009). Approximately 22% of AI/ANs live on reservations or in rural areas and have ready access to IHS facilities (U.S. Department of Health and Human Services Office of Minority Health, 2014). As a result of the issues with budgeting and funding, IHS hospitals offer only basic care, have limited access to diagnostic and therapeutic services, and offer limited preventive care (Thierry et al., 2009).

While the average annual U.S. per capita Medicare budgeting was $9,702 in 2012, the U.S. government budgeted only $2,690 per person for AI/AN health, indicating an important inequity in funding for federally guaranteed health care for AI/ANs (Kaiser Family Foundation, 2012; Warne et al., 2012). Additionally, in 2012 per capita budgeting for the IHS healthcare system was less than what was spent per person nationally (Crowder, Jim, Joseph, & Hayes, 2013). Actual spending from 2010 to 2012 reveals a distinctive disparity in national spending per capita for AI/ANs in the IHS system and spending for Medicare, Medicaid, and the Veterans Administration.

The 2013 budget has dramatically improved funding levels, but the long-term deficit has created dire situations in many IHS service units that will take many years of funding to improve. Furthermore, 60% of AI/ANs live in urban areas and have access to mixed resources (U.S. Department of Health and Human Services Office of Minority Health, 2014). These include using private health insurance, receiving care at Urban Indian Health Centers, or returning to their reservations to access IHS health services. The migratory population of AI/ANs creates additional stress on the IHS system, which does not account for nonresident AI/AN populations in its budget (Holkup, 2002; Warne et al., 2012; U.S. Department of Health and Human Services Office of Minority Health, 2014).

Even with its history of underfunding and misguided federal policies, IHS has proved itself to be effective through the decrease in AI/AN mortality during the past 50 years. Infectious diseases, such as tuberculosis, gastroenteritis, and pneumonia/influenza, have substantially decreased as well (IHS, 2005). Unfortunately, a simultaneous increase has occurred in chronic diseases, such as cancer and diabetes. Currently, IHS serves as a healthcare provider for approximately 2.1 million AI/ANs (IHS, 2013).

Indian Health Service and Oncology Care

Few AI/ANs have private health insurance that can cover the costs of cancer care. Thus, they must rely on funding from IHS or from county, sole community, or university hospitals as appropriate. IHS funding is charged as the payer of last resort, often causing a significant delay in payment. Patients using the IHS system who have a cancer diagnosis are placed on a prioritized list that will direct them to oncology care when funding is available, leading to delays in treatment (Burhansstipanov & Hollow, 2001).

Unfortunately, cancer is a disease that is best treated early and aggressively, so any delay in treatment can increase both morbidity and mortality. The rural nature of most reservations, as well as nonreservation tribal communities, creates poor access to resources. In many instances, AI/ANs live far from cancer centers. Distance to care has been acknowledged to influence cancer outcomes, and AI/ANs have been identified to have the longest travel times to the nearest National Cancer Institute cancer centers in comparison with the overall U.S. population (Onega et al., 2008). Longer travel distance results in a proportionally higher mortality rate from cancer for AI/ANs nationwide. This results in delayed and missed opportunities for cancer screening, as well as missed treatment appointments (Espey et al., 2007; Wilson et al., 2011).

American Indians and Cancer

AI/ANs make up only 1.2% of the U.S. population (U.S. Census Bureau, 2014c), yet as a group they experience considerable health inequities compared to other racial and ethnic groups. AI/AN cancer outcomes are particularly poor; for example, cancer morbidity is surprisingly high and the number of cancer deaths relative to the incidence of cancer is much higher in AI/ANs than in other ethnic groups. In 2006–2010, the age-adjusted average incidence for cancer in AI/ANs was 441.1 males and 372 females per 100,000, and mortality was 191 males and 139 females per 100,000. In contrast, the average incidence for non-Hispanic Whites (NHWs) was 548.6 males and 436.2 females, and mortality was 217.3 males and 153.6 females per 100,000 (Siegel, Ma, Zou, & Jemal, 2014). Despite lower incidence rates for AI/ANs than other ethnic groups, AI/ANs are diagnosed at later stages and have poorer outcomes (Espey et al., 2007).

In 1999–2004, the overall cancer incidence and death rates in the United States for most cancers were lower for AI/AN people compared to NHWs. However, these rates were higher for cancers of the stomach, liver, cervix, kidney, and gallbladder. The overall incidence and death rates conceal variations by geographic region for AI/AN people (Espey et al., 2007). See Figure 11-2 for regions used in cancer incidence analyses for AI/ANs. For instance, high incidence and mortality rates for several cancers, including breast, colorectal, and lung cancers, are noted for AI/AN people living in the Northern and Southern Plains, as well as Alaska. In general, cancer rates were lowest for AI/ANs in the Southwest (Espey et al., 2007).

Regional variations in cancer rates may be a result of differences in screening and risk factors such as

> tobacco use (lung, kidney, and colorectal cancer), obesity (colorectal and breast cancer), low level of physical activity (breast and colorectal cancer), heavy alcohol consumption (breast and liver cancer), and dietary factors, including consumption of large amounts of red meat and inadequate intake of fruits and vegetables (colorectal cancer). (Espey et al., 2007, p. 2142)

AI/ANs are less likely than NHWs to be diagnosed at localized stages for cancers of the breast, colon and rectum, prostate, and cervix (Espey et al., 2007). This is likely due in part to the lower cancer screening prevalence for AI/ANs compared with NHW populations. However, AI/ANs have less favorable socioeconomic status and healthcare access compared with NHWs, which likely contributes to low screening rates. Tobacco control and cancer screening were cited as priorities by Espey et al. (2007), especially in the Northern and Southern Plains and Alaska. Furthermore, continued efforts

Figure 11-2. States and Contract Health Service Delivery Area (CHSDA) Counties, by Indian Health Service Region

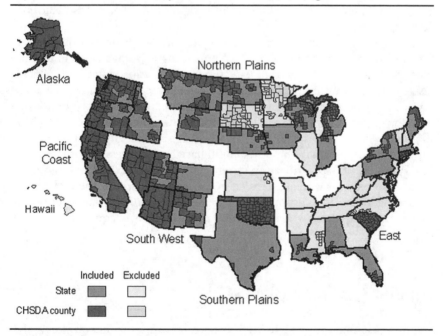

Note. From "Annual Report to the Nation on the Status of Cancer, 1975–2004, Featuring Cancer in American Indians and Alaska Natives," by D.K. Espey, X.-C. Wu, J. Swan, C. Wiggins, M.A. Jim, E. Ward, ... B.K. Edwards, 2007, *Cancer, 110,* p. 2123. doi:10.1002/cncr.23044. Published by the American Cancer Society. This article is a U.S. government work and is in the public domain in the United States of America.

are needed to reduce the cancer burden among AI/AN people (Espey et al., 2007).

IHS is a healthcare delivery system that is able to provide health care for patients within certain specific parameters. When patients are diagnosed, or are suspected of a diagnosis that is outside the treatment expertise or diagnostic capability of the IHS providers' areas of expertise, they must be referred. This system of referral is similar to a patient being referred from a primary care provider to a specialist's care. However, unlike when an insured patient is referred, an IHS patient does not have health insurance that follows him or her to the specialist. Instead, the IHS referral system distributes a limited annual budget to each service unit via the CHS program to provide funds for patients who require out-of-system referrals during that fiscal year (U.S. Department of Health and Human Services, 2013b).

Because the entire IHS system is suffering from substantial financial strain, CHS is rarely able to provide full funding to meet its needs in any year, leaving many patients with serious illness without care as the fiscal year draws to a close. Patient services are prioritized based on need, with highest priority going to lifesaving procedures. Patients with cancer may be denied recommended treatments for their cancer or turned away by their oncology care provider because CHS is notoriously slow with payment (Haozous, 2009).

Another equally troubling consequence of the prioritization of CHS funds is the delay of treatment to patients with early-stage cancers because of the relative low severity of disease. The prioritization system requires patients who are in life-threatening situations to receive highest priority. As some early-stage cancers are considered curable, these patients do not rate as high priority and are forced to wait for funds to become available within the CHS system. Over time, these cancers progress in acuity and become life-threatening or terminal when they could have been successfully treated. The flaw is not with the prioritization system but with the lack of funding for the number of patients who are in need of specialty care within the IHS system, as turning away a patient with a life-threatening condition is as unethical as turning away a patient with a condition that will likely become life-threatening over time due to systematic delays.

Cultural Aspects of Wellness

The resilience with which AI/ANs have recovered from countless physical, historical, and cultural insults is in and of itself a testimony to the vital role that culture plays in the lives of AI/ANs (Grandbois & Sanders, 2009). The traditional way of life practiced by AI/ANs has ensured survival for countless millennia. It is arrogant to expect AI/ANs to give up cultural and religious practices for the sake of healthcare providers' convenience and societal expectations. AI/ANs may act in a manner that may be considered detrimental to their cancer care to preserve their culture and community, but it is important to recognize that many AI/ANs consider the health of their community as a priority over their individual health. When cultural practices are not allowed to be continued, this may negatively affect the well-being of all AI/AN people (Haozous & Knobf, 2013). Such barriers include inflexible hospital visiting regulations and policies controlling diet during hospitalization, which prevent the family from fully supporting the patient.

Cultural values differ among tribes. However, some common values related to wellness are presented here to facilitate understanding of behaviors that oncology healthcare providers may encounter. In this way, healthcare providers may advocate for health policy that supports culturally appropriate care for AI/AN patients with cancer. Cultural aspects of wellness comprise several aspects. These include spirituality, harmony, balance, and generosity.

Spirituality

There is no separation between the AI/AN person and the wholeness of life (Grandbois & Sanders, 2009). Many AI/ANs refer to their strong spiritual values, believing that all of life is sacred and interconnected and that there is a link between spirituality and healing (BigFoot & Schmidt, 2010).

An AI/AN nurse scholar, Dr. Roxanne Struthers, contended that engaging in traditional indigenous healing is one way in which AI/ANs can attain wholeness in the midst of receiving a cancer diagnosis (Struthers, Eschiti, & Patchell, 2004). Even if the patient is not able to overcome the disease, the harmony of spirit obtained by the patient and family from traditional tribal practices is an incredible uplift during a devastating period in family life. Thus, oncology healthcare providers and policy makers need to be supportive of traditional healing practices, even if they do not understand them.

Harmony

AI/AN beliefs in a harmonious cosmos are a deeply embedded part of life. It is unlikely to see AI/AN people berate others for a harm they have incurred at their hands (Gray & Rose, 2012), because it would disturb group harmony and social balance. This is sometimes referred to as *native noninterference* (Stromnes-Elias, 2007). Oncology healthcare providers need to be aware of this cultural value in order to be sensitive to nonverbal cues that a patient or family may not be satisfied with some aspect of care, as it may not be verbalized. For instance, a female AI/AN patient may prefer that a female nursing assistant help her with bathing, but she may not ask for one. If a male nursing assistant offers to provide assistance, the AI/AN patient may decline but not provide the reason. The nurse may need to query the patient or family further to ascertain why the bathing assistance was declined.

Balance

The Medicine Wheel Model of Wellness, Balance, and Healing may be used to illustrate the needed balance between mental, emotional, social, and physical needs of AI/ANs (Gray & Rose, 2012). Social balance is a cultural value for a tribal people who have historically relied on one another for survival. Thus, when providing health care to AI/AN patients, oncology healthcare providers need to maintain a holistic perspective of healing and wellness. Cancer remission may not be considered an indication of healing to the AI/AN patient if the process of cancer treatment financially and emotionally destroys the family.

Generosity

Sharing of all aspects of life is expected and enjoyed in AI/AN culture through the value of generosity (BigFoot & Schmidt, 2010). This includes food, clothing, survival items, money, housing, and even ceremonies and uplifting humor, stories, and blessings of good words. There is no division between one person and another; the community is one in enjoying the bounty of communal life (Brokenleg, n.d.). Thus, oncology healthcare providers and researchers need to advocate for hospital policies to accommodate requests, such as bringing in traditional foods from home for the patient with cancer.

Barriers to Oncology Care

Numerous additional barriers to adequate oncology care exist across the cancer continuum for AI/ANs beyond those already mentioned. These include cultural beliefs that preclude seeking cancer care, mistrust of the medical system, cancer causation beliefs, fear of screening results, insensitivity of healthcare personnel toward AI/AN people, lack of Native providers, unavailability of healthcare facilities, language and communication barriers, lack of transportation, competing priorities, lack of cancer-related knowledge, inadequate financial resources, difficulty understanding treatment options, fragmentation of care, and referral and payment issues among multiple healthcare entities (Filippi et al., 2013; Hodge & Casken, 1999; Petereit et al., 2008). These barriers must be addressed by health policy to eliminate cancer disparities among AI/AN people.

The Affordable Care Act

The ACA, passed in March 2010, introduced sweeping healthcare reform affecting all Americans. Within the ACA is a panoply of new policies intended to radically change the way health care is paid for in the United States. Most important to AI/ANs, the ACA permanently reauthorizes the Indian Health Care Improvement Act, authorizing Congress to fund the IHS budget without periodic presidential reauthorization. This critical piece of legislation makes funding for AI/AN health immune from partisan politics and ushers IHS into the new system of healthcare delivery.

Tribes are working to increase enrollment in the Children's Health Insurance Program (CHIP) and Medicaid, streamline billing and business processes, and consider health insurance obligations as employers (NCAI, 2013a). NCAI, a national policy and advocacy group representing a collective voice of AI/AN tribes, stated,

> Successful and seamless implementation of the ACA will increase health care access for American Indians and Alaska Natives, support the IHS system of care, broaden services provided in rural communities, and strengthen an integral network of providers. In addition, the Administration has proposed and supported improvements in tribal prevention. These programs are designed to be tribally driven, culturally sensitive, and locally provided. (NCAI, 2013a, p. 7)

Beneficial changes for AI/ANs who receive Medicare include provision of some preventive services without charge, such as mammograms and screening colonoscopies. Free wellness visits and coordinated care are additional benefits of the ACA (Medicare.gov, n.d.).

Health Exchange States and the Affordable Care Act

The ACA also introduced health insurance exchanges (referred to as *exchanges*), which are in essence private and public insurance plans made available to individuals and employers at comparable prices. Exchanges are intended to allow consumers to easily compare and select health insurance policies that meet their individual needs. For states that opt out of the federally funded Medicaid expansion, subsidies are provided to protect individuals whose income falls between the Medicaid amount and the lower limit for exchange subsidies (Connolly & Gitlin, 2013). Exchanges also act as information clearinghouses to help direct individuals to available resources, limiting unnecessary private and public expenditures—for example, providing information about state and federally funded programs such as Medicaid or the state's CHIP (Locke & Dixon, 2011).

The country's AI/AN population is most densely distributed across the western United States. Although most western states are participating in Medicaid expansion, at press time, approximately half of U.S. states were either opting out or leaning toward opting out of Medicaid expansion (Advisory Board Company, 2014).

In states with exchanges, tribes have the option to encourage tribal members to enroll in and subsidize exchange plans. With the ACA, Medicaid covers many more AI/ANs, and this in concert with private health insurance billing will create new sources of revenue for tribal and IHS clinics. These funding streams will greatly affect the solvency and ultimately the quality of care that these historically underfunded institutions have been able to provide (Locke & Dixon, 2011).

Implications of the Affordable Care Act on Indian Health

The ACA will have minimal impact on the health of AI/AN people who are enrolled members of federally recognized tribal nations. This is due to the sovereign nature of each AI/AN nation, which is not held to compliance with stipulations of the act (Warne, 2011). Although the ACA mandates minimum coverage for all Americans with penalties for those who opt out of voluntary insurance plans, AI/ANs eligible for IHS benefits were determined to be exempt from minimum-coverage penalties (Irving, 2013). Additionally, for those AI/ANs who purchase health insurance through exchanges, cost sharing and co-payments will be waived for those who meet income-level restrictions (U.S. Department of Health and Human Services, 2013a).

A difficulty facing many AI/ANs is that to get health insurance, they must have filed a tax return (Healthcare.gov, n.d.). Because many have minimal income, they have not had to file tax returns in the past. Such obstacles and possible remedies are currently being discussed as this chapter goes to press. Those AI/ANs who are not enrolled members of federally recognized tribes will have to purchase health insurance or incur penalties.

Because guidelines for Medicaid will be expanded so that more AI/ANs can be insured under the program, providers and facilities serving those AI/ANs will be able to bill Medicaid for services rendered (U.S. Department of Health and Human Services, 2013a). Thus, funding and limited contract health dollars will be saved for use with other AI/AN people who may otherwise be denied care under the IHS system.

At the time of press, the landscape surrounding the ACA and exchanges is rapidly changing. Many of these projections stated here rely heavily on the devoted work of AI/AN and other dedicated advocates working to maintain an AI/AN voice at the policy table.

Urban Indian Cancer Care

Substantial health disparities exist among urban AI/ANs, who suffer from similar cancer disparities as those in rural areas. Health problems of urban AI/ANs are often exacerbated by the lack of family and traditional cultural environments (IHS, 2014). Even though a cancer center may be only several miles from an AI/AN patient's home, one cannot assume the patient has bus fare or access to other transportation. In addition, funding for urban Indian healthcare centers has been decreased over time, while the need for healthcare services, including cancer care, has grown (Urban Indian Health Commission, 2007).

Patient Navigation

One solution that has found solid footing in AI/AN communities is the use of patient navigators to help AI/AN patients as they negotiate the complicated healthcare systems throughout their cancer journey. Cancer navigators are typically lay health workers, often from the patients' community, who have been trained to help a patient navigate through the bureaucratic morass of cancer care (Robinson-White, Conroy, Slavish, & Rosenzweig, 2010). Researchers are finding that services provided by culturally trained navigators may positively influence cancer care received by AI/AN people (Eschiti, Burhansstipanov, & Watanabe-Galloway, 2012). Further research is needed, but it is likely that funds spent for navigators to assist AI/AN people to ascertain care and services are cost-effective over time.

Unfortunately, navigators are not the panacea for the fractured healthcare systems that exist in many AI/AN regions. For example, in northern New Mexico, where AI/AN populations can make up as much as 10%–20% of the general population (U.S. Census Bureau, 2014b), patients with cancer can move between multiple healthcare systems during the course of their cancer trajectory. These systems can include, but are not limited to, skilled nursing facilities, emergency departments, regional and distant cancer care centers, hospitals, and short-term care facilities.

Although navigators and community health workers are an important contributor to bridging these care systems for families and patients, in resource-poor settings, lay health workers such as navigators have become the solution for all care gaps, providing transportation, mental health counseling, resource procurement, patient education, practical support, and companionship. Relying on a navigator to serve these roles is neither appropriate nor ethical, as there is the potential for care provision that is unlicensed and outside the navigator's scope of practice and training. Although navigation in its purest intended form is a clinically useful tool and has particular application in culturally diverse AI/AN communities, it should be kept within the intended role, which is to assist patients with cancer in navigating through the bureaucracies of clinical cancer care during a difficult time (Robinson-White et al., 2010).

Patients' perspectives must be considered when discussing cancer policy, education, health systems, and a holistic view of health care. In the transition to the post-ACA world, the Centers for Medicare and Medicaid Services have funds earmarked for navigators in certain states, recognizing the need for this essential service in patient care (Dixon, 2013).

Alaska Native Care

A common issue in delivery of cancer care in AI/AN communities is negotiating the multiple barriers of care. Nowhere is transportation more of an issue than in Alaska, where the average number of people per square mile is only 1.2, in contrast to the U.S. average of 87.4 (U.S. Census Bureau, 2014a). Not only is the population density in Alaska comparatively low, but the geographic vastness of the state, along with weather and topography that often requires air transportation, makes healthcare delivery particularly challenging.

In a state of this size, having on-site oncology expertise within the sparsely populated villages is impractical, and many patients with cancer have to leave their homes for months at a stretch to receive treatment. Preparing for a months-long absence from home can create delays in treatment as patients prepare their home and family for their departure, having to ensure that caregiving duties for older adults and children are attended to and that food supplies are stocked. Many ANs live off the road system, so any cancer care requires air travel to Anchorage or Seattle, adding economic burdens to care.

For ANs receiving care through the Alaska Native Medical Center, oncology care is delivered in Anchorage and through contract care facilities in Seattle. While subsidies exist for patients who need to travel, long absences incur costs beyond what can be covered by these subsidies, creating tremendous burdens on patients and their families. Patients have to make difficult decisions, weighing the burden of care on their financial future, the future of their families, and their ability to have meaningful quality of life for the duration of their lives given the reality of their diagnosis.

Through innovations in research, barriers in cancer care are being addressed. Clinicians, community leaders, and policy makers are tasked with translating these research innovations to clinical practice. Cancer navigation for AI/AN people is an area that needs considerable research to determine whether it is cost-effective and improves cancer screening rates and outcomes.

Most published projects are descriptive in nature, with limited generalizability (Eschiti et al., 2012). Navigation as cancer policy is a growing field, and funding for cancer navigation in Alaska is included in the ACA (Dixon, 2013).

Telehealth, which is the use of videoconferencing systems to connect patients, healthcare providers, and community members across distances for consultation, education, case conferences, or even support groups, has proved to be particularly effective in AN communities, connecting small tribal villages throughout the state (Doorenbos et al., 2011). Policies that fund expansion of telehealth networks will benefit AI/ANs throughout the nation by connecting expert clinicians to small regional clinics and building networks through existing technology at a low cost burden to the healthcare system.

The National Breast and Cervical Cancer Early Detection Program, a Centers for Disease Control and Prevention–funded project designed to target prevention and early diagnosis of breast and cervical cancer, is a cancer-related policy with widespread implications in rural states such as Alaska. By investing time and funding in screening, prevention, and education, cancers are prevented and diagnosed at early stages, and treatment begins before the cancer has advanced to late stages, when the prognosis is less positive. Implications of policies that target wellness have particular applicability in AI/AN communities, where health-based interventions are considered culturally congruent and more likely to have sustainable success (Brown et al., 2011; Walters & Simoni, 2009).

Existing Tribal Policy Efforts

As stated earlier in this chapter, the policy landscape is rapidly changing at the time of this writing. With the ACA, federal sequestration, and the recent economic downturn, budgets for AI/AN health are being challenged. NCAI gave testimony before the House Appropriations Committee on Interior, Environment, and Related Agencies at an oversight hearing on Indian health, arguing that federal budgeting decisions for IHS should not be affected by the sequestration, as funding is obligated by federal treaties between the government and AI/AN nations (NCAI, 2013b).

Recommendations for Health Policy Change

In a query of federally funded health research within the National Institutes of Health Research Portfolio Online Reporting Tools system (http://projectreporter.nih.gov) using the search terms *health policy*, *Alaska Native*, and *American Indian,* from 2001 to 2013, 72 studies yielded relevant research. Only 33 had mention of health policy within the body of the abstract. Nine studies referred to health policy in the context of research findings having possible implications for future policy change. Only 24 of the 72 studies funded had health policy as an actual feature of the research. Of those abstracts, authors included research on policy advocacy, policy research, and policy education. Granted, the National Institutes of Health is best positioned to fund primary research and not policy research; yet, as the health research hub for American institutions, the paucity of health policy research related to AI/AN health indicates the low priority of health policy in AI/AN health research in current academic research.

A tremendous body of literature exists on interventions that have proven efficacy in AI/AN communities. Policies that fund and implement these interventions are needed to take what has been established in the research and disseminate it into practice, particularly in the realm of cancer survivorship and end-of-life care. As AI/AN tribes and nations are building financial independence through economic development, they are able to determine their own course of action regarding health for their communities. Through collaboration with researchers, implementation and dissemination of research, and a long-term focus on sustainable programs for their populations, tribes are well positioned to make substantive and meaningful changes for their communities and, in particular, their tribal members living with cancer.

Future Directions

National healthcare reform has provided AI/AN nations with unique opportunities for cancer care improvements. The ACA brings with it resources, changing policies, and re-envisioned provision of care for all Americans. Unfortunately, existing health disparities place AI/ANs at a disadvantage from the onset of reform, and few provisions have been included to bring AI/AN health care and cancer care to parity with that of the general population. Without special consideration of these disparities and a concerted push from tribal leaders, thought leaders, and policy makers, the funneling of funds necessary to bring health and cancer care equity to AI/ANs is unlikely.

Conclusion

The cancer care journey for AI/AN people has been shown to be complex and currently undergoing change as a result of the ACA. Cancer incidence and mortality rates are high in parts of the country, in part due to numerous barriers to adequate care along the cancer continuum, as well as a history of provision of culturally incongruent health care from mainstream healthcare providers and institutions. Advocacy on the part of oncology healthcare providers, stakeholders, researchers, and other providers is needed to improve cancer care to AI/AN people in clinical settings, research, and health policy.

The authors express gratitude to the elders who have come before them for the sacrifices they made to preserve the Native way of life for future generations.

References

Advisory Board Company. (2014, September 4). Where the states stand on Medicaid expansion: 27 states, D.C. expanding Medicaid. Retrieved from http://www.advisory.com/daily-briefing/resources/primers/medicaidmap

BigFoot, D.S., & Schmidt, S. (2010). Honoring children, mending the circle: Cultural adaptation of trauma-focused cognitive-behavioral therapy for American Indian and Alaska Native children. *Journal of Clinical Psychology, 66,* 847–856. doi:10.1002/jclp.20707

Brokenleg, M. (n.d.). Native American perspectives on generosity. Retrieved from http://www.altruists.org/f164

Brown, S.R., Nuno, T., Joshweseoma, L., Begay, R.C., Goodluck, C., & Harris, R.B. (2011). Impact of a community-based breast cancer screening program on Hopi women. *Preventive Medicine, 52,* 390–393. doi:10.1016/j.ypmed.2011.02.012

Burhansstipanov, L., & Hollow, W. (2001). Native American cultural aspects of oncology nursing care. *Seminars in Oncology Nursing, 17,* 206–219. doi:10.1053/sonu.2001.25950

Connolly, C., & Gitlin, J. (2013). Executive briefing 1: Health insurance exchanges. *Trustee: The Journal for Hospital Governing Boards, 66*(3), 15–18.

Crowder, C., Jim, R.L., Joseph, A., Jr., & Hayes, G. (2013). *Creating a legacy of honor and trust: Striving for health parity for all American Indians and Alaska Natives. The National Tribal Budget Formulation Workgroup's recommendations on the Indian Health Service fiscal year 2015 budget.* Retrieved from http://www.nihb.org/docs/07112013/FY%202015%20IHS%20budget%20full%20report_FINAL.pdf

Dixon, M. (2013). Information for tribes about navigator funding. Retrieved from http://www.nihb.org/tribalhealthreform/wp-content/uploads/2013/01/Information-for-Tribes-about-Navigator-Funding-Mim-Dixon-5-6-131.pdf

Doorenbos, A.Z., Demiris, G., Towle, C., Kundu, A., Revels, L., Colven, R., ... Buchwald, D. (2011). Developing the Native People for Cancer Control Telehealth Network. *Telemedicine and e-Health, 17,* 30–34. doi:10.1089/tmj.2010.0101

Eschiti, V., Burhansstipanov, L., & Watanabe-Galloway, S. (2012). Native cancer navigation: The state of the science. *Clinical Journal of Oncology Nursing, 16,* 73–82. doi:10.1188/12.CJON.73-82

Espey, D.K., Wu, X.-C., Swan, J., Wiggins, C., Jim, M.A., Ward, E., ... Edwards, B.K. (2007). Annual report to the nation on the status of cancer, 1975–2004, featuring cancer in American Indians and Alaska Natives. *Cancer, 110,* 2119–2152. doi:10.1002/cncr.23044

Filippi, M.K., Ndikum-Moffor, F., Braiuca, S.L., Goodman, T., Hammer, T.L., James, A.S., ... Daley, C.M. (2013). Breast cancer screening perceptions among American Indian women under age 40. *Journal of Cancer Education, 28,* 535–540. doi:10.1007/s13187-013-0499-4

Grandbois, D.M., & Sanders, G.F. (2009). The resilience of Native American elders. *Issues in Mental Health Nursing, 30,* 569–580. doi:10.1080/01612840902916151

Gray, J.S., & Rose, W.J. (2012). Cultural adaptation for therapy with American Indians and Alaska Natives. *Journal of Multicultural Counseling and Development, 40,* 82–92. Retrieved from http://ruralhealth.und.edu/pdf/jmcd_0412_vol40.pdf

Haozous, E.A. (2009). *Exploring cancer pain in Southwest American Indians* (Doctoral dissertation). Available from ProQuest Dissertations and Theses database. (Publication No. 3395766)

Haozous, E.A., & Knobf, M.T. (2013). "All my tears were gone": Suffering and cancer pain in Southwest American Indians. *Journal of Pain and Symptom Management, 45,* 1050–1060. doi:10.1016/j.jpainsymman.2012.06.001

Healthcare.gov. (n.d.). Health coverage for American Indians/Alaska Natives. Retrieved from https://www.healthcare.gov/if-im-an-american-indian-or-alaska-native-what-do-i-need-to-know-about-the-marketplace

Hodge, F.S., & Casken, J.D. (1999). American Indian breast cancer project: Educational development and implementation. *American Indian Culture and Research Journal, 23,* 205–215. Retrieved from http://nursing.ucla.edu/workfiles/CAIIRE/Articles/AI%20breast%20cancer%20project.pdf

Holkup, P.A. (2002). Big changes in the Indian Health Service: Are nurses aware? *Journal of Transcultural Nursing, 13,* 47–53. doi:10.1177/104365960201300108

Indian Health Service. (2005). *Indian Health Service gold book—The first 50 years of the Indian Health Service.* Retrieved from http://www.ihs.gov/newsroom/includes/themes/newihstheme/display_objects/documents/GOLD_BOOK_part1.pdf

Indian Health Service. (2013, April 18). Increase proposed for Indian Health Service budget [Press release]. Retrieved from http://www.ihs.gov/newsroom/pressreleases/2013pressreleases/increaseproposedforindianhealthservicebudget

Indian Health Service. (2014, January). Urban Indian health program. Retrieved from http://www.ihs.gov/newsroom/factsheets/urbanindianhealthprogram

Irving, F. (2013, June 28). HHS affirms American Indian ACA exemptions. *Healthcare Payer News.* Retrieved from http://www.healthcarepayernews.com/content/hhs-affirms-american-indian-aca-exemptions

Kaiser Family Foundation. (2012). The facts on Medicare spending and financing. Retrieved from http://kff.org/medicare/fact-sheet/medicare-spending-and-financing-fact-sheet

Locke, K., & Dixon, M. (2011, March 14). *Tribal planning for health insurance exchanges begins now* (Report prepared for the Tribal Self Governance Advisory Committee). Retrieved from http://www.ndhealth.gov/oehd/Tribal_Planning_for_Exchanges_3-14-11.pdf

McKosato, H. (2013, December 9). Health coverage could improve with Affordable Care Act education. *Indian Country Today Media Network.* Retrieved from http://indiancountrytodaymedianetwork.com/2013/12/09/health-coverage-could-improve-affordable-care-act-education-152601

Medicare.gov. (n.d.). The Affordable Care Act and Medicare. Retrieved from http://www.medicare.gov/about-us/affordable-care-act/affordable-care-act.html

National Congress of American Indians. (2013a). *Securing our futures.* Retrieved from http://www.ncai.org/Securing_Our_Futures_Final.pdf

National Congress of American Indians. (2013b, March 26). *Testimony of the National Congress of American Indians: Oversight hearing Indian Health House Appropriations Subcommittee on Interior, Environment, and Related Agencies,* 113 Cong. Session 1 (2013). Retrieved from http://www.ncai.org/resources/testimony/ncai-testimony-indian-health-affairs-oversight-hearing

Onega, T., Duell, E.J., Shi, X., Wang, D., Demidenko, E., & Goodman, D. (2008). Geographic access to cancer care in the U.S. *Cancer, 112,* 909–918. doi:10.1002/cncr.23229

Petereit, D.G., Molloy, K., Reiner, M.L., Helbig, P., Cina, K., Miner, R., … Roberts, C.R. (2008). Establishing a patient navigator program to reduce cancer disparities in the American Indian communities of Western South Dakota: Initial observations and results. *Cancer Control, 15,* 254–259. Retrieved from http://www.ncbi.nlm.nih.gov/pmc/articles/PMC2556124

Robinson-White, S., Conroy, B., Slavish, K.H., & Rosenzweig, M. (2010). Patient navigation in breast cancer: A systematic review. *Cancer Nursing, 33,* 127–140. doi:10.1097/
NCC.0b013e3181c40401

Schneider, A. (2005). Reforming American Indian/Alaska Native health care financing: The
role of Medicaid. *American Journal of Public Health, 95,* 766–768. doi:10.2105/AJPH.2004
.061317

Shelton, B.L. (2001). Legal and historical basis of Indian health care. In M. Dixon & Y. Roubide-
aux (Eds.), *Promises to keep: Public health policy for American Indians and Alaska Natives in the 21st
century* (pp. 1–28). Washington, DC: American Public Health Association.

Siegel, R., Ma, J., Zou, Z., & Jemal, A. (2014). Cancer statistics, 2014. *CA: A Cancer Journal for Clinicians, 64,* 9–29. doi:10.3322/caac.21208

Stromnes-Elias, K. (2007). *Technical assistance on Native American culture: Improving CWIC services
for Native American SSA beneficiaries with disabilities* (Issues Brief No. 2). Missoula, MT: American Indian Disability Technical Assistance Center.

Struthers, R., Eschiti, V.S., & Patchell, B. (2004). Traditional indigenous healing: Part I. *Complementary Therapies in Nursing and Midwifery, 10,* 141–149. doi:10.1016/j.ctnm.2004.05.001

Thierry, J., Brenneman, G., Rhoades, E., & Chilton, L. (2009). History, law, and policy as a foundation for health care delivery for American Indian and Alaska Native children. *Pediatric
Clinics of North America, 56,* 1539–1559. doi:10.1016/j.pcl.2009.09.018

Transfer Act (Indian Health Facilities Act of 1954, Pub L. No. 568, 68 Stat. 674, codified as
amended at 42 U.S.C. §§ 2001–2005f).

U.S. Census Bureau. (2014a, July). State and county QuickFacts: Alaska. Retrieved from http://
quickfacts.census.gov/qfd/states/02000.html

U.S. Census Bureau. (2014b, October). State and county QuickFacts: New Mexico. Retrieved
from http://quickfacts.census.gov/qfd/states/35000.html

U.S. Census Bureau. (2014c, July). State and county QuickFacts: USA. Retrieved from http://
quickfacts.census.gov/qfd/states/00000.html

U.S. Department of Health and Human Services. (2013a). Fact sheet: The Affordable Care
Act and American Indian and Alaska Native people. Retrieved from http://www.hhs.gov/
healthcare/facts/factsheets/2011/03/americanindianhealth03212011a.html

U.S. Department of Health and Human Services. (2013b). *Fiscal year 2014 Indian Health Service: Justification of estimates for appropriations committees.* Retrieved from http://www.npaihb.
org/images/resources_docs/QBM%20Handouts/2013/April/4B1%20-%20FY2014Budget
Justification.pdf

U.S. Department of Health and Human Services Office of Minority Health. (2014). Profile:
American Indian/Alaska Native. Retrieved from http://minorityhealth.hhs.gov/omh/
browse.aspx?lvl=3&lvlid=62

Urban Indian Health Commission. (2007). *Invisible tribes: Urban Indians and their health in a
changing world.* Retrieved from http://www.uihi.org/wp-content/uploads/2009/09/UIHC_
Report_FINAL.pdf

Walters, K.L., & Simoni, J.M. (2009). Decolonizing strategies for mentoring American Indians and Alaska Natives in HIV and mental health research. *American Journal of Public Health,
99*(Suppl. 1), S71–S76. doi:10.2105/AJPH.2008.136127

Warne, D. (2011). *Affordable Care Act as it affects Native Americans* [Video]. Retrieved from http://
www.natamcancer.org/WorkGroups/DonWarne-pt4.html

Warne, D., Kaur, J., & Perdue, D. (2012). American Indian/Alaska Native cancer policy: Systemic approaches to reducing cancer disparities. *Journal of Cancer Education, 27*(Suppl. 1), S18–
S23. doi:10.1007/s13187-012-0315-6

Wilson, R.T., Giroux, J., Kasicky, K.R., Fatupaito, B.H., Wood, E.C., Crichlow, R., ... Cobb, N.
(2011). Breast and cervical cancer screening patterns among American Indian women at
IHS clinics in Montana and Wyoming. *Public Health Reports, 126,* 806–815. Retrieved from
http://www.publichealthreports.org/issueopen.cfm?articleID=2747

CHAPTER 12

Creation of a Statewide Mammography Surveillance Program

Anne Marie Murphy, PhD, Carol Estwing Ferrans, PhD, RN, FAAN, David Ansell, MD, MPH, and Danielle M. Dupuy, MPH

This work was funded by grants to the Metropolitan Chicago Breast Cancer Task Force by Susan G. Komen and the Avon Foundation for Women, and by National Institutes of Health grant 2P50CA106743 from the National Cancer Institute.

Introduction

During the past two decades, substantial investment has taken place to improve breast cancer detection and treatment in the United States, leading to a significant decrease in breast cancer mortality overall. However, similar to overall improvements in health care nationally, the benefits of these improvements have not been shared equally among all segments of the population (Haynes & Smedley, 1999). Nationally and in Chicago, the breast cancer mortality rate for Caucasian women has been steadily declining since the mid-1990s. In contrast, the breast cancer mortality rate for African American women in Chicago has remained virtually unchanged during this time period (Hirschman, Whitman, & Ansell, 2007) (see Figure 12-1).

A recent study examined the 25 most populous cities in the United States and found that African American women in Chicago have one of the highest breast cancer mortality rates, as well as one of the largest disparities in breast cancer mortality, with African American women being 61% more likely than Caucasian women to die from breast cancer (Whitman, Orsi, & Hurlbert, 2012). Other large cities, such as New York and Baltimore, have seen reduc-

Figure 12-1. Age-Adjusted Breast Cancer Mortality Rates, 1980–2005

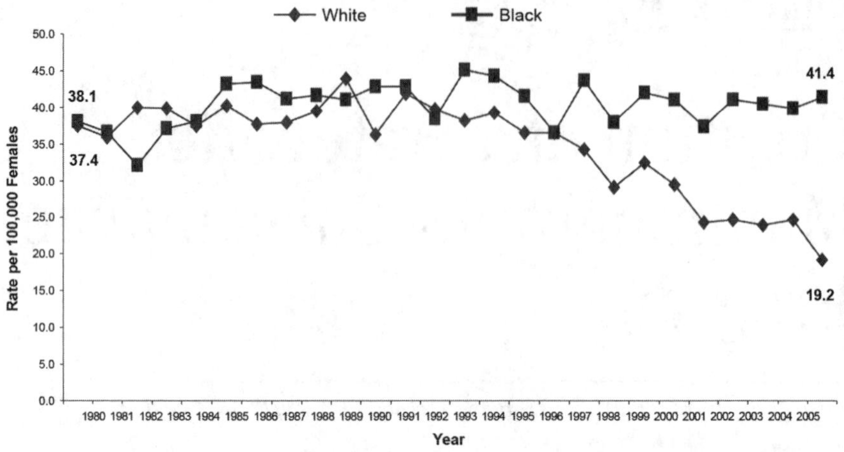

Note. From "A Community Effort to Reduce the Black/White Breast Cancer Mortality Disparity in Chicago," by D. Ansell, P. Grabler, S. Whitman, C. Ferrans, J. Burgess-Bishop, L.R. Murray, … E. Marcus, 2009, *Cancer Causes and Control, 20,* p. 1683. Copyright 2009 by Springer Science + Business Media. Reprinted with permission.

tions in African American mortality rates and concomitant mortality disparities, although not yet complete parity (Whitman et al., 2012). Geographic variations exist, with low African American/Caucasian disparities sometimes due to low mortality for African American women, as in San Francisco, and sometimes due to a high mortality rate for both African American and Caucasian women, as in Detroit (Whitman et al., 2012). This geographic variability in breast cancer mortality suggests that variation in healthcare system factors is a significant driver of disparities. While differences in tumor biology may play a role (Carey et al., 2006; Cunningham, Montero, Garrett-Mayer, Berkel, & Ely, 2010; Ooi, Martinez, & Li, 2011), they cannot explain the widening of the breast cancer mortality disparity over time (Silber et al., 2013), nor can they explain geographic variability in such disparities.

Action in Chicago

Against the backdrop of the publication of the first paper in 2007 showing this disturbing and growing breast cancer disparity in Chicago (Hirschman et al., 2007), a Call to Action Summit took place in Chicago to unite to end this disparity. The summit brought together more than 200 healthcare providers, researchers, and community members, many of whom subsequently participated in three work groups that met repeatedly over six months to identify causes and propose solutions to the disparity problem. These work groups created a comprehensive report titled *Improving Quality and Reducing Disparities in Breast Cancer Mortality in Metropolitan Chicago* (Metropolitan Chicago Breast Cancer Task Force, 2007), presenting 37 recommendations to the city for combating the disparity. These recommendations called for healthcare quality improvement and health system reform, including public funding for healthcare resources for uninsured women, along with widespread public outreach and education to promote breast cancer screening, and improvement of the quality of mammography and treatment. The recommendations were data based and addressed three factors hypothesized as driving the mortality disparity in Chicago, which were that

* African American women receive fewer mammograms
* African American women receive mammograms of inferior quality
* African American women have inadequate access to quality treatment once breast cancer is diagnosed.

A number of Chicago-based researchers provided data to identify causes, as well as the 37 recommendations, based on their completed research. In addition, the first Chicago-wide mammography capacity study was conducted for the report. Results showed that minority populations were less likely to (Ansell et al., 2009; Rauscher, Allgood, Whitman, & Conant, 2012)

* Be screened at academic and private nonacademic institutions
* Receive care at a facility with digital mammography
* Have their mammograms read by a trained breast imaging specialist
* Receive same-day results for diagnostic mammograms.

In addition, a variety of institutions voluntarily shared in-depth data on mammography quality for the report. These data provided preliminary evidence of poor mammography quality in certain safety net venues (Metropolitan Chicago Breast Cancer Task Force, 2007). These findings point to factors contributing to the mortality disparity in Chicago, given that digital mammography has been found to be more effective for women younger than 50 (Pisano et al., 2005); African American women are more likely to get breast cancer at a younger age than Caucasian women (American Cancer Society, 2013); and studies have shown that breast imaging specialists are more effective at finding breast cancers (Sickles, Wolverton, & Dee, 2002). In the time since the report was released, digital mammography has become more readily available in Chicago, but the other factors (e.g., availability of breast imaging specialists, same-day readings) have not improved significantly.

With respect to treatment quality, the Metropolitan Chicago Breast Cancer Task Force (Task Force) also mapped treatment facilities in Chicago, which showed a maldistribution of the highest quality providers. Of the 25 community areas in Chicago with the highest breast cancer mortality rates, 24 at that time were predominantly African American. However, of the 14 programs approved by the American College of Surgeons Commission on Cancer in Chicago, only one was located in a high-mortality community area (Ansell et al., 2009) (see Figure 12-2).

Metropolitan Chicago Breast Cancer Task Force

In light of these findings, the Call to Action Summit report recommended the establishment of an office for the Task Force for the purpose of continued research and quality improvement. In 2008, funding was received from the Avon Foundation for Women to establish the Task Force office and from Susan G. Komen for the Task Force's project, the Chicago Breast Cancer Quality Consortium (the Consortium). The Consortium was creat-

Figure 12-2. Distribution of American College of Surgeons Commission on Cancer–Accredited Comprehensive Care Sites Relative to High-Mortality Areas in Chicago

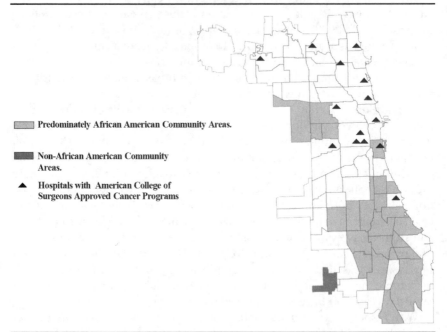

Note. From "A Community Effort to Reduce the Black/White Breast Cancer Mortality Disparity in Chicago," by D. Ansell, P. Grabler, S. Whitman, C. Ferrans, J. Burgess-Bishop, L.R. Murray, ... E. Marcus, 2009, *Cancer Causes and Control, 20,* p. 1684. Copyright 2009 by Springer Science + Business Media. Reprinted with permission.

ed to bring together facilities that screen, diagnose, and treat breast cancer; to share breast cancer quality data to identify deficits; and to collaborate in quality improvement interventions. The Illinois Hospital Association joined the Task Force to start the collaborative effort.

The Consortium is the first project in the nation to address racial health disparities through quality improvement with voluntary provider collaboration across an entire community's health system (Metropolitan Chicago, including Cook and collar counties [the five counties around Cook]). Consortium activities are guided by a steering committee and relevant expert advisory boards, representing 14 area Metropolitan Chicago institutions. These committees generate consensus on the quality metrics to be collected and the benchmarks used to evaluate institution metrics. The expert advisory boards also are involved in the development and implementation of quality improvement initiatives.

Historically, Illinois hospitals and healthcare providers have been reluctant to share quality data because of legal concerns. Recognizing these concerns nationwide, Congress passed the Patient Safety and Quality Improvement Act of 2005 to establish new federal confidentiality protections for organizations whose primary mission is patient safety and quality improvement and that were willing to meet certain standards. The Consortium applied for these federal protections, and approval was granted in September 2009. The Consortium is the first patient safety organization (PSO) in the nation dedicated exclusively to quality improvement for breast cancer services and to elimination of a racial health disparity. The Consortium's PSO status is a key feature to creating a confidential environment for providers so that they can focus on quality improvement without fear of legal repercussions or negative media attention.

To be covered by the confidentiality protections of the Patient Safety Act, a PSO must enter into a data-sharing contractual agreement with each participating provider. Working with a local law firm (pro bono), the Consortium developed these data-sharing agreements. The Consortium also decided to seek institutional review board (IRB) approval for both itself and each participating institution, and Consortium staff developed an IRB protocol template for participating sites. The Rush University Medical Center IRB served the Consortium overall and also was the IRB of record for safety net institutions that did not have IRBs of their own.

Data Collection

Expert advisory working groups formed to develop consensus on the quality metrics to collect for mammography quality and treatment quality, and data collection tools were developed (see www.chicagobreastcancer.org/site/epage/93661_904.htm for tools). For the first year, the sites used a web portal provided by the Illinois Hospital Association, which was similar to the one they used for other state reporting. However, some institutions found the portal difficult to use, so in subsequent years, after discussions with personnel from the Agency for Healthcare Research and Quality PSO staff, sites moved to submitting data on Excel spreadsheets via email. Ease of use was critically important for robust participation, as institutional participation was voluntary.

The Consortium began with separate data collection for mammography quality and treatment quality. We subsequently developed an additional care process analysis project designed to look across the continuum of care from a patient-centered perspective. This care process or environmental scanning captured all the touchpoints from a woman's first call to schedule a screening mammogram through follow-up imaging, diagnostics, and treatment. Twenty-six institutions participated in the care process analysis and, during the first two years, 59 healthcare institutions and their affiliated clinics participated in at least one year of quality data collection.

Because there were no financial incentives originally, personal outreach by the Metropolitan Chicago Breast Cancer Task Force founders and board members was key to engaging healthcare institutions in this original voluntary data collection, as well as that of the Illinois Hospital Association and the three cochairs of the original Call to Action Summit. The three cochairs were the former commissioner of health for the city of Chicago, the former head of Cook County Bureau of Health Services, and the current chief executive officer of the largest federally qualified healthcare center network in Chicago. The Consortium director had also previously served as the state's Medicaid director and thus had relationships with many institutions. In addition, the expert advisory working groups welcomed experts from all participating institutions with broad representation across academic, community, public, and safety net hospitals and hospital systems in metropolitan Chicago. This "big tent" approach, openly encouraging all to participate, was key to garnering widespread participation in an entirely voluntary quality improvement data collection endeavor that relied only on civic responsibility and commitment to reducing disparities and improving breast cancer outcomes.

Metrics

A high-quality screening mammography program should detect breast cancers when present and visible via mammography, should detect them when small and early stage, and should ensure prompt follow-up. Such a program should avoid calling back too many women for unnecessary follow-up imaging or unnecessarily identifying women for biopsies who do not in fact have cancer. The metrics of the Consortium Mammography Expert Advisory Board were designed to measure all of these areas. The measures were as follows.
• **Recall rate:** The proportion of screening mammograms interpreted as abnormal (Breast Imaging Reporting and Data System 0, 4, or 5) (bench-

mark of no less than 5% and no more than 14% of screening mammograms interpreted as abnormal [i.e., requiring recall]).

- **Not lost at imaging:** The proportion of abnormal screening mammograms receiving follow-up diagnostic imaging within 12 months of the screening mammogram (benchmark of 90% and above).
- **Timely follow-up imaging:** The receipt of diagnostic imaging within 30 days of an abnormal screen, among those receiving diagnostic imaging within 12 months of the screen (benchmark of 90% and above).
- **Biopsy recommendation rate:** Proportion of abnormal screening mammograms resulting in a recommendation for biopsy (benchmark of 8%–20%).
- **Not lost at biopsy:** The proportion of women with a biopsy recommendation who received a biopsy within 12 months of the abnormal screen (benchmark of 70% and above).
- **Timely biopsy:** The receipt of a biopsy within 60 days of the abnormal screen, among those receiving a biopsy within 12 months of the screen (benchmark of 90% and above).

The following three measures of the quality of cancer detection were calculated for facilities that reported at least 1,000 screening mammograms during the calendar year.

- **Cancer detection rate:** The number of breast cancers detected following an abnormal screen for every 1,000 screening mammograms performed (benchmark of 3–10 per 1,000).
- **Cancer if abnormal screen (also known as PPV1):** The proportion of abnormal screens that received a breast cancer diagnosis within 12 months of the screen (benchmark of 3%–8%).
- **Cancer if biopsied (also known as PPV3):** The proportion of patients biopsied following an abnormal screen who received a breast cancer diagnosis within 12 months of the screen (benchmark of 15%–40%).

The following two measures of ability to detect breast cancer early were calculated for facilities that reported at least 10 screen-detected breast cancers during the calendar year.

- **Proportion minimal:** The proportion of screen-detected breast cancers that were either in situ or no greater than 1 cm in largest diameter (benchmark of greater than 30%). Breast cancers with unknown minimal status were excluded from both the numerator and denominator of this measure. While the program attempted to collect information on lymph node status for minimal cancers, many institutions were unable to provide this data reliably, so lymph node status was not included in the definition of minimal cancer.
- **Proportion early-stage:** The proportion of screen-detected breast cancers that were either in situ or stage I (benchmark of greater than 50%). Breast cancers with unknown stage were excluded from both the numerator and denominator of this measure.

The metrics collected are reviewed each year and modified when necessary. Most metrics remained consistent over each data collection cycle (see Table 12-1). However, some debate existed with respect to timeliness metrics; these showed some changes between years (see Table 12-1).

A high-quality breast cancer treatment program should ensure that care is provided according to national guidelines. These guidelines change over time, and high-quality treatment programs make adjustments accordingly. The metrics chosen by the Consortium Treatment Advisory Board are based on National Quality Forum and Commission on Cancer standardized measures in breast cancer treatment quality, as well as literature on procedures and outcomes in breast cancer diagnosis and treatment (see Table 12-2). They include the following.

- **Excisional biopsy**
  - Of invasive breast cancers diagnosed at the facility (class 0/1), the percentage for whom diagnostic workup included an excisional biopsy.

Table 12-1. Mammography Measures Collected by Calendar Year (CY)

Measure	CY 2006	CY 2009	CY 2010	CY 2011
Recall rate	X	X	X	X
Lost to follow-up	X	X	X	X
Follow-up imaging 30 days	X		X	X
Follow-up imaging 45 days			X	
Follow-up imaging 60 days		X		
Follow-up imaging 12 months		X	X	X
Recommended biopsy		X	X	X
Biopsy within 60 days		X	X	X
Biopsy within 12 months		X	X	X
PPV1[a]	X	X	X	X
PPV3[b]		X	X	X
Cancer detection rate	X	X	X	X
Proportion minimal	X	X	X	X
Proportion early-stage	X	X	X	X

[a] Proportion of abnormal mammograms resulting in cancer diagnosis

[b] Proportion of biopsies resulting in cancer diagnosis

Table 12-2. Treatment Measures Collected by Calendar Year (CY)[a]

Measure	CY 2006	CY 2009	CY 2010
Number of cancers by stage	X[b]	X[b]	X[b]
Number of cancers by class of case		X[b]	X[b]
Number of cancers by node status		X[b]	X
Age range			X
Of those receiving breast-conserving surgery: % **recommended** for radiation and % who **received** radiation therapy[c]	X[b]	X[b]	X
Of those who tested ER+ or PR+: % **recommended** for hormone therapy and % who **received** hormone therapy[c]	X[b]	X[b]	X
Of those who tested HER2+: % who were **recommended** for trastuzumab and % **who received** trastuzumab	X[b]		X
Type of breast biopsy performed		X	X
Type of lymph node biopsy performed		X	
Proportion with time from diagnosis to treatment ≤ 30 days	X[b]		
Proportion with time from diagnosis to treatment 12 months, 6 months, and ≤ 60 days		X	X
Chemotherapy for node-positive		X	X

[a] CY 2011 data for treatment is to be determined.
[b] Collected for invasive and in situ cancers
[c] Percent recommended and percent receiving collected separately
ER—estrogen receptor; PR—progesterone receptor

- Rationale: Advancements in breast cancer diagnosis have led to the use of needle biopsies as the best and least invasive mode for diagnosing cancer. If a facility is using excisional methods for biopsying too often, further investigation is required to determine whether there is a quality issue.
- **Estrogen receptor (ER) and progesterone receptor (PR) test result available**
  - Of invasive breast cancers treated at the facility (class 1/2), the percentage with ER and PR test results available.
  - Rationale: All breast cancers should be tested for hormonal receptors.

- **Recommended hormone therapy**
  - Of invasive breast cancers treated at the facility that had a positive ER/PR test result, the percentage of patients who are receiving or were recommended hormone therapy.
  - Rationale: If a breast cancer is hormone receptor positive, then in most cases, it should be treated with hormone therapy.
- **HER2 test result available**
  - Of invasive breast cancers treated at the facility (class 1/2) that are stage II, III, or IV, the percentage with a HER2 test result available.
  - Rationale: All breast cancers should be tested for HER2 receptors.
- **Recommended HER2 therapy**
  - Of invasive breast cancers treated at the facility (class 1/2) that are stage II, III, or IV and HER2 positive, the percentage of patients who are receiving or were recommended for HER2 therapy.
  - Rationale: If a breast cancer is HER2 receptor positive, then in most cases, it should be treated with trastuzumab.
- **Treated within 12 months (i.e., not lost to follow-up for treatment)**
  - Of invasive breast cancers treated at the facility, the percentage treated within 12 months of diagnosis (a positive biopsy).
  - Rationale: Breast cancers diagnosed should be treated.
- **Treated within 60 days (i.e., timeliness of treatment)**
  - Of invasive breast cancers treated at the facility within 12 months of diagnosis, the percentage treated within 60 days of diagnosis.
  - Rationale: Literature suggests that poor outcomes are associated with delays in treatment beyond 60 days of diagnosis.
- **Recommended radiation after breast-conserving surgery**
  - Of invasive breast cancers among females aged 18–69 treated at the facility with breast-conserving surgery, the percentage receiving or recommended for radiation.
  - Rationale: Most breast cancers that are treated through lumpectomy or partial mastectomy should receive radiation treatment afterward.
- **Completed radiation after breast-conserving surgery**
  - Of invasive breast cancers treated among females aged 18–69 at the facility with breast-conserving surgery, the percentage receiving or recommended radiation who completed radiation within one year of diagnosis.
  - Rationale: Most breast cancers that are treated through lumpectomy or partial mastectomy should receive and complete radiation treatment afterward.
- **Recommended chemotherapy**
  - Of node-positive invasive breast cancers treated at the facility, the percentage receiving or recommended for chemotherapy.
  - Rationale: Most patients with breast cancer who have tested positive for cancer in their lymph nodes should be treated with chemotherapy.

While the data collected are based generally on commonly known American College of Radiology and National Quality Forum measures, for simplicity of data collection, there was some deviation from the national metrics. This was done because of the concern about low-resource facilities' ability to collect some of the data. However, this led to some discontent from institutions that were already collecting data for the national quality data efforts, because they now had to collect data in additional ways.

Because of the nuances of data collection and to ensure collection was as accurate as possible, the Consortium provided training to site staff to ensure that data were collected and submitted appropriately. Each year, the Consortium held multiple webinar trainings to provide this instruction. Still, in some instances, sites required more than a training module to be able to collect the data. As an all-inclusive initiative, the Consortium has both high- and low-resource institutions participating; some sites have sophisticated mammography tracking systems integrated into their electronic health records, while other sites track mammography patients using paper-based systems. Some institutions were unable to collect the data on their own because of data system limitations, limited staff availability, and limited understanding of data collection methods. Because the goal was complete participation, the Consortium offered data collection assistance to sites that requested it.

Results

The report on the first year of data collection received a great deal of media attention because it was the first of its kind in Chicago. This report focused on screening and treatment data from calendar year 2006 and was released in the fall of 2010 (Metropolitan Chicago Breast Cancer Task Force, 2010). Both the *Chicago Sun-Times* and the *Chicago Tribune* carried front-page stories ("Chicago Hospitals' Grade on Breast Cancer," 2010; Shelton, 2010). The *Sun-Times* story was aptly titled "Not Good Enough" and reported that only about one-third of Chicago hospitals were able to detect breast cancer in its earliest stages or provide treatment within 30 days of diagnosis. While some members of the Task Force and Consortium advisory boards had worried that this kind of media attention would result in reluctance to continue participation in the quality improvement efforts, the reaction was generally the opposite. The media coverage focused attention on the problem and generated more resolve to move forward to tackle it.

Results from 2009 and 2010 yielded interesting findings, particularly in the area of mammography quality. Eleven screening measures were analyzed in both years, and 26%–74% of facilities could not demonstrate that they met screening benchmarks in 2009. This range improved slightly in 2010, with 17%–73% unable to meet screening benchmarks. Specifically, there was a decrease in the proportion of facilities meeting benchmarks among three of the 11 quality measures (recall rate, timely biopsy, and cancers detected among abnormal screens). However, there was an increase in the proportion that could demonstrate that they met benchmarks among the remaining eight measures. These findings could indicate either an improvement in facilities quality or an improvement in their ability to demonstrate quality collected data from year to year. To account for this challenge, the Consortium has worked to improve data collection processes each year. Collection of multiple years of data will enable more reliable interpretation of the data moving forward.

In terms of treatment quality, a smaller proportion of participating facilities were unable to demonstrate that they met benchmarks. In 2009, 0%–30% of facilities could not demonstrate they met benchmarks; this increased slightly to 0%–33% in 2010. From 2009 to 2010, fewer facilities demonstrated meeting benchmarks among four of the eight quality measures (percentage of excisional biopsy, percentage of no biopsy, recommended for hormone therapy among ER/PR-positive cancers, and radiation therapy among those receiving breast-conserving surgery). No change occurred in the proportion of facilities that met benchmarks among two of the measures: ER/PR results available and loss to follow-up at treatment. A slight increase was noted in the proportion of sites demonstrating they met the remaining two benchmarks: receipt of chemotherapy and timely treatment.

One challenge in interpreting these results for the community as a whole is the lack in diversity in types of institutions participating in treatment data collection. Most that do submit data are the academic health centers, which are American College of Surgeons–accredited, high-resource centers. As the program moves forward, considerable effort will be made to incorporate lower-resource facilities in collection of treatment data.

The Consortium is recognized as an unprecedented initiative and therefore has no project or organization that it can look to for successful approaches to accomplishing goals. Because of its focus on quality improvement in a dynamic field where new methods in breast care are constantly being developed, the Consortium has adopted a philosophy of regular process review and improvement. The Consortium will continue to review and revise not only its approaches in data collection, but also analysis, interpretation, and the quality improvement plans and projects it carries out based on evidence in the literature, practical feedback from participating sites, and new developments in breast care.

Reducing Breast Cancer Disparities Act of 2009

At the same time that the Consortium was getting started, members of the Task Force, along with the Public Policy Committee of the Susan G. Komen Chicagoland affiliate, initiated efforts to pass legislation in Illinois to address areas identified as contributing to breast cancer disparities in the Task Force's original report. The legislation, known as the Reducing Breast Cancer Disparities Act of 2009 (Public Act 95-1045), made changes to Illinois Medicaid law and also to Illinois insurance law.

The Medicaid changes put into law included mammography coverage for women younger than 40 who had a family history of breast cancer, prior personal history of breast cancer, a positive genetic test for *BCRA1* or *BCRA2*, and other factors. It also statutorily required coverage of ultrasound screening by Medicaid if a mammogram finds heterogeneous or dense breast tissue. Illinois Medicaid mammography screening rates have historically been extremely low. Compared to other state Medicaid programs, Illinois' Medicaid mammography screening rates as measured by HEDIS (the Healthcare Effectiveness Data and Information Set), which measure the proportion of women aged 40–69 who have had a mammogram in the past two years, has been well below the 50th percentile.

The Task Force Call to Action work groups suggested that providers are reluctant to engage in outreach to Medicaid clients, and some mammography providers refuse to enroll in Medicaid because the reimbursement rates are so low. The Medicaid rate for the technical component of a bilateral digital mammogram at the time was $53.20, compared to Medicare's Chicago rate of $109.77. The Medicaid rate for the professional component of the same digital bilateral screening mammogram was $17.98, compared to Medicare's Chicago rate of $37.37. It was also suggested that providers who perform a large volume of mammography for Medicaid enrollees are financially hurt by so doing and have fewer resources for quality improvement, new equipment, staff training, and hiring of breast imaging specialists rather than general radiologists. Therefore, the new Reducing Breast Cancer Disparities Act legislation required Illinois Medicaid to pay Medicare rates for mammography.

To address mammography quality, the legislation required the Medicaid agency to convene an expert panel to including representatives of hospitals, freestanding mammography facilities, and doctors (including radiologists) to establish mammography quality standards. Based on these standards, the Illinois Medicaid program would provide bonus payments to mammography facilities meeting these standards for screening and diagnosis that would be at least 15% higher than the Medicare rates for mammography. To further address access issues, the Illinois Medicaid department was required to establish a rate methodology for mammography that was performed at federally qualified health centers and other facilities that receive a Medicaid encounter rate. These facilities were encouraged to collaborate with other hospital-based mammography facilities.

Recognizing that low screening rates are not only a product of inadequate outreach by mammography facilities but also arise from many other factors, the Reducing Breast Cancer Disparities Act also required the Illinois Medicaid program to establish a methodology to remind women enrolled in Medicaid who are age-appropriate for screening mammography but have not received a mammogram within the previous 18 months of the importance and benefit of screening mammography. The legislation also directed the Medicaid agency to establish a pay-for-performance program for primary care providers who meet a certain level of mammography screening among their age-appropriate female patient population.

Finally, with respect to Medicaid provisions, the Task Force was aware of research being carried out by John Ayanian's group in Massachusetts. This research was looking at the positive effect of case management included in the National Breast and Cervical Cancer Early Detection Program with respect to decreasing delays in time between abnormal mammography and diagnosis and the lack of such decrease in delays with respect to treatment when patients were then navigated into the non–case-managed Massachusetts Medicaid program. This work was later published (Lobb, Allen, Emmons, & Ayanian, 2010). This spurred inclusion of a legislative requirement with the Reducing Breast Cancer Disparities Act that Illinois Medicaid initiate patient navigation pilots.

In addition to the Medicaid provisions, the Reducing Breast Cancer Disparities Act also modified the Illinois insurance code to require state-regulated health insurers to cover pain therapy and pain medication when medically appropriate for patients with breast cancer. Additionally, it eliminated cost sharing for mammography. This last provision was also included later in the federal Patient Protection and Affordable Care Act.

The legislation as originally drafted required mammography facilities to accept self-referrals for mammography, as the Task Force town hall meetings suggested that requiring a physician's order for a screening mammogram was a barrier to access. However, the final bill did not include this provision.

After the legislation was signed into law in April 2009, the insurance-related provisions were promptly put into place. Some of the Medicaid provisions for coverage of ultrasounds or mammography for certain women younger than 40 codified current practice and therefore did not require implementation. The primary care pay-for-performance bonus provision was implemented, along with a variety of other pay-for-performance programs for providers. However, with a new governor and changes in agency personnel, the Medicaid provisions increasing mammography rates and establishing an expert panel to develop quality metrics and quality bonuses required additional pressure to implement. On October 18, 2010, Governor Quinn announced the establishment of the Breast Cancer Quality Screening and Treatment Advisory Board, which would assist the Medicaid agency (Department of Healthcare and Family Services) in implementing the statutory provisions in the legislation. The Medicaid agency suggested that its mission would be to

- Identify gaps in screening and diagnostic mammogram services throughout the state.
- Recommend the availability and use of digital mammography.
- Recommend common quality standards for Medicaid, the Illinois Breast and Cervical Cancer Program, and healthcare providers, regardless of payer.
- Recommend best practices for effective outreach to reduce racial disparities in breast cancer mortality.
- Monitor the navigation pilot projects being established.

Some of these provisions were outside the scope of the legislation, but the components related to quality standards and the navigation pilots were clearly linked to the original legislation. Eleven of the 19 board members appointed were associated with the Task Force. A series of meetings took place, eventually reaching consensus to use the quality metrics already being collected through the Task Force's Chicago Breast Cancer Quality Consortium project. The director of the Illinois Department of Healthcare and Family Services overseeing Illinois Medicaid was unwilling to implement a straight increase in mammography reimbursement rates, but instead suggested passing further legislation to tie the increase in mammography reimbursement rates to Medicare's rate, conditional on a provider submitting mammography quality data to the Medicaid agency. This would be consistent with the agency's focus on improving healthcare quality. The director also suggested eliminating the 15% bonus above the Medicare rate for those that met certain metrics, as there was no current consensus on what it meant to meet the benchmarks and there was concern that paying for Medicaid services at a rate that is higher than Medicare might not receive federal approval. With agreement from the Task Force and other interested parties, subsequent legislation ("An Act Concerning Public Aid," Public Act 97-0638) was passed and signed into law on December 16, 2011.

Challenges of Implementing a Statewide Mammography Quality Surveillance Program

Because the Consortium had been collecting and analyzing mammography quality data for several years and had an established expert advisory board for mammography quality with representation from many of the area providers, the Medicaid agency delegates this project to the Consortium by way of a grant. The statewide mammography quality measurement program was established in 2012 after administrative rules were passed by the Illinois administrative body charged with overseeing legislative rules.

With establishment of this program, Illinois would become the first state in the nation to have a mammography quality surveillance program that is more rigorous than the federal standards contained in the Mammography Quality Standards Act (MQSA). However, the first initial implementation ran into challenges with respect to limitations in the Illinois Medicaid claims processing system. Mammography is generally reimbursed in two parts: a mammography facility receives a technical component reimbursement for the costs of having a machine and operating a facility, and a radiologist receives a reimbursement for reading the mammogram. Under the legislation, both would be eligible for the increased reimbursement if mammography quality data were being submitted to the Consortium project. However, the Illinois Medicaid claims processing system was unable to associate specific radiologist claims with the facility at which the mammogram was originally performed. Many radiologists read at multiple facilities. If some of those facilities participated but others did not, it was impossible to know which claims would mandate that radiologists be paid at a higher rate. In an attempt to resolve this, the Medicaid agency required global billing. Indeed the general trend in health care is to move to global billing and bundled or capitated payments. However, in this particular instance, the global billing would be limited to mammography services. Under such a scenario, a facility would sign up for the mammography quality program and would receive an enhanced Medicare-level global payment and would then be responsible for paying the radiologist. For most facilities, this was not practical. It would require setting up separate accounting for mammography alone, with maintenance of the separate billing for other radiology services. Therefore, under this iteration of the program, participation was low.

To address this challenge, the program was revised in 2013. Global billing as a requirement was eliminated. Instead, a quality survey was developed for radiologists based off a prior survey developed by the Breast Cancer Surveillance Consortium and funded by the National Cancer Institute. Under the new program, facilities would sign an agreement with the state to submit their mammography quality data and a mammography facility capacity survey. The radiologists would sign a separate agreement with the state and submit a radiologist quality survey. Because the collection of data is now linked with a state quality improvement initiative, an IRB is no longer required, therefore reducing some of the burden on sites' participation. This program is currently recruiting providers and participation has been significantly more robust than the initial rollout. We anticipate 50%–70% participation (by Medicaid mammography volume) by the end of the first year.

Conclusion

It is hoped that this program can inform the nation as a whole. Mammography quality has been a thorny issue going back to the 1980s (Gray,

1994); these original problems gave rise to passage of the federal MQSA in 1992. Congress asked the National Cancer Policy Board (NCPB) in 2005 to review the adequacy of MQSA, which was due for reauthorization in 2007. The NCPB published a report in 2005 through the Institute of Medicine that recommended a series of improvements to strengthen and standardize audits with respect to the quality of mammography imaging and reading (Nass & Ball, 2005). These inadequacies in federal law allow for widespread variation, as demonstrated in Metropolitan Chicago. The NCPB report and the literature all support collection of certain mammography quality elements to assess and improve quality. We hope this project will demonstrate that such collection is feasible and is in fact necessary to eliminate variation in mammography quality. Allowing such variability undermines the public health message of promoting prevention and early detection screening and also fosters racial health disparities.

References

American Cancer Society. (2013). *Breast cancer facts and figures 2013–2014*. Retrieved from http://www.cancer.org/research/cancerfactsstatistics/breast-cancer-facts-figures

An act concerning public aid, Section 5-5 of The Illinois Public Aid Code (305 ILCS 5/5-5 as amended by P.A. 97-0638, effective January 1, 2012).

Ansell, D., Grabler, P., Whitman, S., Ferrans, C., Burgess-Bishop, J., Murray, L.R., ... Marcus, E. (2009). A community effort to reduce the black/white breast cancer mortality disparity in Chicago. *Cancer Causes and Control, 20*, 1681–1688. doi:10.1007/s10552-009-9419-7

Carey, L.A., Perou, C.M., Livasy, C.A., Dressler, L.G., Cowan, D., Conway, K., ... Millikan, R.C. (2006). Race, breast cancer subtypes, and survival in the Carolina Breast Cancer Study. *JAMA, 295*, 2492–2502. doi:10.1001/jama.295.21.2492

Chicago hospitals' grade on breast cancer: Not good enough. (2010, October 21). *Chicago Sun-Times*. Retrieved from http://www.suntimes.com

Cunningham, J.E., Montero, A.J., Garrett-Mayer, E., Berkel, H.J., & Ely, B. (2010). Racial differences in the incidence of breast cancer subtypes defined by combined histologic grade and hormone receptor status. *Cancer Causes and Control, 21*, 399–409. doi:10.1007/s10552-009-9472-2

Gray, J.E. (1994). Mammography (and radiology?) is still plagued with poor quality in photographic processing and darkroom fog. *Radiology, 191*, 318–319. doi:10.1148/radiology.191.2.8153299

Haynes, M.A., & Smedley, B.D. (Eds.). (1999). *The unequal burden of cancer: An assessment of NIH research and programs for ethnic minorities and the medically underserved*. Retrieved from http://www.nap.edu/catalog.php?record_id=6377

Hirschman, J., Whitman, S., & Ansell, D. (2007). The black:white disparity in breast cancer mortality: The example of Chicago. *Cancer Causes and Control, 18*, 323–333. doi:10.1007/s10552-006-0102-y

Lobb, R., Allen, J.D., Emmons, K.M., & Ayanian, J.Z. (2010). Timely care after an abnormal mammogram among low-income women in a public breast cancer screening program. *Archives of Internal Medicine, 170*, 521–528. doi:10.1001/archinternmed.2010.22

Mammography Quality Standards Act, Pub. L. 102-539, 106. Stat. 3547 (1992).

Metropolitan Chicago Breast Cancer Task Force. (2007, October). *Improving quality and reducing disparities in breast cancer mortality in metropolitan Chicago*. Retrieved from http://www.chicagobreastcancer.org/site/epage/93672_904.htm

Metropolitan Chicago Breast Cancer Task Force. (2010, October 21). *Annual report back to the community*. Retrieved from http://www.chicagobreastcancer.org/site/files/904/100588/352277/506545/October_2010_Event_Report_Final.pdf

Nass, S., & Ball, J. (Eds.). (2005). *Improving breast imaging quality standards*. Retrieved from http://www.nap.edu/catalog.php?record_id=11308

Ooi, S.L., Martinez, M.E., & Li, C.I. (2011). Disparities in breast cancer characteristics and outcomes by race/ethnicity. *Breast Cancer Research and Treatment, 127,* 729–738. doi:10.1007/s10549-010-1191-6

Patient Protection and Affordable Care Act, Pub. L. 111-148, 124 Stat. 119 (2010).

Patient Safety and Quality Improvement Act of 2005, Pub. L. 109-41, 42 U.S.C. ch. 6A subch. VII pt. C.

Pisano, E.D., Gatsonis, C., Hendrick, E., Yaffe, M., Baum, J.K., Acharyya, S., … Rebner, M. (2005). Diagnostic performance of digital versus film mammography for breast-cancer screening. *New England Journal of Medicine, 353,* 1773–1783. doi:10.1056/NEJMoa052911

Rauscher, G.H., Allgood, K.L., Whitman, S., & Conant, E. (2012). Disparities in screening mammography services by race/ethnicity and health insurance. *Journal of Women's Health, 21,* 154–160. doi:10.1089/jwh.2010.2415

Reducing Breast Cancer Disparities Act, Section 5-5 of The Illinois Public Aid Code (305 ILCS 5/5-5 as amended by P.A. 95-1045, effective March 27, 2009).

Shelton, D.L. (2010, October 20). Study: Quality of breast cancer care in Chicago area isn't uniform. *Chicago Tribune*. Retrieved from http://articles.chicagotribune.com/2010-10-20/health/ct-met-mammogram-quality-20101020_1_breast-cancer-chicago-hospital-screening

Sickles, E.A., Wolverton, D.E., & Dee, K.E. (2002). Performance parameters for screening and diagnostic mammography: Specialist and general radiologists. *Radiology, 224,* 861–869. doi:10.1148/radiol.2243011482

Silber, J.H., Rosenbaum, P.R., Clark, A.S., Giantonio, B.J., Ross, R.N., Teng, Y., … Fox, K.R. (2013). Characteristics associated with differences in survival among black and white women with breast cancer. *JAMA, 310,* 389–397. doi:10.1001/jama.2013.8272

Whitman, S., Orsi, J., & Hurlbert, M. (2012). The racial disparity in breast cancer mortality in the 25 largest cities in the United States. *Cancer Epidemiology, 36,* e147–e151. doi:10.1016/j.canep.2011.10.012

CHAPTER 13

Lessons in Cancer Activism From the Breast Cancer and Prostate Cancer Movements

Karen M. Kedrowski, PhD, and Marilyn Stine Sarow, PhD

Introduction

La plus que ça change, plus c'est la même chose—the old French proverb that the more things change, the more they stay the same—describes the state of affairs of the breast cancer and prostate cancer movements today. Significant research on the effectiveness of screening protocols for both diseases has modified diagnostic practices; however, many grassroots survivors' organizations (GSOs) still cling to the message that early diagnosis saves lives. Federal funding remains essentially stable for both diseases despite debates about the lack of medical breakthroughs. Critics of the use of cause-related marketing to fund GSOs cite the emphasis on raising money rather than focusing on treatments and causes. Changes in media usage fueled by the rise of social networking enable organizations to talk more directly to their constituencies, but it also means that donors can respond in kind. Some say the pink and blue ribbons, symbols of the movements, are beginning to lose their impact. Meanwhile, our neighbors to the north in Canada are taking a different approach to these issues.

In the book *Cancer Activism: Gender, Media, and Public Policy*, we documented and compared the development and success of the breast cancer and prostate cancer movements in the 1980s and 1990s. We found that the breast cancer movement entered the public consciousness through popular media and benefited from increased public policy attention as a result. The prostate cancer movement sought to pattern itself after the breast cancer movement, yet failed to achieve the same degree of success (Kedrowski & Sarow, 2007).

Our analysis essentially ended in 1998. What has happened to these two movements in the ensuing 15 years? How do the movements in the United States compare to those in Canada? These are the central questions of this chapter. We argue that both movements have matured and now seek to maintain their positions of relative strength. Much is similar in terms of media coverage, policy attention, the roles of women as leaders in both movements, and government investment in research.

Background

Breast and prostate cancer remain major health threats in the United States, especially to older men and women. The American Cancer Society (ACS) estimated that 40,290 women and 440 men will die of breast cancer in 2015 (ACS, 2015). The morbidity and mortality rates are higher among women older than 40. ACS estimated that 42% of new diagnoses of invasive breast cancer occur in women older than 64 (ACS, 2013).

For 2015, ACS estimated 220,800 new cases of prostate cancer with 27,540 deaths (ACS, 2015). About 56% of cases are diagnosed in men older than 65 (ACS, 2015).

Breast and prostate cancer remain national public health priorities. The long-range planning document for the health of the nation, *Healthy People 2020* (U.S. Department of Health and Human Services, 2013), called for a target reduction of prostate cancer deaths from 23.5 per 100,000 population in 2007 (baseline) to 21.9 deaths (age-adjusted) in 2020 (U.S. Department of Health and Human Services, 2013). The report also called for a reduction of deaths from late-stage female breast cancer from 43.2 per 100,000 in 2007 (baseline year) to 41 per 100,000 in 2020, and a 10% decrease in the death rate from breast cancer from 22.9 cancer deaths per 100,000 in 2007 to 20.6 deaths per 100,000 (U.S. Department of Health and Human Services, 2013).

Effective Advocacy

The significant role of advocacy organizations in shaping and molding public policy is called *agenda setting*. As Cobb and Elder (1972) noted, agenda setting may be viewed in terms of the media agenda, the public agenda, and the policy agenda.

To influence public policy (i.e., government attention and public funding), organizations must seize the public's attention through events and activities that, in turn, capture the attention of the media and give an issue salience. Through the scope and amount of media coverage of a particular issue and the framing of that issue, the public, policy leaders, and other interested groups evaluate its significance. Thus, as an issue gains attention and legitimacy in the media, it becomes part of the public agenda and eventually may come under consideration for government action (Shaw & McCombs, 1997).

GSOs are the drivers behind increasing public attention through both direct and indirect subsidies. Information sent directly from an organization to the public is referred to as *direct subsidies*, whereas information filtered through the media before it reaches the public is known as *indirect subsidies*. Emails, blogs, Twitter feeds, and other forms of social media are direct subsidies.

Aside from the media agenda, issues reach the policy agenda when they rise to the awareness of the "attentive public." GSOs are attentive publics. Cobb and Elder (1972) defined this group as "a generally informed and interested stratum of the population. Though not homogeneous, the attentive public tends to be relatively stable in composition and comes disproportionately from the more educated and higher income groups" (p. 107).

Criteria for the Success of Grassroots Survivors' Organizations

Powerful GSOs have learned how to help frame national health policy debates and lobby for the need for public funding by influencing media coverage. Such coverage lends credibility to the cause while encouraging others at the grassroots level to become active participants.

We found the following seven criteria to be fundamental to the success of the breast and prostate cancer movements.

- Both diseases are long-term illnesses with a high rate of survival.
- Both diseases have an activist tradition encouraged, in part, by the training and tactics of the AIDS movement (Altman, 1996; Casamayou, 2001).
- Both breast cancer and prostate cancer survivors are not afraid to tell their stories or "to offer themselves as evidence."
- Both groups benefit from an educated, activated populace.
- Both organizations use the media and the courts to keep their stories alive and in the public agenda.
- Women are important drivers in supporting the movements.
- Both depend on financial and promotional support from a variety of types of organizations (Kedrowski & Sarow, 2007).

Barkhorn, Huttner, and Blau (2013) identified nine conditions to successful advocacy campaigns. They include the power of external events that often drive demand and the organizational power and resources of advocates who can persuade decision makers to come to a solution. These conditions also are readily apparent in successful GSOs.

The Breast Cancer Movement

The breast cancer advocacy movement traces its origins to ACS's Reach to Recovery program, founded in 1952. It currently provides support and advice for patients with breast cancer and their families through face-to-face or telephone contact (ACS, 2014a). This program has evolved over the years. In its earliest years, patient-to-patient outreach was unheard of, and Reach to Recovery founder Térèse Lasser encountered significant opposition from doctors who saw hospital visits by volunteers as a threat to the sanctity of the doctor-patient relationship (Olson, 2002). In the 1970s, Reach to Recovery came under criticism by feminist writer Audre Lorde, who saw its emphasis on looking "normal" after a mastectomy disempowering and sexist (Lorde, 1980). Yet Reach to Recovery was the forerunner of support groups that are ubiquitous today.

In the 1970s, Rose Kushner, a consumer activist, feminist writer, and patient with breast cancer, rose to prominence with campaigns against the Halsted, or radical, mastectomy and in support of informed consent. As the surgical practice of radical mastectomies began to fade in the 1980s and informed consent requirements were adopted by state legislatures (Berman, 1994; Montini, 1996, 1997), two new national organizations were formed: the Susan G. Komen Foundation (now known as Susan G. Komen), based on the power of local activists working through affiliates to tell their stories and influence public officials, and the National Alliance of Breast Cancer Organizations (NABCO), providing information and referrals to people with breast cancer and especially targeting lesbians or men with breast cancer. NABCO dissolved in 2004 (Kedrowski & Sarow, 2007).

In 1991, local and national organizations formed the National Breast Cancer Coalition (NBCC), which has become a powerful force in mobilizing congressional support for federal funding of breast cancer research. The early leaders of the group were skilled activists with roots in the civil rights and women's movements (Altman, 1996; Ferraro, 1993). Today, NBCC works to maintain breast cancer as a national priority, accelerate the research process, and ensure that treatment is available for all women (NBCC, n.d.).

The Avon Walk for the Cure and Susan G. Komen have been highly successful in securing media attention through their annual race events. Komen is the largest private donor, outside of the federal government, for breast cancer research. The organization claims to have raised more than $2.5 billion to fund research, community health outreach, advocacy, and programs in more than 50 countries (Susan G. Komen, n.d.). The Susan G. Komen Advocacy Alliance, the policy wing of the organization, brands itself as the voice of advocacy working to ensure that government funding for research is a priority among policy makers in Washington, DC, and across the country.

However, the movement also has its critics. Breast Cancer Action (BCA), for example, has more than 50,000 members and is a strong proponent of breast cancer environmental research. Its late leader, Barbara Brenner, was one of the first advocates to question the "pinkwashing" of the disease, or the number of pink ribbons and products carrying labels promoting their contributions to breast cancer research (Grady, 2013). BCA's "Think Before You Pink" campaign demands transparency in corporate giving (BCA, n.d.). This critique was echoed by Samantha King (2006), who argued that the social marketing and feel-good corporate involvement lead the public to forget that breast cancer is not "pretty" but is a disease that kills millions.

Another critic of the movement, Peggy Orenstein, herself a breast cancer survivor, argues,

> All that well-meaning awareness has ultimately made women *less* conscious of the facts: obscuring the limits of screening, conflating risk with disease, compromising our decisions about health care, celebrating "cancer survivors" who may never require treating. And ultimately, it has come at the expense of those whose lives are at most risk. (Orenstein, 2013, p. 70)

The Prostate Cancer Movement

The prostate cancer movement began almost a decade later than the breast cancer movement. In the 1980s, the American Prostate Society, Patient Advocates for Advanced Cancer Treatment, and Prostate Cancer Education Council were established. In addition, the Men's Health Network, founded in 1992, became a counterpart to the women's health movement. This organization continues to advocate for an Office of Men's Health in the U.S. Department of Health and Human Services, to parallel the Office of Women's Health established in 1991. The Prostate Cancer Foundation (originally known as CaP CURE) promotes itself as the leading foundation for prostate cancer research, with global research funding of $80 million (Prostate Cancer Foundation, n.d.).

In 1996, prostate cancer forces joined together to form the National Prostate Cancer Coalition (NPCC). The organization, modeled after NBCC, was created to pull together grassroots groups, corporate sponsors, and state coalitions to increase federal funding for prostate cancer research. In 2008, NPCC became ZERO—The End of Prostate Cancer, or Generation ZERO, with the goal of wiping out prostate cancer in future generations. ZERO seeks to create a grassroots movement with a nationwide "Dash for Dad" race and other fund-raising efforts to support medical research (ZERO, n.d.). However, lobbying and advocacy efforts are now under the leadership of the Prostate Cancer Roundtable, which is a coalition of several GSOs, including ZERO, UsTOO, the Prostate Cancer Foundation, Men's Health Network, Malecare, and other organizations.

The agenda of the Prostate Cancer Roundtable mirrors that of the NBCC by focusing on increasing government funding for cancer research, creating the Office of Men's Health, developing initiatives to eliminate the "epidemic" of prostate cancer among African American men, and establishing a Prostate Cancer Scientific Advisory Board within the U.S. Food and Drug Administration (Prostate Cancer Roundtable, 2014).

The prostate cancer movement also receives funding from corporate sources, including Major League Baseball, but has been less successful than the breast cancer movement in raising corporate funds. Name changes and the reorganization and reorientation of organizations have given prostate cancer–related groups less long-term name recognition and public presence.

The Media Agenda

In *Cancer Activism*, we reported our findings on the power of the media to set the policy agenda, using a database of 4,246 news stories on breast and prostate cancer from 1980 to 1998 from five newspapers and three television networks. Breast cancer dominated the news with 85% of the identified stories (Kedrowski & Sarow, 2007).

Media coverage of prostate cancer increased from 1980 to 1998, but breast cancer coverage increased as well. Coverage often ebbed and flowed with scientific discoveries, controversial practices, and personality stories linked to high-profile individuals who had the disease.

In the early 1980s, prostate cancer received essentially no coverage, whereas breast cancer generated 20–40 stories a year in these media outlets. By 1985, the number of breast cancer stories had increased slightly with the coverage of medical discoveries related to improved treatments. Coverage increased gradually in the early 1990s until 1994, when the reporting of fraud in government-funded trials and the silicone breast implant controversy increased coverage to 465 stories. Coverage of breast cancer declined again until 1998, the year our study ended (Kedrowski & Sarow, 2007).

Prostate cancer coverage experienced several peaks during the period of our study. In 1987, there were 28 stories concerning personalities with prostate cancer; the coverage declined again until 1991, when then-Senators Alan Cranston (D-CA) and Bob Dole (R-KS) were diagnosed with the disease. Prostate cancer stayed on the media agenda and then peaked again in 1998 (the year our study ended) with 132 stories (Kedrowski & Sarow, 2007).

The subject matter of breast cancer stories compared to that of prostate cancer stories varied significantly. Almost half (43%) of prostate cancer stories centered on personalities, while breast cancer stories were dominated (34%) by medical discoveries (Kedrowski & Sarow, 2007).

For this chapter, we replicated a portion of our analysis to see whether news coverage of breast and prostate cancer has changed since our previous study. Our analysis demonstrates that relatively little has changed in the past 15 years. We counted the number of news stories in the *Washington Post* on selected diseases (breast cancer, prostate cancer, lung cancer, lymphedema, and flu) from 2001–2012. We chose the *Washington Post* because of its heavy readership among members of Congress and the policy community, and we chose lymphedema, the flu, and lung cancer as comparisons because each of these topics was in the news during the past decade and we believe they received substantial news coverage.

In *Cancer Activism*, we reported that breast and prostate cancer both saw significant gains in news media attention starting in 1991 (Kedrowski & Sarow, 2007). In this analysis, we saw that this trend did not continue in the 2000s. While prostate cancer stories averaged about 200 per year, breast cancer averaged about 500 stories per year until 2010. Coverage of breast cancer outpaced that of all other cancers, while coverage of lung cancer paralleled prostate cancer's coverage.

Notably, news coverage for both prostate and breast cancer declined in the 2000s, demonstrating that these diseases have lost some of their urgency and newsworthiness. Instead, coverage of the flu rose through most of the decade and peaked in 2012 with the avian flu (H5N1) and swine flu (H1N1) epidemics in 2003–2004 and 2009–2010, respectively (see Figure 13-1).

What is the content of these stories? In the 1980s and 1990s, prostate cancer news stories were dominated by stories about prominent individuals, with less about public policy issues or scientific discoveries. Breast cancer news still featured a number of personalities, yet also emphasized policy and scientific discovery (Kedrowski & Sarow, 2007). To see whether the content had changed since 1998, one author subscribed to Google Alerts for six months in 2013, with the terms *breast cancer politics* and *prostate cancer politics*. Google Alerts provides a news digest service drawing from online news sources worldwide. This exercise with the Google Alerts algorithm demonstrated that little has changed since the 1990s. The prostate cancer alerts yielded a few dozen news stories. They focused on prominent personalities with the disease: an Australian parliamentarian, a best-selling author, a governmental minister in Canada, and a late president of Ghana. There were a few stories about drug approvals. Just one set of stories

Figure 13-1. *Washington Post* **News Stories of Selected Diseases by Year**

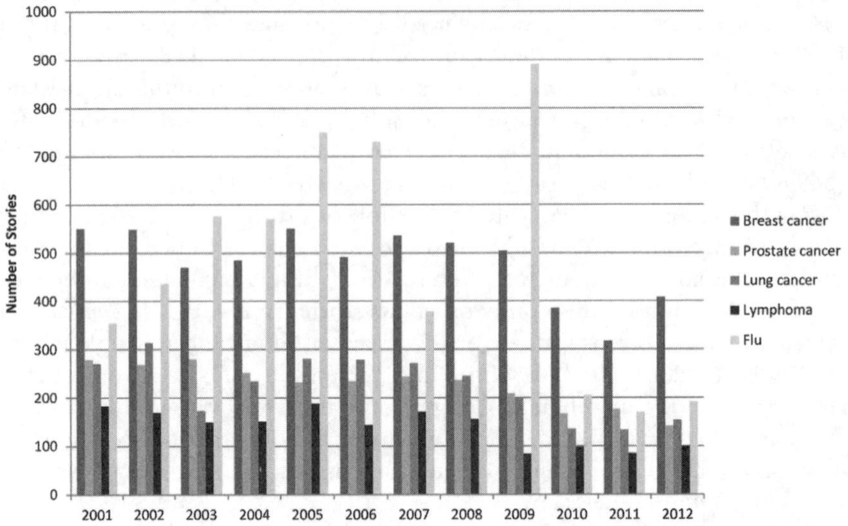

Note. Data compiled by authors.

concerned policy; these were reprints of a news release about the creation of a bipartisan Congressional Men's Health Caucus (e.g., Runyan, 2013).

In contrast, the alerts for *breast cancer politics* yielded more plentiful and diverse results—ones that reflect how breast cancer remains at the center of public consciousness and public policy debates. Actress Angelina Jolie's decision to have a double mastectomy and reconstructive surgery after learning she has a mutated version of the breast cancer gene led to a flurry of articles, blog posts, and opinion pieces. Another large group of stories focused on the business and health ramifications of the U.S. Supreme Court decision that corporations could not patent human genes. Other stories discussed a lower court ruling that schools could not ban plastic bracelets designed to raise breast cancer awareness, even if those bracelets carry off-color messages; and a series of stories was published on a state legislator's attempt to link abortion to breast cancer. In short, these policy stories were really about civil liberties, the limits of corporate power, and abortion politics instead of breast cancer. Breast cancer was simply the vehicle used to bring these other concerns to the table (e.g., Feran, 2013; Jolie, 2013; Mears, 2013; Shulman, 2013). Taken together, these analyses demonstrate that little has changed in two decades. As the breast and prostate cancer movements have matured, prostate cancer still struggles for attention, while breast cancer basks in it and has even entered the political mainstream, becoming entwined with many other important issues on the public agenda.

Social Media

Since the 1990s, major differences in the media environment have changed both private and public communication. They include the decline of traditional media and the rise of Internet-based communication, particularly social media.

Social media's power rests in its ability to bring a different communication experience to the user. No longer is information presented in a top-down (media being the expert), one-way, sender-driven, or time-specific way; users now exercise control over both product and process. The media elite, including GSOs, as illustrated later in this chapter, have less and less control over content. Media scholars Chaffee and Metzger (2001) noted that "in addition to allowing a greater variety of voices and views into public discourse, the interactive capacity of the new media creates new ways of grassroots organizing and coalition building" (p. 370). From an organizational perspective, social media enables organizations to build relationships with their followers and encourage dialogic, or two-way, communication.

The Pew Research Center's Internet and American Life Project found that 72% of online adults use social networking sites. Usage was higher among those in the 18–29 age range (89%) and the 30–49 age range (78%) (Brenner & Smith, 2013). In terms of social media usage among those who are chronically ill, the Pew Research Center reported that 1 in 5 created online health content, including commenting on a blog or in a forum, posting a review of a hospital or physician, and categorizing or tagging health-related content (Fox & Purcell, 2010).

For example, Prostate Cancer International brands its social network as the "New" Prostate Cancer InfoLink Social Network. It lists as one of its primary goals: "to help newly diagnosed men to come to the best possible decision *for them* about a specific course of action" (Prostate Cancer International, n.d.). The site includes more than 20 interest groups, blogs, and links to the organization's Facebook page and Twitter feed.

GSOs are well attuned to the need to use social media tools to build relationships with a broad range of constituencies. They also understand that messages need to be framed to reach a particular audience. GSOs have learned, sometimes painfully, that information presented to the public needs to be accurate. Social media audiences are quick to respond to information they believe is inaccurate. In a qualitative study of email messages sent by Susan G. Komen for the Cure and the Komen Advocacy Alliance, Weberling (2012) noted that e-news messages cited "the latest scientific breakthroughs, typically delivered alongside a photo of the organization's chief scientific advisor, Dr. Eric P. Winer, MD" (p. 113), as well as information about the organization and its outreach efforts. However, Komen's fundraising messages were more emotional, emphasized the race against time, and attempted to put a public face on the breast cancer survivor. By contrast, policy messages used a political approach, urging receivers of the message to help in the fight against breast cancer by contacting their legislators (Weberling, 2012).

Although the power to immediately share a message with a particular targeted audience is valuable for organizations, once the message is shared, the organization has little control over how it is received or framed by competitive interests or even by its own supporters. Thousands of people are able to express their opinions at will, creating a groundswell of public opinion (Gates, 2012). A whole new group of stakeholders has emerged, sometimes referred to as *netizens*, or online publics. These individuals are not just online but are willing to express themselves "in ways that represent their moral compass so to speak—their feelings for what is right and wrong, or good or bad" (Sheldrake, 2011, p. 23). Such individuals understand the value and influence of public communication.

Organizations unprepared to handle the impact of social media, particularly in crisis situations, risk losing their reputation and funding support. Susan G. Komen experienced the power of social media to shape a message in fall 2011, when it announced that it would no longer extend grant funding to Planned Parenthood for breast cancer screening. The original five-year grant of approximately $700,000 had enabled Planned Parenthood to conduct 170,000 breast cancer screenings, or 4% of its examinations performed nationwide (CNN Wire Staff, 2012).

Komen's rationale centered on a federal inquiry into Planned Parenthood, initiated by Representative Cliff Stearns (R-FL), questioning whether the organization had violated federal law by using federal dollars to fund abortions (Crary, 2012). Because of this inquiry, pro-life members of Komen's board and leaders in the movement voted to withdraw support from Planned Parenthood (Harris & Belluck, 2012). While this was the stated rationale for the board's decision, pro-life groups, including the Catholic Church, among others, had previously publicly criticized Komen for funding Planned Parenthood (Sulik, 2011). Although Komen's leadership attempted to reframe its actions as apolitical and the result of decisions on how grants were to be awarded (Roan, 2012), the public outcry began to threaten Komen's fund-raising efforts (see Watt, 2012, for an analysis of the rhetoric used in the controversy).

As Gayle Sulik (2011) concluded in her book, *Pink Ribbon Blues*,

> Komen has, in some ways, been used as a pawn to fuel the anti-choice/pro-life agenda. . . . Mammograms have become symbolic of a vital women's health service (despite their limitations and inaccurate labeling as a preventive measure), so questioning Planned Parenthood's role in providing them is an increasingly common strategy for delegitimizing the network as a primary care provider. (p. xlii)

Komen's decision became public in late January 2012, when the Associated Press broke the story. In its response to the public announcement, Planned Parenthood Federation of America accused Komen of succumbing to political pressure. Planned Parenthood president Cecile Richards noted that when Komen broke the news, it was done as an announcement, not as a two-way conversation (Crary, 2012). Planned Parenthood continued to frame all of its public response to the Komen announcement in terms of how the action politicized the women's healthcare movement.

Komen's decision drew immediate public reaction from people on social media sites. National Public Radio reported that its original story about the Komen decision drew more than 400 comments the first day, including responses by celebrities and public figures (Memmott, 2012). Within 24 hours, donations to Planned Parenthood poured in, including $400,000 from online donors (Kliff & Sun, 2012). A post published by *The Lede* (the *New York Times* news blog) in February 2012 reported that Twitter responses were overwhelmingly in support of Planned Parenthood. It also reported that Planned Parenthood had used its misfortune to post an open letter that was shared by more than 19,000 people in less than 24 hours, and that it was actively seeking donations through its Twitter account (Preston, 2012).

This immediate public outcry created dissent among Komen's board members and some affiliates. On February 3, 2012, Komen president Nancy Brinker said,

> We want to apologize to the American public for recent decisions that cast doubt upon our commitment to our mission of saving women's lives. We have been distressed at the presumption that the changes made to our funding criteria were done for political reasons or to specifically penalize Planned Parenthood. They were not. (as cited in Khan, 2012)

Brinker noted that for future decisions, "disqualifying investigations must be criminal and conclusive in nature and not political" (Brinker, 2012, para. 2).

The *New York Times* noted the power of social media to rapidly mobilize public opinion. It reported that on February 2, 2012, Planned Parenthood and Komen were the subject of 460,000 posts; the next day, Brinker's announcement drew 1.3 million tweets (Belluck, Preston, & Harris, 2012).

Banyan Branch, a social media consulting group, analyzed the impact of social media on the organizations. It found that before the crisis, Komen had an average of 52.4 likes and 17.5 comments per post on its Facebook page. However, in the time between Komen's decision and its reversal, "comments increased by 31,417% (5,515.4 per post), likes decreased by 99% (0.3 likes per comment), and likes on user comments increased by 288% (6.6 per comment)" (Fleming & O'Connor, 2012). In terms of Twitter, Komen saw an average of 457,301 mentions a day from January 31 through February 7, an increase of 32,731% from its previous daily average of 1,399 (Fleming & O'Connor, 2012).

Six months after the crisis, Komen realized that its brand and image were still tarnished. It redirected its traditional advertising campaign, which was designed to raise support for its October Race for the Cure, to one that highlighted survivors' stories. According to *Advertising Age* (Bruell, 2012), however, Komen's donations were down about 30%, according to multiple executives familiar with the matter. In addition, cause-marketing experts reported receiving questions from their clients on whether they should continue their relationships with the organization (Bruell, 2012).

The lesson of this controversy is that the people who support breast cancer organizations support women's health issues in general. Casting Komen's decision in a political light forced women to make a choice, and in this case many chose Planned Parenthood over Komen (Baralt & Weitz, 2012).

Public Policy: Congressional Action and National Cancer Institute Funding

In *Cancer Activism*, we found that the increased media coverage in the 1990s was mirrored by increased public policy attention. The number of bills introduced in Congress began to rise in 1991–1992 for both breast and prostate cancer. Federal investment in breast and prostate cancer funding also grew. What, if anything, has changed in terms of public policy attention during the past two decades? We repeated our analysis of congressional activity, starting with this increase in 1992 (Kedrowski & Sarow, 2007).

Figure 13-2 shows the number of bills mentioning breast cancer or prostate cancer introduced into the U.S. Congress in the 102nd (1991–1993) through 112th Congresses (2011–2013) and the number of hearings on either disease (102nd–112th Congresses). The bills and hearings were identified using THOMAS (now Congress.gov), the U.S. Congress site maintained by the Library of Congress.

Figure 13-2 shows that breast cancer continues to receive more attention from policy makers than does prostate cancer. However, the number of breast cancer bills introduced has declined fairly steadily over time, while prostate cancer bills have been fairly level. Also, more breast cancer hearings than prostate cancer hearings take place in any given Congress. Yet compared to 1980–1998, when only three hearings were held in 19 years, prostate cancer now averages about 15 hearings per two-year Congress (Kedrowski & Sarow, 2007). Hearings were identified using keyword searches.

The declining number of bills introduced implies that advocates see little new work that needs to be done, or that the agenda is shifting to new policy priorities. The gaping holes—Medicare coverage of cancer screening and mammography standards—were addressed in the 1990s. Titles of bills intro-

Figure 13-2. Legislative Activity of 102nd–112th Congresses (1991–2013)

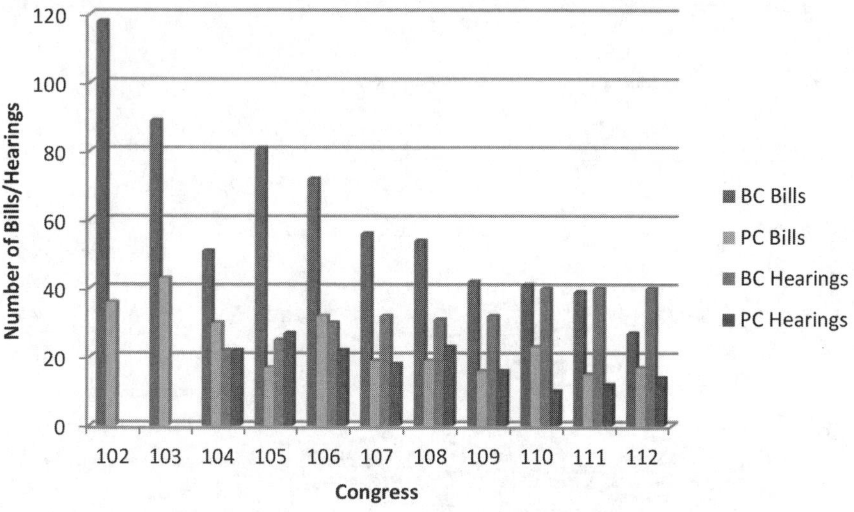

BC—breast cancer; PC—prostate cancer

Note. Data compiled by authors.

duced between 1992 and 2012 suggest much of the same. Bills such as the Mammography Quality Standards Reauthorization Act indicate that advocates seek to ensure the innovations they sought in the early 1990s remain in law.

An analysis of published National Cancer Institute (NCI) funding data tell a similar story. Each year, NCI releases total funding by cancer type. In *Cancer Activism*, we described how the share of NCI research dollars awarded to breast and prostate cancer projects started to increase in the early 1990s and remained comparatively high throughout that decade (Kedrowski & Sarow, 2007). Breast cancer continues to receive a larger percentage of NCI funds than any other cancer or AIDS, or about 12% of all NCI funds. This was approximately $600 million in 2011, the most recent year available (see Figure 13-3). NCI funding for AIDS declined from 1992 to 2011, and that disease now receives a smaller share of NCI funding than breast cancer, prostate cancer, or lung cancer and about the same amount as allocated for colorectal cancer. Prostate cancer funding held steady at around 6% of all NCI funds (or about $300 million in 2011). For much of this time, prostate cancer was second only to breast cancer (NCI, n.d.).

These results suggest that breast and prostate cancer are now part of politics as usual. As government policy rarely changes dramatically, breast and prostate cancer advocates only had to maintain current levels of funding in order to keep their diseases at the top of the NCI agenda.

Figure 13-3. National Cancer Institute Funding by Cancer, by Year

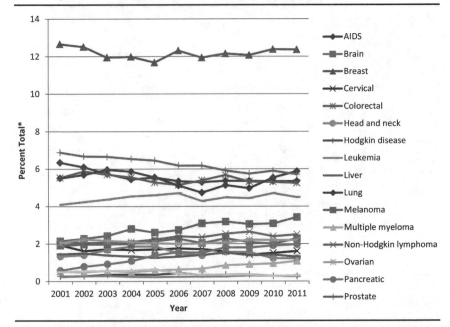

* Percentages do not add to 100% because awards may be allocated to more than one cancer type. It also does not include funding provided by other institutes in the National Institutes of Health.

Note. Data compiled by authors from tables published in the *NCI Fact Book*, various years. Retrieved from http://obf.cancer.gov/financial/factbook.htm.

The Patient Protection and Affordable Care Act

There are limits to GSOs' political power. The Patient Protection and Affordable Care Act—or the Affordable Care Act (ACA)for short—is a landmark piece of health legislation signed into law by President Obama in 2010. For decades, breast and prostate cancer organizations promoted early screening as the way to fight their respective diseases. But scientific evidence and subsequent government policy directives have led breast and prostate cancer GSOs to modify their messages concerning cancer screening. The result is often confusion and frustration among activists and the public in general. Questions concerning when to use screening tests surfaced again during public debates on the ACA.

The U.S. Preventive Services Task Force (USPSTF) is an independent panel of volunteer experts who make medical treatment recommendations based on current medical evidence. Members are appointed by the director of the Agency for Healthcare Quality and Research and are prescreened to ensure they have no conflicts of interest (USPSTF, 2014). In 2009, USPSTF recommended (a) women aged 50–74 should receive biennial mammography screening, (b) clinicians should not teach breast self-examination, and (c) the appropriateness of mammography screening for women younger than age 50 should be decided by the patient and her doctor. The task force also concluded it could not assess the relative costs and benefits of clinical breast examinations (USPSTF, 2009). Many disease-related groups did not agree with these recommendations (see Newman, 2012). ACS disagreed with the task force's finding concerning the advisability of screening for women aged 40–50. In a public statement, ACS agreed with most of the USPSTF findings, stating that "mammography has limitations . . . some cancers will be missed; and some women will undergo unnecessary treatment. . . . But the limitations do not change the fact that breast cancer screening using mammography starting at age 40 saves lives" (ACS, 2009, para. 3). This position was also endorsed by the American Society of Breast Surgeons (2011).

The USPSTF report was issued at the height of the ACA debate—and was seized on by Republican members of Congress as an attempt at healthcare rationing. As a result, the ACA now does not follow the USPSTF mammography guidelines. Instead, it requires health plans to cover yearly mammograms for women starting at age 40.

NBCC was an early supporter of the ACA but was unhappy that the legislation did not follow the USPSTF's recommendations. NBCC has long held that mammography does not prevent breast cancer, leads to false positives and overdiagnosis, and in its current state of development "can prevent women from being diagnosed with later stages of breast cancer" (NBCC, 2010).

In the case of prostate cancer diagnostic tools, the evidence seems to spark less public disagreement. Although the prostate-specific antigen (PSA) test was once widely used to diagnose prostate cancer, neither the USPSTF nor NCI recommend the test for routine use. Studies have found that elevated PSA is unreliable in determining whether a man has the disease. Medicare, however, does cover an annual PSA test for all Medicare-eligible men age 50 and older. The ACA does not mandate private insurers to cover this test (NCI, 2012).

The Prostate Cancer Roundtable noted in May 2012 that physicians, and in turn patients, would be confused by conflicting guidelines from the American Urological Association, USPSTF, American College of Physicians, and National Comprehensive Cancer Network. The roundtable cited the lack of reliable data offering "incontrovertible evidence" about prostate cancer screening and the failure of the medical community to provide uniform and consistent guidance for patients and their families (Moyer, 2013; Prostate Cancer Roundtable, 2013).

ACS urges men to decide about PSA screening after consulting with their physicians. This position is shared by the American College of Physicians, which recommends that patients be informed about the risks, benefits, and harms of screening, their general health and life expectancy, and the fact that they have choices. The American College of Physicians does not recommend the test for patients "who do not express a clear preference for screening" (Qaseem, Barry, Denberg, Owens, & Shekelle, 2013, p. 761).

The Canadian Movement Comparison

The Canadian breast cancer movement evolved about the same time as its American counterpart, in the 1980s and early 1990s. Today, however, it may be a harbinger of the U.S. movement's future, with a shifting focus to younger women and to environmental causes.

The Canadian Breast Cancer Foundation (CBCF) is probably the earliest breast cancer fund-raising organization in that country. It was founded in 1986 by a group of volunteers who sought to raise funds for breast cancer research (CBCF, n.d.). CBCF hosts an annual Run for the Cure, which is sponsored by a major bank and has races in multiple sites around Canada. After CBCF, two additional groups were founded in rapid succession. Breast Cancer Support Services in Burlington, Ontario, founded in 1988, was likely the first support group established in Canada (P. Kelly, personal communication, April 13, 2010). The second group is Breast Cancer Action Montreal (BCAM). Initially, BCAM sought to bring breast cancer into public consciousness, engage in political advocacy, and build a network of activists (Batt, 1994).

In 1992, the Canadian House of Commons turned its attention to the issue of breast cancer through a series of parliamentary hearings (Greene, 1992). This led Health Canada, the Canadian national public health agency, to convene the National Forum on Breast Cancer, in Montreal in 1993 (Health Canada, 1994). This conference led to the establishment of the Canadian Breast Cancer Research Initiative, later renamed the Canadian Breast Cancer Research Alliance (CBCRA). Funded through a combination of public and private funds, CBCRA aimed to fund medical research on breast cancer in Canada (Birdsell, 1997). Although it was disbanded in 2010, CBRCA donated more than $192 million to breast cancer research during its life span (D. Ermel, personal communication, March 24, 2010).

The principal Canadian government agency for medical research funding is the Canadian Institutes of Health Research. The Institute of Cancer Research (ICR) is one of 13 research networks focusing on strategic research initiatives. ICR provided about $125 million (Canadian dollars) in research funding in 2010. However, ICR does not report funding amounts by cancer type (ICR, 2012). Medical research funding is also available through the 11 provincial and territorial governments and private foundations, such as the Canadian Cancer Society (ICR, 2014).

Many parallels exist between the U.S. and Canadian breast cancer movements. For instance, BCAM took its name, with permission, from Breast Cancer Action in San Francisco and drew inspiration for its earliest activities from NBCC (S. Batt, personal communication, April 23, 2010). Likewise, CBCF is analogous to Susan G. Komen. It holds races, uses the pink ribbon as its symbol, and claims to be the largest breast cancer charity in Canada (CBCF, n.d.). Similarly, the CURE Foundation, another Canadian breast cancer organization, also raises funds for research and projects. Its major event is Denim Day, which is patterned after the U.S. event Lee Denim Day. In both cases, employees at participating firms may donate $5 to breast cancer research in exchange for the right to wear jeans to work one day (J. Braun, personal communication, February 3, 2010; Lee National Denim Day, 2014). Finally, like the American Breast Cancer Foundation—a small, Maryland-based charity that provides free breast cancer screenings to low-income women (American Breast Cancer Foundation, n.d.)—the Breast Cancer Society of Canada is a small, family-run charity with a highly focused mission to provide funding for research and special projects (M. Davidson, personal communication, March 31, 2010).

Yet, the two movements have important differences. The first is that several Canadian breast cancer groups have consciously focused on environmental issues. Embodying Barbara Ley's thesis in her book, *From Pink to Green*, these Canadian organizations call attention to environmental health threats that could lead to breast cancer (Ley, 2009). Most notable of these is FemmeToxic, an initiative sponsored by BCAM, which calls attention to chemicals and hormones in household cleaning products, cosmetics, and foods that can mimic estrogen in the body. These groups also lobby for more stringent controls on ingredients for cosmetics and toiletries sold in Canada. One U.S. breast cancer organization, Breast Cancer Action in San Francisco, makes the same connection. However, the environmental movement is not as integrated into the U.S. breast cancer movement as it is in Canada.

The second important difference is the Canadian movement's conscious efforts to reach young women and girls and to draw them into the fold. FemmeToxic, for instance, seeks to reach girls as young as 12 (BCAM, n.d.). Ontario-based Rethink Breast Cancer provides support for women with breast cancer who are younger than age 40 (Rethink Breast Cancer, n.d.). Team Shan is dedicated to educating young people that breast cancer also affects young women (Team Shan, 2010). The Pink Tulip Foundation engages in public education and public awareness efforts with the Girl Guides (the Canadian version of Girl Scouts), targeting girls aged 9–18. Both FemmeToxic and the Pink Tulip Foundation base their public education efforts on the premise that breast cancers may be related to a lifetime of unhealthy habits, whether it is alcohol and diet or the use of poorly regulated cosmetics (L. White, personal communication, May 10, 2010; BCAM, n.d.). In at least one case, these efforts are designed to help perpetuate the organization. Many BCAM leaders had been involved with the organization since its founding, and they wanted to step away. They developed FemmeToxic, in part, to draw younger women into their organization who would then become its future leaders (D. Delusey-Apel, personal communication, January 18, 2010).

In contrast, this type of outreach is in its earliest stage in the United States. For instance, the Young Survival Coalition and Bright Pink were among the first groups to focus on young women exclusively. The Young Survival Coalition is an advocacy group for women younger than 40 diagnosed with breast cancer (Young Survival Coalition, 2014). Bright Pink focuses on genetic predispositions for breast, cervical, and ovarian cancers (Bright Pink, n.d.). In addition, Susan G. Komen, which once referred to breast cancer as "your mother's disease," now visits college campuses and works with the Girl Scouts to raise breast cancer awareness in young women and girls. Yet, none of these efforts focus on educating girls and young women about the importance of a lifetime of healthy habits.

Conclusion

The breast and prostate cancer advocacy movements in the United States continue to be influential forces in shaping the health policy agenda. However, media coverage and public funding show little change during the past decade. Social media may force these organizations to be more transparent and responsive to their constituencies. As these movements mature, they face challenges. One is dissension, especially on issues related to the efficacy of current detection methods. Another is the need to reach beyond their current base to bring in the next generation of activists. The Canadian breast cancer movement may offer a glimpse into the future agenda of the breast and prostate cancer movements in the United States.

The authors thank Travis Whisenant for his research assistance and Kathryn Wilson for her copy editing and formatting assistance.

References

Altman, R. (1996). *Waking up, fighting back: The politics of breast cancer.* Boston, MA: Little, Brown.
American Breast Cancer Foundation. (n.d.). About ABCF: ABCF mission. Retrieved from http://www.abcf.org/ABCF-Mission.htm

American Cancer Society. (2009, November 16). American Cancer Society responds to changes in USPSTF mammography guidelines [Press release]. Retrieved from http://pressroom .cancer.org/index.php?s=43&item=201

American Cancer Society. (2013). *Breast cancer facts and figures 2013–2014*. Retrieved from http:// www.cancer.org/acs/groups/content/@research/documents/document/acspc-042725.pdf

American Cancer Society. (2014). Reach to Recovery. Retrieved from http://www.cancer.org/ treatment/supportprogramsservices/reach-to-recovery

American Cancer Society. (2015). *Cancer facts and figures 2015*. Retrieved from http://www. cancer.org/research/cancerfactsstatistics/index

American Society of Breast Surgeons. (2011, August 15). Position statement on screening mammography. Retrieved from https://www.breastsurgeons.org/statements/PDF_Statements/ Screening_Mammography.pdf

Baralt, L., & Weitz, T.A. (2012). The Komen–Planned Parenthood controversy: Bringing the politics of breast cancer advocacy to the forefront. *Women's Health Issues, 22,* e509–e512. doi:10.1016/j.whi.2012.07.008

Barkhorn, I., Huttner, N., & Blau, J. (2013, Spring). Assessing advocacy. *Stanford Social Innovation Review,* pp. 59–64. Retrieved from http://www.ssireview.org/articles/entry/assessing_advocacy

Batt, S. (1994). *Patient no more: The politics of breast cancer*. Charlottetown, Prince Edward Island, Canada: Gynergy Books.

Belluck, P., Preston, J., & Harris, G. (2012, February 3). Cancer group backs down on cutting off Planned Parenthood. *New York Times*. Retrieved from http://www.nytimes .com/2012/02/04/health/policy/komen-breast-cancer-group-reverses-decision-that-cut -off-planned-parenthood.html?pagewanted=all

Berman, M. (1994). The politics of breast cancer: A state representative takes aim at her colleagues. *Detroit Monthly, 17*(7), 50–51.

Birdsell, J.M. (1997). *Policy making in the Canadian Breast Cancer Research Initiative: An institutional analysis* (Doctoral dissertation, University of Calgary). Retrieved from http://hdl.handle .net/1880/26865

Breast Cancer Action. (n.d.). Mission, vision, values. Retrieved from http://www.bcaction.org/ about/mission-vision-values

Breast Cancer Action Montreal. (n.d.). FemmeToxic. Retrieved from http://www.bcam.qc.ca/ content/femmetoxic

Brenner, J., & Smith, A. (2013, August 5). 72% of online adults are social networking site users. Pew Research Center's Internet & American Life Project. Retrieved from http://www .pewinternet.org/2013/08/05/72-of-online-adults-are-social-networking-site-users

Bright Pink. (n.d.). About us. Retrieved from http://www.brightpink.org/about-us

Brinker, N.G. (2012, February 3). Statement from Susan G. Komen Board of Directors and Founder and CEO Nancy G. Brinker [News release]. Retrieved from http://ww5.komen .org/News/Statement-from-Susan-G–Komen-Board-of-Directors-and-Founder-and-CEO -Nancy-G–Brinker.html

Bruell, A. (2012, September 3). Komen bows campaign in bid to restore blemished brand. *Advertising Age*. Retrieved from http://adage.com/article/news/komen-bows-campaign-bid -restore-blemished-brand/236996

Canadian Breast Cancer Foundation. (n.d.). About us. Retrieved from http://www.cbcf.org/ central/AboutUsMain/Pages/default.aspx

Casamayou, M.H. (2001). *The politics of breast cancer*. Washington, DC: Georgetown University Press.

Chaffee, S.H., & Metzger, M.J. (2001). The end of mass communication? *Mass Communication and Society, 4,* 365–379. doi:10.1207/S15327825MCS0404_3

CNN Wire Staff. (2012, February 4). Komen Foundation reverses funding decision of Planned Parenthood. Retrieved from http://www.cnn.com/2012/02/03/politics/planned-parenthood -komen-foundation

Cobb, R.W., & Elder, C.D. (1972). *Participation in American politics: The dynamics of agenda building*. Baltimore, MD: Johns Hopkins University Press.

Crary, D. (2012, January 31). Komen for the Cure halts grants to Planned Parenthood. *Huffington Post*. Retrieved from http://www.huffingtonpost.com/2012/01/31/komen-for-the-cure-halts-_n_1245320.html

Feran, T. (2013, June 24). State Rep. Ron Hood links abortion and breast cancer in legislation. *Cleveland Plain Dealer*. Retrieved from http://www.politifact.com/ohio/statements/2013/jun/24/ron-hood/state-rep-ron-hood-links-abortion-and-breast-cance

Ferraro, S. (1993, August 15). The anguished politics of breast cancer. *New York Times Magazine*, pp. 24–27, 58, 61–62.

Fleming, M., & O'Connor, A. (2012, February 10). *Tracking a social media crisis: Susan G. Komen for the Cure and Planned Parenthood*. Retrieved from https://web.archive.org/web/20120222154331/http://www.banyanbranch.com/social-blog/tracking-a-social-media-crisis-susan-g-komen-for-the-cure-and-planned-parenthood

Fox, S., & Purcell, K. (2010, March 24). Chronic disease and the Internet: Social media and health. Pew Research Center's Internet & American Life Project. Retrieved from http://www.pewinternet.org/2010/03/24/social-media-and-health

Gates, M. (2012, February 9). Social media plays major role in Komen, Planned Parenthood controversy. *USA Today College*. Retrieved from http://www.usatodayeducate.com/staging/index.php/pulse/social-media-plays-major-role-in-komen-planned-parenthood-controversy

Grady, D. (2013, May 20). Barbara Brenner, breast cancer iconoclast, dies at 61. *New York Times*. Retrieved from http://nytimes.com/2013/05/21/us/barbara-brenner-breast-cancer-iconoclast-dies-at-61.html?_=0

Greene, B. (1992). *Breast cancer: Unanswered questions* (Report of the Standing Committee on Health and Welfare, Social Affairs, Seniors and the Status of Women). Ottawa, Ontario, Canada: House of Commons.

Harris, G., & Belluck, P. (2012, February 1). Uproar as breast cancer group ends partnership with Planned Parenthood. *New York Times*. Retrieved from http://www.nytimes.com/2012/02/02/us/uproar-as-komen-foundation-cuts-money-to-planned-parenthood.html?pagewanted=all

Health Canada. (1994). *Report on the National Forum on Breast Cancer*. Ottawa, Canada: Minister of Supply and Services.

Institute of Cancer Research. (2012, September 26). ICR research funding. Retrieved from http://www.cihr-irsc.gc.ca/e/25551.html

Institute of Cancer Research. (2014). ICR useful links. Retrieved from http://www.cihr-irsc.gc.ca/e/24077.html

Jolie, A. (2013, May 14). My medical choice. *New York Times*. Retrieved from http://www.nytimes.com/2013/05/14/opinion/my-medical-choice.html?_r=1&

Kedrowski, K.M., & Sarow, M.S. (2007). *Cancer activism: Gender, media, and public policy*. Urbana, IL: University of Illinois Press.

Khan, H. (2012, February 3). Susan G. Komen apologizes for cutting off Planned Parenthood funding. *ABC News*. Retrieved from http://abcnews.go.com/blogs/politics/2012/02/susan-g-komen-apologizes-for-cutting-off-planned-parenthood-funding

King, S. (2006). *Pink ribbons, Inc.: Breast cancer and the politics of philanthropy*. Minneapolis, MN: University of Minnesota Press.

Kliff, S., & Sun, L.H. (2012, February 1). Planned Parenthood says Komen decision causes donation spike. *Washington Post*. Retrieved from http://www.washingtonpost.com/national/health-science/planned-parenthood-says-komen-decision-causes-donation-spike/2012/02/01/gIQAGLsxiQ_story.html

Lee National Denim Day. (2014). What is Denim Day? Retrieved from https://www.denimday.com/Movement/About

Ley, B.L. (2009). *From pink to green: Disease prevention and the environmental breast cancer movement*. New Brunswick, NJ: Rutgers University Press.

Lorde, A. (1980). *Cancer journals*. San Francisco, CA: Spinsters Ink/Aunt Lute.

Mammography Quality Standards Reauthorization Act, Pub. L. 108-365, 118 Stat. 1738 (2004).

Mears, B. (2013, June 13). Court: Human genes cannot be patented. Retrieved from http://www.cnn.com/2013/06/13/politics/scotus-genes

Memmott, M. (2012, January 31). Furor erupts over Susan G. Komen halt of grants to Planned Parenthood. National Public Radio. Retrieved from http://www.npr.org/blogs/thetwo-way/2012/01/31/146177902/furor-erupts-over-susan-g-komen-halt-of-grants-to-planned-parenthood

Montini, T. (1996). Gender and emotion in the advocacy for breast cancer informed consent legislation. *Gender and Society, 10*, 9–12. doi:10.1177/089124396010001002

Montini, T. (1997). Resist and redirect: Physicians respond to breast cancer informed consent legislation. *Women and Health, 26*(1), 85–105. doi:10.1300/J013v26n01_06

Moyer, C.S. (2013, July 22). Men say doctors often don't give in-depth advice on PSA test. Amednews.com. Retrieved from www.amednews.com/article/20130722/health/130729976/4/?utm_source=nwltr&utm

National Breast Cancer Coalition. (n.d.). NBCC's 2014 legislative and public policy priorities. Retrieved from http://www.breastcancerdeadline2020.org/get-involved/public-policy/public-policy.html

National Breast Cancer Coalition. (2010, September 17). Public submission: Comments on the interim final rules for group health plans and health insurance issuers relating to coverage of preventive services under the Patient Protection and Affordable Care Act. Retrieved from https://fdms.erulemaking.net

National Cancer Institute. (n.d.). *NCI fact book*. Retrieved from http://obf.cancer.gov/financial/factbook.htm

National Cancer Institute. (2012, July 24). Fact sheet: Prostate-specific antigen (PSA) test. Retrieved from http://www.cancer.gov/cancertopics/factsheet/detection/PSA

Newman, D.H. (2012, November 28). Ignoring the science on mammograms. *The Agenda: Health.* Retrieved from http://well.blogs.nytimes.com/2012/11/28/ignoring-the-science-on-mammograms/?_r=0

Olson, J.S. (2002). *Bathsheba's breast: Women, cancer and history*. Baltimore, MD: Johns Hopkins University Press.

Orenstein, P. (2013, April 28). The problem with pink. *New York Times Magazine*, pp. 36–43, 68–71.

Patient Protection and Affordable Care Act, Pub. L. No. 111-148, 124 Stat. 119 (2010).

Preston, J. (2012, February 1). Komen split with Planned Parenthood draws fire online. *New York Times*. Retrieved from http://thelede.blogs.nytimes.com/2012/02/01/komen-split-with-planned-parenthood-draws-uproar-online

Prostate Cancer Foundation. (n.d.). About PCF. Retrieved from http://www.pcf.org/site/c.leJRIROrEpH/b.5780287/k.E064/About_PCF.htm

Prostate Cancer International. (n.d.). *The "New" Prostate Cancer InfoLink Social Network—A service of Prostate Cancer International*. Retrieved from http://prostatecancerinfolink.ning.com

Prostate Cancer Roundtable. (2013, May 23). Professionals and patients increasingly confused by guidance on screening for risk of prostate cancer [Press release]. Retrieved from http://www.prostatecancerroundtable.net/media/media-release-5-23-13

Prostate Cancer Roundtable. (2014). Policy agenda. Retrieved from http://www.prostatecancerroundtable.net/agenda

Qaseem, A., Barry, M.J., Denberg, T.D., Owens, D.K., & Shekelle, P. (2013). Screening for prostate cancer: A guidance statement from the Clinical Guidelines Committee of the American College of Physicians. *Annals of Internal Medicine, 158*, 761–769. doi:10.7326/0003-4819-158-10-201305210-00633

Rethink Breast Cancer. (n.d.). How we (re)think. Retrieved from http://rethinkbreastcancer .com/about-rethink/old-think-vs-rethink

Roan, S. (2012, February 2). Susan G. Komen for the Cure founder defends Planned Parenthood decision. *Los Angeles Times.* Retrieved from http://articles.latimes.com/2012/feb/02/ health/la-he-komen-backlash-20120203

Runyan, J. (2013, June 29). Digital Journal—Bi-partisan support for the Congressional Men's Health Caucus. Project Vote Smart. Retrieved from http://votesmart.org/public-statement/ 796262/digital-journal-bi-partisan-support-for-the-congressional-mens-health-caucus# .UxpR8f4o7PQ

Shaw, D.L., & McCombs, M.E. (1997). *The emergence of American political issues: The agenda-setting function of the press.* St. Paul, MN: West.

Sheldrake, P. (2011). *The business of influence: Reframing marketing and PR for the digital age.* Chichester, West Sussex, United Kingdom: John Wiley & Sons.

Shulman, J. (2013, August 16). Circuit court sent clear message in "Boobies" case." *Constitution Daily.* Retrieved from http://blog.constitutioncenter.org/2013/08/circuit-court-sent-clear-message-in-boobies-case

Sulik, G.A. (2011). *Pink ribbon blues: How breast cancer culture undermines women's health.* New York, NY: Oxford University Press.

Susan G. Komen. (n.d.). About us. Retrieved from http://ww5.komen.org/AboutUs/AboutUs .html

Team Shan. (2010). Team Shan. Retrieved from http://www.teamshan.ca

U.S. Department of Health and Human Services. (2013). Cancer DATA2020. Healthy People 2020. Retrieved from http://www.healthypeople.gov/2020/Data

U.S. Preventive Services Task Force. (2009). Screening for breast cancer. Retrieved from http:// www.uspreventiveservicestaskforce.org/uspstf/uspsbrca.htm

U.S. Preventive Services Task Force. (2014). About the USPSTF. Retrieved from http://www .uspreventiveservicestaskforce.org/about.htm

Watt, S.S. (2012). A postfeminist apologia: Susan G. Komen for the Cure's evolving response to the Planned Parenthood controversy. *Journal of Contemporary Rhetoric, 2*(3/4), 65–79. Retrieved from http://contemporaryrhetoric.com/articles/watt5_2.pdf

Weberling, B. (2012). Framing breast cancer: Building an agenda through online advocacy and fundraising. *Public Relations Review, 38,* 108–115. doi:10.1016/j.pubrev.2011.08.009

Young Survival Coalition. (2014). Press kit. Retrieved from http://www.youngsurvival.org/ sites/default/files/docs/MediaKit2014.pdf

ZERO—The End of Prostate Cancer. (2013). About. Retrieved from http://www.zerocancer .org

CHAPTER 14

The Cancer Survivorship Movement Exemplar of Cancer Activism

Mandi Pratt-Chapman, MA

Introduction

This chapter provides an overview of policy efforts that have influenced cancer survivorship, including policy and advocacy at the federal, organizational, and individual levels. Key forces behind the survivorship movement are discussed, along with legislative accomplishments affecting cancer survivors, current legislative proposals specific to survivorship, new quality metrics that will influence long-term outcomes, and experimental payment structures to compensate quality cancer care. The chapter ends with challenges, opportunities, and practice implications for cancer survivorship advocacy.

In the United States, nearly 14.5 million cancer survivors were alive as of January 1, 2014, and the number is growing, with 64% living five or more years after diagnosis (American Cancer Society [ACS], 2014). With improved early detection methods and better treatments, by 2024 the number of cancer survivors will grow to nearly 19 million (ACS, 2014). Access to high-quality, comprehensive post-treatment care, care coordination, tertiary prevention, and health promotion is critical given the impact of cancer treatment and the risk of recurrence. Oeffinger et al. (2006) discovered that 73.4% of childhood cancer survivors who were 30 years past diagnosis had acquired a chronic health condition, and 42.4% of conditions were severe, disabling, or life-threatening. Compounding significant morbidity, the economic burden of cancer is substantial. Not accounting for indirect costs or lost productivity, the annual direct cost of cancer care is projected to increase from $124.5 billion in 2010 to $157.8 billion in 2020 if incidence, survival, and healthcare costs remain constant, or $172.8 billion if healthcare delivery costs continue to increase by 2% annually (Yabroff, Lund, Kepka, & Mariotto, 2011).

Given the significant physical, psychosocial, and economic impact of cancer, policy makers are increasingly turning their attention to cancer survivorship. While no federal legislation has been passed by Congress that focuses specifically on the comprehensive needs of cancer survivors, policies can have a real impact on survivorship, not simply in federal and state legislatures but in other branches of the government and at the organizational level. Likewise, advocacy is not simply an activity conducted on Capitol Hill; a patient's ability to self-advocate can contribute significantly to the quality of their care and the outcomes they experience. Finally, it is difficult to divorce policies focused on access and quality of care during treatment from survivorship, as access to high-quality cancer care and psychosocial support has a direct impact on survivors' physical and mental health outcomes, as well as long-term quality of life. This chapter outlines major policy successes and ongoing advocacy in cancer survivorship.

The Cancer Survivorship Movement: Organizational Advocacy

Awareness of cancer survivorship as a distinct phase of cancer care emerged in the 1980s and 1990s. In 1986, 21 individuals assembled to raise awareness about cancer survivors' needs and inaugurated the National Coalition for Cancer Survivorship (NCCS). In 1988, the National Cancer Institute (NCI) expanded its focus on the prevention, cause, diagnosis, and treatment of cancer to include rehabilitation from cancer as part of its legislative mandate through the Health Omnibus Programs Extension Act of 1988. And in April 1996, Dr. Richard Klausner announced the formation of the Office of Cancer Survivorship within NCI in direct response to a consensus paper adopted at the First National Congress on Cancer Survivorship on November 13, 1995. In a pivotal paper, *Imperatives for Quality Cancer Care*, Clark et al. (1996) issued a Declaration of Principles that created a call to action for addressing the physical and psychosocial long-term and late effects of cancer survivors while defining quality cancer care.

The formation of the NCI Office of Cancer Survivorship resulted in the first dedicated office committed to research focused on survivors' quality of life and long-term and late effects of treatment. The Declaration of Principles in the NCCS consensus paper laid the groundwork for policies enacted years later through the Patient Protection and Affordable Care Act (ACA) of 2010, such as eliminating preexisting condition exclusions, as well as increasing the focus on quality of life, quality of care, a multidisciplinary approach to care, shared decision making, survivorship standards of care, shared care models, distress screening, and advancing clinical trials. Many of the contributors to *Imperatives for Quality Cancer Care* have been leading researchers and advocates pushing cancer survivorship science forward, despite the dearth of policies or payment structures providing incentives for quality, longitudinal care.

The Institute of Medicine (IOM), another important nonlegislative body driving policy changes, has released a variety of reports that have bolstered attention regarding the needs of cancer survivors. Its 2003 report, *Childhood Cancer Survivorship: Improving Care and Quality of Life,* outlined seven key recommendations to improve care for the 270,000 pediatric cancer survivors in the United States (Hewitt, Weiner, & Simone, 2003). The report noted that the lack of standardized clinical practice guidelines impeded health insurance reimbursement for quality survivorship care. The authors identified four key areas in which pediatric cancer survivors need support, which were

• Psychological implications of treatment
• School transitions
• Insurance
• Employment and transitions to adult systems of care.

The report also called for a minimum set of standards for follow-up care, supported enhanced professional education and training on the management of cancer survivors, emphasized the importance of access to insurance and adequate networks of providers for children with special healthcare needs, and supported federal investments in research to prevent and ameliorate the impacts of cancer (Hewitt et al., 2003).

Another 2006 report, *From Cancer Patient to Cancer Survivor: Lost in Transition,* served as a call to action for cancer programs across the country to address the longitudinal needs of all cancer survivors (Hewitt, Greenfield, & Stovall, 2006). The key recommendations from that report included

• The establishment of survivorship as a distinct phase in the cancer continuum
• The provision of survivorship care plans and reimbursement for care planning
• The development of evidence-based clinical practice guidelines for survivorship care
• Expansion of education to help clinicians provide quality care to cancer survivors
• Elimination of employment discrimination for survivors
• Access to adequate and affordable health insurance.

Other IOM reports have focused on quality of care (Hewitt & Simone, 1999; IOM, 2001), the persistence of cancer disparities (Smedley, Stith, & Nelson, 2003), and the psychosocial needs of patients with cancer(Adler & Page, 2008). IOM also has convened a series of workshops relevant to survivorship and quality cancer care, including Implementing Cancer Survivorship Care Planning (Hewitt & Ganz, 2007), Assessing and Improving Value in Cancer Care (Schickedanz, 2009), and Patient-Centered Cancer Treatment Planning: Improving the Quality of Oncology Care (Patlak, Balogh, & Nass, 2011). IOM has been a leading force in demanding access to quality care for the most vulnerable populations.

Several key advocacy organizations and professional societies have been instrumental in advancing IOM recommendations. The Children's Oncology Group (COG) spearheaded the development of comprehensive clinical practice guidelines for pediatric-onset cancer survivors in 2003 (COG, 2008). In 2004, the Lance Armstrong Foundation (now the Livestrong Foundation) partnered with the Centers for Disease Control and Prevention (CDC) to issue the *National Action Plan for Cancer Survivorship: Advancing Public Health Strategies*. This plan served as the basis for funding the National Cancer Survivorship Resource Center, collaboratively launched in 2010 by ACS and the George Washington University Cancer Institute through a cooperative agreement with the CDC. In 2013, the resource center, along with the American Society of Clinical Oncology (ASCO) and the National Comprehensive Cancer Network, leveraged the expertise of leading researchers and clinicians to develop a number of complementary post-treatment clinical practice guidelines. ASCO also led the development of survivorship care plan templates, included the provision of treatment summaries in its Quality Oncology Practice Initiative (Moy et al., 2011), and has worked to develop health information technology standards that may assist with the generation of treatment summaries (ASCO, n.d.-b). Further, ASCO and NCCS established the Cancer Quality Alliance, which created the *Blueprint for a Better Cancer Care System* (Rose, Stovall, Ganz, Desch, & Hewitt, 2008). The blueprint assesses five case studies using six quality indicators identified by the Committee on Quality of Health Care in America of the IOM (2001) to elevate the quality of care for survivors.

Table 14-1 summarizes significant milestones in cancer survivorship affecting research, clinical care delivery, and public health.

Key Legislation Affecting Cancer Survivors

Little in the way of legislation has focused specifically on post-treatment cancer issues. However, nonlegislative government bodies and broader legislative changes have affected survivorship care delivery and payment. The Centers for Medicare and Medicaid Services (CMS) issued survivorship-specific Healthcare Common Procedure Coding System codes for cancer treatment planning and care coordination effective April 1, 2012. These codes describe a common set of services to help payers track managed care and formulate new payment strategies (NCCS, 2012). While not survivorship-

Table 14-1. Significant Milestones in Cancer Survivorship

Year	Event
1986	National Coalition for Cancer Survivorship (NCCS) assembly convenes to raise awareness of cancer survivor needs.
1988	National Cancer Institute (NCI) expands its focus on prevention, cause, diagnosis, and treatment of cancer to include rehabilitation from cancer as part of its legislative mandate (Health Omnibus Programs Extension Act of 1988).
1988	Cancer Survivors' Bill of Rights is written by Natalie Davis Spingarn (Spingarn, 1995).
1990	Americans With Disabilities Act provides civil rights protections to those with disabilities.
1995	NCCS First National Congress on Cancer Survivorship results in *Imperatives for Quality Cancer Care* (Clark et al., 1996).
1996	Dr. Richard Klausner announces formation of the Office of Cancer Survivorship within NCI (CancerNetwork 1996).
1996	Health Insurance Portability and Accountability Act limits preexisting condition exclusions.
1997	State Children's Health Insurance Program provides health insurance coverage for children not eligible for Medicaid; reauthorized in 2009 as CHIP (Children's Health Insurance Program Reauthorization Act of 2009).
1998	The Women's Health and Cancer Rights Act requires health insurance to cover reconstructive surgery and other benefits following mastectomy, including prostheses and lymphedema care.
1998	THE MARCH—Coming Together to Conquer Cancer brings advocacy groups together in Washington, DC.
1999	Institute of Medicine (IOM) publishes the report *Ensuring Quality Cancer Care*.
2001	IOM publishes *Crossing the Quality Chasm: A New System for the 21st Century*.
2003	IOM publishes *Unequal Treatment: Confronting Racial and Ethnic Disparities in Health Care*.
2003	Children's Oncology Group develops long-term follow-up guidelines for pediatric-onset cancers: www.survivorshipguidelines.org.
2003	IOM publishes *Childhood Cancer Survivorship: Improving Care and Quality of Life*.
2004	President's Cancer Panel issues *Living Beyond Cancer: Finding a New Balance* (Reuben, 2004).

(Continued on next page)

Table 14-1. Significant Milestones in Cancer Survivorship *(Continued)*

Year	Event
2004	Livestrong Foundation (formerly the Lance Armstrong Foundation) and the Centers for Disease Control and Prevention (CDC) release the *National Action Plan for Cancer Survivorship: Advancing Public Health Strategies.*
2006	IOM publishes *From Cancer Patient to Cancer Survivor: Lost in Transition.*
2008	IOM publishes *Cancer Care for the Whole Patient: Meeting Psychosocial Health Needs.*
2010	Patient Protection and Affordable Care Act provides expanded access to health insurance coverage and protections for special populations.
2010	National Cancer Survivorship Resource Center is founded by the American Cancer Society and the George Washington University Cancer Institute through a cooperative agreement with CDC.
2011	Livestrong Foundation publishes *The Essential Elements of Survivorship Care* (Rechis et al., 2011).
2012–2014	American College of Surgeons Commission on Cancer requires accredited programs to begin to integrate survivorship care planning by 2015, with full implementation by 2019.
2013	National Comprehensive Cancer Network (www.nccn.org) issues symptom-based survivorship guidelines for anxiety and depression, cognitive function, exercise, fatigue, immunizations and infections, pain, sexual function, and sleep disorders.
2013	IOM publishes *Delivering High-Quality Cancer Care: Charting a New Course for a System in Crisis* (Levit et al., 2013).
2013–2014	American Society of Clinical Oncology (2014) issues survivorship guidelines on fertility preservation, anxiety and depression, fatigue, and chemotherapy-induced peripheral neuropathy in patients with cancer.
2014	American Cancer Society publishes prostate cancer survivorship guidelines (Skolarus et al., 2014).

specific, the importance of broader federal laws providing protections for those with disabilities and the impact of the ACA cannot be overstated.

Several federal laws provide limited employment and benefits protection for cancer survivors. The Americans With Disabilities Act (ADA) of 1990 provides significant civil rights protections for cancer survivors. Prior to the ADA, the Rehabilitation Act of 1973 provided some antidiscrimination protection. This law still applies to employers with fewer than 15 employees who receive federal contracts or federal financial assistance, as well as some government employees. The Family and Medical Leave Act of 1993 applies to employers with 50 or more employees and provides limited job protection for those who need to take time off for serious illness or as a caregiver. The Employee Retirement Income Security Act of 1974 prohibits discrimination regarding employee benefits for those with a history of cancer. Additionally, the Genetic Information Nondiscrimination Act of 2008, the ADA, and the Health Insurance Portability and Accountability Act (HIPAA) of 1996 provide limited protections against discrimination in the workplace due to genetic history. Hoffman (2005) provided a helpful summary of federal policies prior to the enactment of the ACA that affect cancer survivors, and ACS (2012) also provides useful information on its website specific to the ADA.

The ADA provides civil rights protections for those with disabilities who work for employers with 15 or more employees, or who work for local, state, or federal government. This is important for cancer survivors, many of whom work through and beyond treatment. Employment is most obviously important for patients' financial health; however, other important factors drive survivors' need to work. In the United States, a large portion of health insurance is employer-provided. Employment also serves a social function and provides a sense of purpose, which can contribute to self-esteem. The ADA protects those with disabilities, those who have a record of disability, and those who are regarded as having a disability. Because many cancer survivors have limitations in performing activities of daily living, many are considered to have a disability under the ADA. The law prohibits employers from not hiring, firing, or providing unequal working conditions, pay, or benefits to a cancer survivor who is able to meet the essential job functions of a position. Employers are also required to provide reasonable accommodation, such as flexible hours, time to rest, or the ability to work from home, which could be helpful to survivors to comply with cancer treatment and follow-up schedules (Hoffman, 2005).

In 2010, the ACA provided important enhancements to existing protections and services for cancer survivors. Major goals of the ACA are to improve coverage, fairness, affordability, efficiency, and quality of care. The expansion of healthcare insurance coverage through the ACA is critical for those at risk for and those who are diagnosed with cancer, given the high costs of cancer treatment. Young survivors sometimes choose to delay care (51%) or do not obtain needed care (44%) or needed prescriptions (31%) because of the cost of care (Hewitt et al., 2006). According to an American Cancer Society Cancer Action Network (ACS CAN) poll, 16% of households affected by cancer indicated that a preexisting condition exclusion prevented them from obtaining insurance prior to the implementation of the ACA, and 59% indicated they could not afford insurance (ACS CAN, 2010). Under the ACA, young survivors immediately benefit from the extension of dependent care coverage on parent plans through age 26, and individuals younger than 19 benefit from a ban on preexisting condition exclusions.

Broader protections under the ACA include complete coverage for preventive and screening services that have a U.S. Preventive Services Task Force recommendation of A or B, such as mammograms, colonoscopies, Pap tests, and pelvic examinations (Virgo et al., 2013).

Some protections of the ACA are being phased in. The ban on preexisting condition exclusions was expanded to adults who were previously denied coverage and uninsured for at least six months when the Preexisting Condition Insurance Plans came into existence in 2010 (Virgo et al., 2013). It then applied to all adults starting in 2014 when the state health exchanges went into effect, expanding prior limited protections under HIPAA and significantly benefiting cancer survivors—particularly those who have previously experienced a gap in insurance coverage. The ACA also bans lifetime limits on coverage for essential health benefits (Rosenbaum, Lee, Chapman, & Patierno, 2011) such as

- Outpatient services
- Emergency services
- Hospitalization
- Mental health services
- Prescription drugs
- Rehabilitation and habilitation services
- Preventive services
- Chronic disease management.

Furthermore, coverage cannot be rescinded except in cases of fraud, protecting cancer survivors from debilitating healthcare expenses in the future. Challenges remain, however, for cancer survivors with extensive prescriptions. While the ACA reduces out-of-pocket prescription costs for Medicare beneficiaries, the cost of cancer drugs may still feel out of reach for seniors who have hit the *donut hole*, the coverage gap under Medicare Part D (Thorpe & Philyaw, 2010).

Going forward, patients with cancer and others will benefit from coverage of routine patient care costs associated with clinical trials and expansion of affordable insurance options with defined essential benefits through the American Health Benefit Exchanges. Tax credits and out-of-pocket maximums will further reduce costs for low-income individuals. Additionally, state Medicaid programs are given incentives to expand eligibility, increasing the accessibility of coverage for previously uninsured populations. However, states are only encouraged to provide coverage for routine care costs of clinical trials under the expanded Medicaid option, keeping the most cutting-edge research potentially out of reach for the most vulnerable (Rosenbaum et al., 2011). Moreover, the Supreme Court decision to make Medicaid expansion optional for states further limits the reach of the law (Kaiser Family Foundation, 2013). See Chapter 15 for a detailed analysis of the ACA specific to cancer care. Virgo et al. (2013) provided another excellent and succinct summary of the implications of the ACA for patients with cancer.

Core challenges that remain for survivorship care delivery are the capacity of the workforce to care for survivors and payment structures to provide incentives for quality care and care coordination. The demand for cancer care is far outpacing the supply of providers (Association of American Medical Colleges Center for Workforce Studies, 2007). The ACA helps by reauthorizing programs for health workforce training, investing in public health infrastructure, allowing for health workforce analysis and planning, and funding new public health programming (Rosenbaum et al., 2011). However, ensuring an adequate workforce and equipping clinicians with the knowledge and skills to provide optimal care to cancer survivors will require a long-term investment. The law also (Moy et al., 2011)

- Increases funding for community health centers
- Provides for community-based collaborative care networks
- Encourages integrated and coordinated care with primary care providers through community health teams
- Increases federal matching for Medicaid providers coordinating care for those with chronic diseases through medical homes
- Provides incentives for coordinated care through accountable care organizations (ACOs).

Implementation of the ACA is ongoing. The active monitoring and collaboration of healthcare professionals, treatment facilities, payers, advocacy organizations, and patients will be critical to optimize the benefits afforded through the law.

Pending Legislative Proposals and Cancer Survivorship

In 2013, several key legislative proposals were being considered in the House and Senate that would affect cancer survivors if passed. On June 25, 2013, Congresswoman Lois Capps (D-CA) and Congressman Charles Boustany (R-LA) introduced the Planning Actively for Cancer Treatment (PACT) Act of 2013, formerly named the Comprehensive Cancer Care Improvement Act. Representative Capps has championed the legislation in four Congresses. PACT supports written cancer care planning and improved coordination of care within the Medicare program, which would be a huge step forward, given that more than half of all cancer diagnoses occur among Medicare beneficiaries (ACS CAN, 2013b). The act draws from various IOM reports, recognizing the importance of shared decision making and affirming the need for coordinated psychosocial services and symptom management, including management for pain, nausea, vomiting, fatigue, and depression. NCCS has been a major advocate for this legislation, stating that it would "strengthen Medicare physician payment while improving patient care" (NCCS, 2013, para. 6). Sixteen advocacy organizations—including

ASCO, ACS CAN, the Cancer Support Community, the Livestrong Foundation, the Leukemia & Lymphoma Society, and the Susan G. Komen Advocacy Alliance—as well as 15 cancer centers officially support the legislation (NCCS, 2013).

ACS CAN has been the leading force for improved palliative care education and research through the Patient-Centered Quality Care for Life Act of 2013 (H.R. 1666) and workforce planning through the Palliative Care and Hospice Education and Training Act of 2013 (S. 641 and H.R. 1339). The Cancer Support Community has also endorsed H.R. 1666. Introduced by Congressman Emanuel Cleaver (D-MO) on April 23, 2013, H.R. 1666 supports a team-based approach to palliative care to relieve symptoms, pain, and stresses for patients who are seriously ill and improve the quality of life for patients and their families. The act mandates the convening of a Patient-Centered Health Care and Quality of Life Stakeholder Summit, composed of federal agencies, health professional organizations, patient nonprofit associations, clinicians, and representatives from the faith community. The act would also establish grants for quality-of-life education and workforce training to catalyze the delivery of patient-centered care and symptom management, as well as support research that addresses quality of life and survivorship. H.R. 1339 and S. 641, the Palliative Care and Hospice Education and Training Act, introduced by Congressman Eliot Engel (D-NY) and Senator Ron Wyden (D-OR), respectively, on March 21, 2013, complements H.R. 1666 by supporting development of faculty careers in academic palliative medicine. The act provides grants to support the career development of residents, fellows, and advanced practice nurses in palliative care, as well as continuing education for healthcare professionals who provide palliative care. ACS CAN (2013a) is leading a parallel advocacy effort at the state level to advance pain control for patients with cancer.

The Oncology Nursing Society and the Cancer Support Community have endorsed the Improving Cancer Treatment Education Act of 2013. This act, introduced by Congressman Steve Israel (D-NY) on April 19, 2013, would improve cancer patient education for Medicare beneficiaries and support research to improve cancer symptom management. The act aims to remedy insufficient education to patients by paying for a one-hour patient treatment education session delivered by an RN prior to treatment that would include a written summary about the course of treatment, responsibilities of patients, and ways to address symptoms and side effects. The act also supports enhanced research on cancer symptom management and nursing interventions.

Companion bills currently focusing on pediatric cancer survivor needs are the Childhood Cancer Survivors' Quality of Life Act, introduced by Congresswoman Jackie Speier (D-CA) on May 20, 2013, and the Pediatric, Adolescent, and Young Adult Cancer Survivorship Research and Quality of Life Act, introduced by Senator Jack Reed (D-RI) on June 27, 2013. Both bills would provide grants to pilot survivorship models of care, as well as support training programs, quality-of-life programs, and transition programs for pediatric survivors. The act would also mandate a report on workforce competencies, models, services, and curricula for pediatric cancer survivorship care.

Table 14-2 summarizes the title, sponsors, purpose, and current status of proposed legislation directly affecting cancer survivors at the time of publication of this book. Most of these bills have a small chance of getting out of committee to the full House or Senate for a vote; however, they do represent the ongoing, diligent efforts of advocacy groups to raise awareness among legislators regarding the needs of cancer survivors. The table does not reflect important legislation at the state level that affects cancer survivors, such as California's Assembly Bill No. 912, passed in 2013, which ensures insurance coverage for fertility preservation services when medical treatments,

Table 14-2. Current Legislative Proposals Being Considered by the House and Senate

Bill and Sponsor	Purpose and Status
Cancer Drug Coverage Parity Act of 2013 H.R. 1801 Sponsor: Rep. Higgins (D-NY)	To provide for coverage of oral anticancer drugs on terms no less favorable than coverage provided for anticancer medications administered by a healthcare provider. *Status:* Referred to House Committees on Education and the Workforce: Health, Employment, Labor, and Pensions (7/23/2013).
Childhood Cancer Survivors' Quality of Life Act of 2013 H.R. 2058 Sponsor: Rep. Speier (D-CA)	To improve and enhance research and programs on childhood cancer survivorship. *Status:* Referred to House Subcommittee on Health (5/24/2013).
Improving Cancer Treatment Education Act of 2013 H.R. 1661 Sponsor: Rep. Israel (D-NY)	To amend Title XVIII of the Social Security Act to provide comprehensive cancer patient treatment education under the Medicare program and to provide for research to improve cancer symptom management. *Status:* Referred to the House Subcommittee on Health (6/23/2013).
Palliative Care and Hospice Education and Training Act of 2013 H.R. 1339 and S. 641 Sponsors: Rep. Engel (D-NY); Sen. Wyden (D-OR)	To amend the Public Health Service Act to increase the number of permanent faculty in palliative care at accredited allopathic and osteopathic medical schools, nursing schools, and other programs to promote education in palliative care and hospice and to support the development of faculty careers in academic palliative medicine. *Status:* Read twice and referred to the Senate Committee on Health, Education, Labor, and Pensions (3/21/2013).

(Continued on next page)

Table 14-2. Current Legislative Proposals Being Considered by the House and Senate *(Continued)*

Bill and Sponsor	Purpose and Status
Patient-Centered Quality Care for Life Act of 2013 H.R. 1666 Sponsors: Reps. Cleaver (D-MO) and Bachus (R-AL) S. 2800; Sen. Begich (D-AK)	To create a patient-centered quality of care initiative for seriously ill patients through the establishment of a stakeholder strategic summit, quality-of-life education and awareness initiative, healthcare workforce training, an advisory committee, and palliative care-focused research. *Status:* Referred to the House Subcommittee on Health (4/23/2013). Introduced and referred to Senate Committee on Health, Education, Labor, and Pensions (9/11/2014).
Pediatric, Adolescent, and Young Adult Cancer Survivorship Research and Quality of Life Act of 2013 S. 1247 Sponsor: Sen. Reed (D-RI)	To improve and enhance research and programs on childhood cancer survivorship. *Status:* Read twice and referred to the Senate Committee on Health, Education, Labor, and Pensions (6/27/2013).
Planning Actively for Cancer Treatment (PACT) Act of 2013 H.R. 2477 Sponsors: Reps. Capps (D-CA) and Boustany (R-LA)	To amend Title XVIII of the Social Security Act to provide for coverage of cancer care planning and coordination under the Medicare program. *Status:* Referred to the House Subcommittee on Health (7/23/2013).

such as those for cancer, might put future fertility at risk. Another state-level success is the adoption of oral chemotherapy parity bills by 34 states and the District of Columbia, making treatment more accessible for some patients; however, these laws do little to reduce the exorbitant cost of oral cancer drugs and will likely result in cost-shifting that will raise overall premiums (Wang, Joffe, & Kesselheim, 2014). A summary of state legislative activity not specific to survivorship is available in the ACS CAN (2013a) report *How Do You Measure Up? A Progress Report on State Legislative Activity to Reduce Cancer Incidence and Mortality.*

Legislative advocacy requires diligence in not simply asking for what is best for cancer survivors, but also opposing policies that may have an unintended negative impact. One legislative proposal currently opposed by most cancer groups is the Medicare Patient Access to Cancer Treatment Act introduced by Representatives Mike Rogers (R-MI) and Doris Matsui (D-CA) on July 31, 2013. This bill supports increased payments for outpatient physician offices for chemotherapy administration by decreasing reimbursement to hospital outpatient departments. While improving outpatient payments would seem to be beneficial at first glance, the Association of Community Cancer Centers (ACCC) has voiced concern that the bill inadequately accounts for higher overhead and more complex cases seen in the hospital setting (Abbott, 2013a). In addition to ACCC, the American Hospital Association (2013) opposes the bill.

Institutional Policies: New Quality Standards and Payment Reform

Arguably, one of the greatest forces driving improved cancer survivorship care has come not from federal or state legislation, but from new accreditation standards from the American College of Surgeons Commission on Cancer (CoC). The CoC's *Cancer Program Standards* include previous standards requiring cancer patient access to psychosocial, rehabilitation, and nutrition services, as well as new patient-centered care standards and quality metrics, including the following (American College of Surgeons CoC, n.d., 2012).
- Standard 2.4, Palliative Care Services, which requires availability of palliative care either on site or by referral
- Standard 3.1, Patient Navigation Process, which requires accredited institutions to formalize a patient navigation process responsive to a community needs assessment that addresses identified barriers to care, either on site or via referral
- Standard 3.2, Distress Screening, which requires the cancer committee to implement, integrate, and monitor a distress screening process, including screening at a minimum of one pivotal medical visit. The CoC indicates a preference for distress screening at the time of diagnosis or during a time of transition, where distress might be higher, including the transition off treatment.
- Standard 3.3, Survivorship Care Plan, which requires institutions to develop, implement, and monitor a process to "disseminate a comprehensive care summary and follow-up plan to patients with cancer who are completing cancer treatment" (American College of Surgeons CoC, 2012, p. 78).

Standard 2.4 is required now, and CoC recently issued clarification statements for Standards 3.1, 3.2, and 3.3. Standards 3.1 and 3.2 are expected to be fully implemented by January 1, 2015 (American College of Surgeons CoC, 2014a). The CoC expects cancer centers seeking accreditation to implement a pilot survivorship care plan process that involves at least 10% of eligible patients to fulfill Standard 3.3 for 2015. The CoC recently instituted a tiered requirement for cancer centers to provide care plans to an increasing percentage of patients with nonmetastatic cancer who have been treated with curative intent, with full implementation for all eligible patients to be in place by January 1, 2019 (American College of Surgeons CoC, 2014b). Once implemented, these new requirements will have a significant impact on how care is delivered at CoC-accredited facilities, which treat more than 70% of newly diagnosed patients with cancer (American College of Surgeons CoC, n.d.).

These new performance metrics put greater pressure on healthcare providers at a time when workforce capacity is strained. Providers, payers, and legislators are exploring alternative payment structures to the traditional fee-for-service model to provide incentives for quality care. President Obama reinforced this by focusing on quality of care rather than number of tests as the standard for payment in his 2013 State of the Union address (Whitehouse.gov, 2013). The Oncology Patient–Centered Medical Home has demonstrated promise in some settings as an alternative model. Sprandio (2012) reported reduced emergency department visits and hospitalizations, shorter lengths of stay for hospitalized patients, fewer outpatient visits, and overall cost savings with improvements to care through the Oncology Patient–Centered Medical Home Model. With the increasing numbers of survivors requiring care and the decreasing pool of providers, replicating efficient, effective treatment and follow-up care models will be critical to sustainably improve the quality of care for cancer survivors.

In August 2013, the House Energy and Commerce Committee unanimously approved the Medicare Patient Access and Quality Improvement Act of 2013, replacing the Medicare Sustainable Growth Rate (SGR) formula with increased payments for exceeding quality measures beginning in 2019. Physicians can opt out of the program if they participate in a patient-centered medical home or ACO. On March 14, 2014, the bill was reported to the House and passed as the SGR Repeal and Medicare Provider Payment Modernization Act of 2014. A companion bill (S.R. 2000) was introduced on February 6, 2014, and the House bill was received in the Senate on March 24, 2014. A final vote on the bill has not yet occurred as of the time of this writing. The underlying problem with the SGR formula is that the increase in expenses for each Medicare patient cannot exceed growth of the gross domestic product. This causes drastic instability to provider payments. While the bill being considered in the Senate mitigates this problem with stable payments and incentives to providers, ACCC is concerned that the bill will not sufficiently achieve provider reimbursement increases because it does not require CMS to reinvest savings realized from the act into cancer services to adequately finance the fix (Abbott, 2013b).

Finding sustainable payment models for quality cancer care has critical implications for long-term survivorship. Payment for cancer care should be linked to quality metrics that are aligned with evidence of improved outcomes and responsive to survivor preferences and priorities for care. To better understand what is currently being delivered in the way of survivorship care, who is providing it, how they are providing it, and whether care delivery corresponds with what patients deem most important, George Washington University is conducting a study to evaluate cancer survivorship care models in collaboration with the CoC, the Livestrong Foundation, the Cancer Support Community, and ACS (Patient-Centered Outcomes Research Institute, 2013). Funded by the Patient-Centered Outcomes Research Institute, findings may inform future accreditation requirements and provide important information as to which care models optimally influence survivor outcomes.

An Exemplar: Empowered Survivors

The federal laws, pending legislative proposals, and new quality standards outlined in this chapter would not have been possible without the efforts of cancer survivors driving legislative and institutional change. Societal awareness about the needs of cancer survivors and the reduction of stigma around a cancer diagnosis are attributable, in large part, to two advocacy organizations: NCCS and the Livestrong Foundation. Since its first meeting in 1986, NCCS has vigorously advocated for cancer survivorship research and legal protections for cancer survivors. The now ubiquitous yellow Livestrong bracelet donned by survivors, caregivers, and friends of survivors is a testament to the impact of a simple message of empowerment and strength. Numerous other advocacy organizations have also provided lifesaving resources, support, and strength to the growing number of survivors in the United States today.

In addition to advocacy at the federal, state, local, and institutional levels, advocacy also happens at the individual level. In August 2013, the evolution of survivorship from stigma to celebration was exemplified by the first-ever National Women's Survivors Convention (now called SURVIVORville) in Nashville, Tennessee, headlined by musical, athletic, and media celebrities talking about their personal experiences as cancer survivors and co-survivors (Women Survivors Alliance, 2013). Olympic gold medalists Shannon Miller and Scott Hamilton, television personality Tabitha Coffey, singer Martina McBride, and numerous other celebrity survivors and co-survivors, as well as internationally renowned researchers, championed this inaugural celebration of survivorship—not for healthcare professionals or researchers, but for survivors themselves. Stories from everyday cancer survivors were displayed on a wall of words at the convention, testifying to the resilience of those who have experienced cancer and their successful efforts to advocate for themselves and others. Themes from these survivor stories included hope, optimism, purpose, courage, resolve, celebration, and faith. Testaments also reflected grief, disfigurement, loss of fertility, and acceptance that not everything is always happy. Underlying each experience was the strength to self-advocate and to accept help from others. Numerous stories reflected the proliferation of nonprofits and support groups to help others who are embarking on the same journey.

Cancer survivors can significantly shape their personal healthcare experience and outcomes with strong self-advocacy skills. As Clark and Stovall (1996) articulated in "Advocacy: The Cornerstone of Cancer Survivorship," knowing how to communicate, make decisions, solve problems, and negotiate are important skills for cancer survivors. NCCS's Cancer Survival Toolbox provides guidance on these topics and others, such as how to pay for cancer care (NCCS, n.d.). Survivors can be their own best medical and wellness advocates by

- Exercising
- Eating nutritiously
- Managing stress
- Creating and using a support network
- Asking questions
- Seeking reliable information
- Asking about eligibility for clinical trials
- Requesting information about their individual risks and symptoms to watch for
- Requesting a survivorship care plan
- Choosing providers who will give them the information they need and deserve.

Survivors can have an impact on quality-of-care improvements by initiating and participating in patient and family advisory councils for cancer programs and providing feedback on their care to improve the experience of others. Finally, survivors can advocate at the institutional, local, state, and federal levels for policies that support quality standards and funding for survivorship research and programs.

Challenges and Opportunities

Cancer survivorship as a field has benefited from the dedication of pioneering researchers and clinicians, the commitment of numerous cancer advocacy organizations, and the vision of lawmakers who have sponsored legislation protecting cancer survivors in the United States. Despite these advances, challenges remain. Policies that protect the most vulnerable patients, provide incentives for survivorship workforce expansion, support an expanded data infrastructure, integrate long-term outcomes into clinical trials, and ensure dissemination of findings are key to addressing the needs of cancer survivors.

While the ACA will expand insurance eligibility for many, the June 28, 2012, Supreme Court ruling in *National Federation of Independent Business v.*

Sebelius deemed it unconstitutional to punish states for not expanding their Medicaid programs, so individuals in some states may not benefit from expanded access. Additionally, the poor still may not access health care due to inability to pay premiums or co-payments and the limited availability of qualified healthcare providers. Poor patients may not be able to prioritize the costs of cancer care above other life needs. Some patients face structural barriers to care, such as transportation to treatment or inability to take time off from work. These barriers may persist after treatment, when follow-up care is needed to optimize length and quality of life.

Furthermore, although providing incentives for state expansion of Medicaid programs is an important stride forward, without an adequate pool of providers who are skilled and willing to provide care to cancer survivors reliant on Medicaid, access will remain a major obstacle to care. Continuing medical education programs focused on cancer survivorship, such as the National Cancer Survivorship Resource Center's Cancer Survivorship e-Learning Series for Primary Care Providers (National Cancer Survivorship Resource Center, n.d.), as well as integration of cancer survivorship knowledge into medical and nursing schools, are key to ensuring that providers are comfortable and qualified to provide survivorship care.

Another challenge is the lack of a comprehensive, coordinated data infrastructure for cancer survivors. Despite increased integration of electronic health records (EHRs), electronic data capture is limited and communication across data systems is difficult and often impossible. Individual organizations have built registries to link survivors to researchers, such as the Dr. Susan Love Research Foundation's Army of Women and the Cancer Support Community's Cancer Experience Registry (Cancer Support Community, n.d.; Dr. Susan Love Research Foundation, n.d.). The CoC's new Rapid Quality Reporting System aims to improve quality of data and provides for more timely data on which to base quality improvements (American College of Surgeons CoC, 2011). Finally, ASCO has championed standards to improve EHR interoperability (ASCO, n.d.-b) and has successfully piloted its CancerLinQ system, which is intended to capture data from individuals treated nationwide and provide real-time quality feedback to clinicians with decision support (ASCO, n.d.-a). A coordinated approach to data collection is required to track and assess long-term outcomes of survivors and provide evidence-based policy recommendations.

Also, diminishing resources for research, as well as its historical focus on the elimination of disease at the expense of health-related quality of life, threaten researchers' ability to build the evidence needed for responsible policies related to survivorship. Funders have an opportunity to influence the outcomes of cancer survivors by creating incentives for the integration of quality-of-life and long-term outcomes measures into clinical trials. New mechanisms for dissemination and implementation of research will encourage the practical application of research findings and their translation to a broader population of patients (Glasgow et al., 2012). A lot is known about how to treat cancer, and there is more to be learned, but there is a huge opportunity right now to apply what is known and make equitable care accessible to all people.

However, with fewer dollars available for research, fragmentation within the cancer community is a threat to progress on the legislative front. Uncoordinated and varying requests by cancer advocacy organizations may result in the cancer community getting less rather than more. One Voice Against Cancer (OVAC), launched in 2000, helps by coordinating efforts across nonprofit organizations to advocate for federal support for cancer research and programs (OVAC, n.d.). Given ever-diminishing resources, the cancer community also will need to collaborate with other disease groups to ensure that legislation has the greatest public health impact on the nation. ACS CAN has set an example in coalition building for their national-, federal-, and state-level palliative care initiative, focusing on the importance of pain relief for all patients with serious illness, rather than just patients with cancer.

Practice Implications

Patients with cancer require and deserve access to a full range of supportive care services, including
- Symptom management
- Psychosocial support
- Palliation from pain
- Interventions for fatigue and nausea
- Dietary counseling and nutrition support
- Survivorship care planning and ongoing follow-up
- Impairment-driven rehabilitation
- Early access to hospice services.

Furthermore, healthcare professionals have an opportunity to reduce post-treatment impairments by providing interventions to increase functionality prior to the start of treatment, also called *prehabilitation* (Silver, Baima, & Mayer, 2013). Finally, care should be equitable, evidence based, and coordinated, and providers should be paid according to the quality rather than the number of procedures.

Equitable access to care and quality of care are paramount to optimize survivor outcomes. While the ACA does much to expand coverage and protections for survivors and the CoC is demanding quality measures for accredited programs, sustainability of access and quality requires adequate and appropriate payment structures for care that is delivered, sufficient training for providers, and an investment in research to build the evidence for the best institutional and legislative policies. Trends reflect a move away from traditional fee-for-service models toward pay-for-performance models, but providers, payers, and legislators are still looking for the right algorithm. New payment structures may include expanded clinical pathway programs, bundled payments for episodes of care, and replication of patient-centered medical homes. Building and sustaining an adequate workforce to care for survivors will require multiple approaches, including continuing healthcare professional education, incorporation of survivorship care standards in professional schools, and recruitment of diverse students to provide quality survivorship care for future patients with cancer. Finally, research must include long-term outcomes to provide evidence-based policies for cancer survivorship in the future.

Advocacy occurs at the federal, state, organizational, and individual levels, and clinicians play an important role at all of these levels. At the federal and state level, healthcare professionals can respond to calls for action from advocacy groups and ensure that legislators are informed on the realities of clinical practice. Collaborating with other providers, across advocacy organizations, and with other disease groups will optimize chances of success. At the organizational level, clinicians and researchers can develop and implement standards of care, test new payment structures for sustainability, participate in real-time quality reporting systems, and deliver quality care for cancer survivors. Given increasing demands and a growing patient population, providers should leverage the numerous advocacy organizations and nonprofits available to support their patients—many of which are led and staffed by cancer survivors or caregivers who are committed to making the cancer journey easier for those who follow in their footsteps.

Conclusion

This chapter has provided an overview of the cancer survivorship movement through organizational and legislative advocacy while highlighting the power of individual advocacy. The power of the word *survivorship* is that it forces patients, family members, friends, healthcare providers, and researchers to think about the future—to expect a future for the patient. The cancer survivorship movement has come a long way in a few decades. Harnessing the power of researchers, advocacy organizations, government agencies, legislators, payers, providers, and patients will ensure continued progress in the decades to come.

The author would like to thank Ellen Stovall, Elizabeth Clark, Rebecca Kirch, Mark Gorman, and Linda House for feedback on this chapter. Special thanks also to Megan Matheny for her administrative support.

References

Abbott, S. (2013a, August 5). Capitol Hill update: HR 2869—Medicare Patient Access to Treatment Act. *ACCCBuzz*. Retrieved from http://acccbuzz.wordpress.com/2013/08/05/capitol-hill-update-hr-2869-medicare-patient-access-to-treatment-act

Abbott, S. (2013b, August 7). Is SGR replacement in sight? *ACCCBuzz*. Retrieved from http://acccbuzz.wordpress.com/2013/08/07/is-sgr-replacement-in-sight

Adler, N.E., & Page, A.E.K. (Eds.). (2008). *Cancer care for the whole patient: Meeting psychosocial health needs.* Retrieved from http://books.nap.edu/openbook.php?record_id=11993

American Cancer Society. (2012, October 31). Americans With Disabilities Act: Information for people facing cancer. Retrieved from http://www.cancer.org/treatment/findingandpayingfortreatment/understandingfinancialandlegalmatters/americans-with-disabilities-act

American Cancer Society. (2014). *Cancer treatment and survivorship facts and figures 2014–2015.* Retrieved from http://www.cancer.org/research/cancerfactsstatistics/survivor-facts-figures

American Cancer Society Cancer Action Network. (2010). *A national poll: Facing cancer in the health care system.* Retrieved from http://acscan.org/ovc_images/file/mediacenter/ACS_CAN_Polling_Report_7.27.10_FINAL.pdf

American Cancer Society Cancer Action Network. (2013a, August). *How do you measure up? A progress report on state legislative activity to reduce cancer incidence and mortality* (11th ed.). Retrieved from http://www.acscan.org/content/wp-content/uploads/2013/08/HDYMU-2013.pdf

American Cancer Society Cancer Action Network. (2013b). *Lifeline: Why cancer patients depend on Medicare for critical coverage.* Retrieved from http://www.acscan.org/content/wp-content/uploads/2013/06/2013-Medicare-Chartbook-Online-Version.pdf

American College of Surgeons Commission on Cancer. (n.d.). About CoC accreditation. Retrieved from http://www.facs.org/cancer/coc/whatis.html

American College of Surgeons Commission on Cancer. (2011). Rapid Quality Reporting System (RQRS). Retrieved from https://www.facs.org/quality-programs/cancer/ncdb/qualitytools/rqrs

American College of Surgeons Commission on Cancer. (2012). *Cancer program standards 2012: Ensuring patient-centered care* [v.1.2.1, released January 2014]. Retrieved from http://www.facs.org/cancer/coc/programstandards2012.pdf

American College of Surgeons Commission on Cancer. (2014a). Accreditation Committee clarifications for Standards 3.1 Patient Navigation Process and 3.2 Psychosocial Distress Screening. Retrieved from https://www.facs.org/publications/newsletters/coc-source/special-source/standard3132

American College of Surgeons Commission on Cancer. (2014b). Accreditation Committee clarifications for Standard 3.3 Survivorship Care Plan. Retrieved from https://www.facs.org/publications/newsletters/coc-source/special-source/standard33

American Hospital Association. (2013, August). Letter to Congress. Retrieved from http://www.aha.org/advocacy-issues/letter/2013/130801-let-cancertrxhr2869.pdf

American Society of Clinical Oncology. (n.d.-a). CancerLinQ™. Retrieved from http://www.instituteforquality.org/cancerlinq

American Society of Clinical Oncology. (n.d.-b). Data interoperability standards. Retrieved from http://www.asco.org/practice-research/data-interoperability-standards

American Society of Clinical Oncology. (2014). Survivorship guidelines. Retrieved from http://www.asco.org/guidelines/survivorship

Americans With Disabilities Act of 1990, Pub. L. No. 101-336, 104 Stat. 328.

Association of American Medical Colleges Center for Workforce Studies. (2007, March). *Forecasting the supply of and demand for oncologists: A report to the American Society of Clinical Oncology*

(ASCO) from the AAMC Center for Workforce Studies. Retrieved from http://www.asco.org/sites/default/files/oncology_workforce_report_final.pdf

Cancer Drug Coverage Parity Act of 2013, H.R. 1801, 113th Cong.

CancerNetwork. (1996, December 1). New cancer programs, Office of Cancer Survivorship announced. Retrieved from http://www.cancernetwork.com/articles/new-cancer-programs-office-cancer-survivorship-announced

Cancer Support Community. (n.d.). Cancer Experience Registry. Retrieved from http://www.cancersupportcommunity.org/MainMenu/ResearchTraining/Cancer-Experience-Registry.html

Centers for Disease Control and Prevention & Lance Armstrong Foundation. (2004, April). *A national action plan for cancer survivorship: Advancing public health strategies*. Retrieved from http://www.cdc.gov/cancer/survivorship/pdf/plan.pdf

Childhood Cancer Survivors' Quality of Life Act of 2013, H.R. 2058, 113th Cong.

Children's Health Insurance Program Reauthorization Act of 2009, Pub. L. No. 111-3, 123 Stat. 8.

Children's Oncology Group. (2008, October). *Long-term follow-up guidelines for survivors of childhood, adolescent, and young adult cancers, version 3.0*. Retrieved from http://www.survivorshipguidelines.org/pdf/LTFUGuidelines.pdf

Clark, E.J., & Stovall, E.L. (1996). Advocacy: The cornerstone of cancer survivorship. *Cancer Practice, 4*, 239–244.

Clark, E.J., Stovall, E.L., Leigh, S., Sui, A.L., Austin, D.K., & Rowland, J.H. (1996). *Imperatives for quality cancer care: Access, advocacy, action, and accountability*. Retrieved from http://www.canceradvocacy.org/wp-content/uploads/2013/01/NCCS_Imperatives_8-96.pdf

Dr. Susan Love Research Foundation. (n.d.). Army of Women. Retrieved from https://www.armyofwomen.org

Employee Retirement Income Security Act of 1974, Pub. L. No. 93-406, 88 Stat. 829.

Family and Medical Leave Act of 1993, Pub. L. No. 103-3, 107 Stat. 6.

Genetic Information Nondiscrimination Act of 2008, Pub. L. No. 110-233, 122 Stat. 881.

Glasgow, R.E., Vinson, C., Chambers, D., Khoury, M.J., Kaplan, R.M., & Hunter, C. (2012). National Institutes of Health approaches to dissemination and implementation science: Current and future directions. *American Journal of Public Health, 102*, 1274–1281. doi:10.2105/AJPH.2012.300755

Health Insurance Portability and Accountability Act of 1996, Pub. L. No. 104-191, 110 Stat. 1936.

Health Omnibus Programs Extension Act of 1988, Pub. L. No. 100-607, 102 Stat. 3054.

Hewitt, M., & Ganz, P.A. (2007). *Implementing cancer survivorship care planning: Workshop summary*. Retrieved from http://books.nap.edu/openbook.php?record_id=11739

Hewitt, M., Greenfield, S., & Stovall, E. (Eds.). (2006). *From cancer patient to cancer survivor: Lost in transition*. Retrieved from http://books.nap.edu/openbook.php?record_id=11468

Hewitt, M., & Simone, J.V. (Eds.). (1999). *Ensuring quality cancer care*. Retrieved from http://books.nap.edu/openbook.php?record_id=6467

Hewitt, M., Weiner, S.L., & Simone, J.V. (Eds.). (2003). *Childhood cancer survivorship: Improving care and quality of life*. Retrieved from http://books.nap.edu/openbook.php?record_id=10767

Hoffman, B. (2005). Cancer survivors at work: A generation of progress. *CA: A Cancer Journal for Clinicians, 55*, 271–280. doi:10.3322/canjclin.55.5.271

Improving Cancer Treatment Education Act of 2013, H.R. 1661, 113th Cong.

Institute of Medicine. (2001). *Crossing the quality chasm: A new health system for the 21st century*. Retrieved from http://books.nap.edu/openbook.php?record_id=10027

Kaiser Family Foundation. (2013, December). *A closer look at the uninsured eligible for Medicaid and CHIP*. Retrieved from https://kaiserfamilyfoundation.files.wordpress.com/2013/12/8533-a-closer-look-at-the-uninsured-eligible-for-medicaid-and-chip.pdf

Levit, L.A., Balogh, E.P., Nass, S.J., & Ganz, P.A. (Eds.). (2013). *Delivering high-quality cancer care: Charting a new course for a system in crisis.* Retrieved from http://books.nap.edu/openbook.php?record_id=18359

Medicare Patient Access and Quality Improvement Act of 2013, H.R. 2810, 113th Cong.

Medicare Patient Access to Cancer Treatment Act of 2013, H.R. 2869, 113th Cong.

Moy, B., Polite, B.N., Halpern, M.T., Stranne, S.K., Winer, E.P., Wollins, D.S., & Newman, L.A. (2011). American Society of Clinical Oncology policy statement: Opportunities in the Patient Protection and Affordable Care Act to reduce cancer care disparities. *Journal of Clinical Oncology, 29,* 3816–3824. doi:10.1200/JCO.2011.35.8903

National Cancer Survivorship Resource Center. (n.d.). Cancer survivorship e-learning series for primary care providers. Retrieved from https://cancersurvivorshipcentereducation.org

National Coalition for Cancer Survivorship. (n.d.). The Cancer Survival Toolbox. Retrieved from http://www.canceradvocacy.org/toolbox

National Coalition for Cancer Survivorship. (2012, January 12). NCCS applauds establishment of cancer treatment planning and care coordination reimbursement codes [Press release]. Retrieved from http://www.canceradvocacy.org/policy-comments/nccs-applauds-establishment-of-cancer-treatment-planning-and-care-coordination-reimbursement-codes

National Coalition for Cancer Survivorship. (2013). PACT Act: Medicare reform for quality cancer care. Retrieved from http://www.canceradvocacy.org/pact-act-medicare-reform-for-quality-cancer-care

National Federation of Independent Business v. Sebelius, 132 S. Ct. 2566 (2012).

Oeffinger, K.C., Mertens, A.C., Sklar, C.A., Kawashima, T., Hudson, M.M., Meadows, A.T., ... Robison, L.L. (2006). Chronic health conditions in adult survivors of childhood cancer. *New England Journal of Medicine, 355,* 1572–1582. doi:10.1056/NEJMsa060185

One Voice Against Cancer. (n.d.). Home. Retrieved from http://www.ovaconline.org

Palliative Care and Hospice Education and Training Act of 2013, H.R. 1339, 113th Cong.

Palliative Care and Hospice Education and Training Act of 2013, S. 641, 113th Cong.

Patient-Centered Outcomes Research Institute. (2013). Evaluating cancer survivorship care models. Retrieved from http://www.pcori.org/research-results/2013/evaluating-cancer-survivorship-care-models

Patient-Centered Quality Care for Life Act of 2013, H.R. 1666, 113th Cong.

Patient Protection and Affordable Care Act, Pub. L. No. 111-148, 124 Stat. 119 (2010).

Patlak, M., Balogh, E., & Nass, S. (2011). *Patient-centered cancer treatment planning: Improving the quality of oncology care: Workshop summary.* Retrieved from http://books.nap.edu/openbook.php?record_id=13155

Pediatric, Adolescent, and Young Adult Cancer Survivorship Research and Quality of Life Act of 2013, S. 1247, 113th Cong.

Planning Actively for Cancer Treatment (PACT) Act of 2013, H.R. 2477, 113th Cong.

Rechis, R., Beckjord, E.B., Arvey, S.R., Reynolds, K.A., & McGoldrick, D. (2011, December). *The essential elements of survivorship care: A Livestrong brief.* Retrieved from http://images.livestrong.org/downloads/flatfiles/what-we-do/our-approach/reports/ee/EssentialElementsBrief.pdf

Rehabilitation Act of 1973, Pub. L. No. 93-112, 87 Stat. 355.

Reuben, S.H. (2004). *Living beyond cancer: Finding a new balance. President's Cancer Panel 2003–2004 annual report.* Retrieved from http://deainfo.nci.nih.gov/advisory/pcp/annualReports/pcp03-04rpt/Survivorship.pdf

Rose, C., Stovall, E., Ganz, P.A., Desch, C., & Hewitt, M. (2008). Cancer Quality Alliance: Blueprint for a better cancer care system. *CA: A Cancer Journal for Clinicians, 58,* 266–292. doi:10.3322/CA.2008.0012

Rosenbaum, S., Lee, J., Chapman, M.P., & Patierno, S.R. (2011). Cancer survivorship and national health reform. In M. Feuerstein & P.A. Ganz (Eds.), *Health services for cancer survivors* (pp. 355–372). doi:10.1007/978-1-4419-1348-7_17

Schickedanz, A. (2009). *Assessing and improving value in cancer care: Workshop summary.* Retrieved from http://books.nap.edu/openbook.php?record_id=12644

SGR Repeal and Medicare Provider Payment Modernization Act of 2014, H.R. 4015, 113th Cong.

Silver, J.K., Baima, J., & Mayer, R.S. (2013). Impairment-driven cancer rehabilitation: An essential component of quality care and survivorship. *CA: A Cancer Journal for Clinicians, 63,* 295–317. doi:10.3322/caac.21186

Skolarus, T.A., Wolf, A.M.D., Erb, N.L., Brooks, D.D., Rivers, B.M., Underwood, W., III., … Cowens-Alvarado, R.L. (2014). American Cancer Society prostate cancer survivorship care guidelines. *CA: A Cancer Journal for Clinicians, 64,* 225–249. doi:10.3322/caac.21234

Smedley, B.D., Stith, A.Y., & Nelson, A.R. (Eds.). (2003). *Unequal treatment: Confronting racial and ethnic disparities in health care.* Retrieved from http://www.nap.edu/openbook.php?record_id=10260

Spingarn, N.D. (1995). Anatomy of a bill of rights. *Illness, Crisis, and Loss, 5,* 88–91.

Sprandio, J.D. (2012). Oncology patient–centered medical home. *Journal of Oncology Practice, 8*(Suppl. 3), 47s–49s. doi:10.1200/JOP.2012.000590

Thorpe, K.E., & Philyaw, M. (2010). Impact of health care reform on Medicare and dual Medicare-Medicaid beneficiaries. *Cancer Journal, 16,* 584–587. doi:10.1097/PPO.0b013e3181ff3156

Virgo, K.S., Bromberek, J.L., Glaser, A., Horgan, D., Maher, J., & Brawley, O.W. (2013). Health care policy and cancer survivorship. *Cancer, 119,* 2187–2199. doi:10.1002/cncr.28066

Wang, B., Joffe, S., & Kesselheim, A.S. (2014). Chemotherapy parity laws: A remedy for high drug costs? *JAMA Internal Medicine, 174,* 1721–1722. doi:10.1001/jamainternmed.2014.4878

Whitehouse.gov. (2013, February 12). *The 2013 State of the Union Address* (enhanced version) [Video file]. Retrieved from http://www.whitehouse.gov/state-of-the-union-2013

Women Survivors Alliance. (2013). SURVIVORville 2013 guest speakers. Retrieved from http://www.survivorville.org/2013-guest-speakers

Women's Health and Cancer Rights Act of 1998, Pub. L. No. 105-277, 112 Stat. 2681.

Yabroff, K.R., Lund, J., Kepka, D., & Mariotto, A. (2011). Economic burden of cancer in the United States: Estimates, projections and future research. *Cancer Epidemiology, Biomarkers and Prevention, 20,* 2006–2014. doi:10.1158/1055-9965.EPI-11-0650

CHAPTER 15

Oncology Implications of the Patient Protection and Affordable Care Act

Janice M. Phillips, PhD, RN, FAAN, Barbara D. Powe, PhD, RN, FAAN, and Mandi Pratt-Chapman, MA

Introduction

The Patient Protection and Affordable Care Act (2010), commonly referred to as the ACA, promises to have a lasting impact on cancer care delivery and related outcomes across the cancer continuum. Policy makers, cancer advocates, consumers, patients with cancer, and other stakeholders no doubt will be waiting to witness the impact this broad, sweeping legislation has on improving the nation's cancer profile. Thus, the purpose of this chapter is to highlight selected provisions of the ACA, namely: access, quality, and research and their related implications for informing cancer care.

Cancer Incidence, Mortality, and Survival

Cancer continues to be a leading global public health concern, accounting for approximately one in four deaths in the United States. The American Cancer Society (ACS) has estimated approximately 1.7 million new cancer diagnoses in the United States in 2015. This estimate does not consider carcinomas in situ of any site (except urinary bladder) or basal and squamous cell cancers of the skin. Prostate, lung/bronchus, and colorectal cancers are the most commonly diagnosed cancers in men, accounting for nearly 50% of cancers, while breast, lung/bronchus, and colorectal cancers are the leading diagnoses in women, accounting for about 50% of diagnosed cancers (ACS, 2015).

Turning to mortality, ACS estimated 589,430 cancer deaths in the United States in 2015. This equates to more than 1,600 deaths each day. Similar to the projections in new cancer cases, the most common causes of cancer death in men are cancers of the lung/bronchus, prostate, and colon/rectum. In women, most cancer deaths are from cancers of the lung/bronchus, breast, and colon/rectum (ACS, 2015).

Thanks to advancements in cancer diagnosis and treatment, the five-year relative survival rate increased from 49% in 1975–1977 to 68% in 2004–2010. African Americans, however, continue to have the poorest survival rates when compared to Caucasians or other population groups. These poor outcomes are attributed, in part, to the late stage at diagnosis, differences in comorbidities, and inequalities in access to cancer care (ACS, 2015).

While advancements in cancer care and outcomes have been greatly enhanced by our ability to discover and apply scientific breakthroughs, some of the advancements in cancer care have been influenced, in part, by advocacy and political activism that have resulted in legislative action. Over the years, a growing number of passionate cancer survivors, powerful grassroots and professional organizations, and committed stakeholders have successfully advocated for a substantial number of public policies that have affected cancer care and cancer outcomes. Legislation and public policies focused on increasing funding for the National Cancer Institute, enhancing tobacco control, and improving access to early detection and treatment represent a few examples where stakeholders advocated to improve the cancer profile and outcomes of the nation. No doubt legislative action will remain a cornerstone in any effort to conquer cancer. The recent passage of the ACA represents a major legislative milestone that promises to have broad, sweeping implications for all Americans, including patients with cancer.

The ACA is a complex and comprehensive piece of legislation with provisions far too numerous to describe here. This chapter will provide a brief overview of select ACA provisions and related implications for cancer care, highlighting key issues including access to cancer care, healthcare quality, and cancer research. The U.S. Department of Health and Human Services (DHHS) provides a detailed discussion on the entire law and related provisions (see U.S. DHHS, 2013a).

The Patient Protection and Affordable Care Act

Not without controversy, the enactment of the ACA in 2010 (Public Law 111-148) was the nation's most significant health legislation since the passage of Medicare and Medicaid in 1965 (Feldman, 2012). Numerous factors underscored the need for such sweeping legislation, including the growing number of uninsured individuals, unsustainably high healthcare costs, the ongoing disparities in health outcomes, and a predominant emphasis on treatment versus prevention, along with a host of health system challenges requiring a major overhaul.

Efforts to achieve some aspect of healthcare reform date back to 1912–1914, when President Theodore Roosevelt was in office. Throughout history, subsequent presidents have tried to establish some form of health reform, but to no avail (Teitelbaum & Wilensky, 2013). Although President Lyndon B. Johnson passed legislation to establish Medicaid and Medicare in 1965, this did not constitute universal coverage or comprehensive health reform (Teitelbaum & Wilensky, 2013).

It is perhaps no surprise that the ACA was met with political resistance and efforts to repeal it. However, it was signed into legislation on March 23, 2010, and was upheld by the Supreme Court on July 28, 2012. Provisions outlined in this historic law include a focus on expanding access to health care and enhancing benefits and consumer protections through a number of insurance reform efforts. The push for improved quality and efficiency in health care, a stronger workforce, and an increased focus on prevention will occur through a number of health system reform efforts. While provisions of the ACA offer a broad approach to insurance and health system reform, these provisions have potentially enormous implications for cancer care and oncology providers. These broad implications transcend the entire cancer continuum in the areas of access, consumer protection, cost, and quality. In fact, ACS (2010) noted that approximately 160 provisions in the ACA will affect millions of Americans who are living with a cancer diagnosis, those at risk for developing cancer, survivors, and those in remission. Figure 15-1 provides a snapshot of key provisions affecting patients with cancer and survivors.

Expanding Access to Care

The potential impact of the ACA on expanding access to care and ensuring consumer protection for patients with cancer promises to be substantive. This impact is projected to be major, given that 46.3 million Americans lacked health insurance prior to its enactment, a critical impetus for such legislation (Schoen, Collins, Kriss, & Doty, 2008). Expanded access to care, coupled with provisions to help ensure consumer protection, is especially important for patients with cancer who have experienced considerable difficulty gaining access to lifesaving cancer care because of access and cost barriers. The need to address such barriers was perhaps best underscored in a previous study conducted by ACS.

Prior to enactment of the ACA, ACS commissioned a study to explore the experience of patients with cancer accessing the healthcare system. A representative sample of 1,011 adults with a personal diagnosis of cancer or reported history of having a household member with a history of cancer completed the survey between May 21 and June 2, 2010. This time period occurred shortly after the passage of the ACA, far too soon to evaluate any impact from the new law. Key findings from this bipartisan study pointed to a number of issues regarding access to and affordability of cancer care services (ACS Cancer Action Network, 2011).

For example, for those younger than 65 diagnosed with cancer, 66% were insured during the entire time of their diagnosis, while 34% were uninsured (ACS Cancer Action Network, 2011). Securing and maintaining insurance

---

Figure 15-1. The New Healthcare Reform Law Through the Cancer Lens: Key Provisions Affecting Patients With Cancer and Survivors

---

Approximately 160 provisions in the final healthcare legislation will directly impact the millions of Americans who have or will face cancer. The following is a list of the most important provisions for the cancer community.

I. Immediate Investments
- Provides immediate access to coverage for uninsured people with a serious preexisting condition through high-risk pools (Sec. 1101)
- No lifetime limits for all plans; phaseout of annual limits by 2014 (Sec. 2711)
- No rescissions except in the case of fraud or intentional misrepresentation (Sec. 2712)
- Coverage of preventive health services (beginning next plan year) (Sec. 2713)
- Dependent coverage extended until age 26 (Sec. 2714)
- Reduction in Medicare Part D prescription drug coverage gap (i.e., the "donut" hole) (Sec. 3301–3315)

II. Enhancing the Role of Disease Prevention and Early Detection
- Guarantees coverage and eliminates out-of-pocket costs for U.S. Preventive Services Task Force (USPSTF) prevention services with an "A" or "B" rating and mammography coverage for all women aged 40 and over. (Sec. 2713)
- Establishes a National Prevention Interagency Council and Strategy (Sec. 4001)
- Establishes a fund, to be administered through the Office of the Secretary at the Department of Health and Human Services (HHS), to provide for an expanded and sustained national investment in prevention and public health programs (Sec. 4002)
- Provides grant funding for state, local, and community-based prevention programs and services (Sec. 4201–4202)
- Strengthens the primary care workforce through student financing, additional primary care residency programs at teaching health centers, and training in cultural competency, prevention, and public health (Sec. 5301–5605)
- Significantly increases community health center funding (Sec. 10503)

(Continued on next page)

Figure 15-1. The New Healthcare Reform Law Through the Cancer Lens: Key Provisions Affecting Patients With Cancer and Survivors *(Continued)*

III. Meaningful Coverage: Availability, Affordability, Adequacy, and Administrative Simplification
A. Private insurance
   • Availability
      – Provides immediate access to coverage for uninsured people with a serious preexisting condition through the high-risk pool, affording a transition coverage until full implementation of the legislation (Sec. 1101)
      – Eliminates preexisting condition medical restrictions for most private insurance plans by 2014 (Sec. 2704)
      – Prohibits all plans from rescinding coverage except in instances of fraud or misrepresentation (Sec. 2712)
      – Guarantees availability and renewability of coverage (Sec. 2702–2703)
   • Affordability
      – Limits insurance premium variation to family structure, geography, the actuarial value of the benefit, age (limited to a ratio of 3 to 1), and tobacco use (limited to a ratio of 1.5 to 1) (Sec. 2701)
      – Creates refundable tax credits to provide premium assistance for individuals and families up to 400% of the federal poverty level for coverage under a qualified health plan (Sec. 1401–1415)
      – Limits out-of-pocket maximums for individuals and families enrolling in qualified health plans (Sec. 1302)
   • Adequacy
      – Eliminates lifetime and annual limits for most plans (Sec. 2711)
      – Requires coverage of preventive health services (Sec. 2713)
      – Requires insurance plans to cover essential health benefits (Sec. 1302)
   • Administrative simplicity
      – Develops and encourages utilization of uniform explanation of coverage documents and standardized definitions (Sec. 2715)
      – Assists consumers with coverage appeals and educates consumers on their rights and responsibilities (Sec. 2719)
B. Medicaid
   • Gives states the option to expand eligibility for individuals with income below 133% of the federal poverty level (FPL) and optional coverage for those above 133% of FPL (Sec. 2001)
   • Generally prohibits states from reducing or dropping breast and cervical cancer treatment eligibility during transition period until 2014 (Sec. 2001)
   • Increases access to tobacco cessation prescription medications and over-the-counter tobacco cessation products (Sec. 2502)
   • Offers incentives for coverage of preventive services for eligible adults in Medicaid (Sec. 4106)
   • Mandates coverage of comprehensive tobacco cessation services for pregnant women in Medicaid (Sec. 4107)
   • Uses incentives to encourage enrollees to participate in chronic disease prevention programs (Sec. 4108)
   • Simplifies enrollment in Medicaid (Sec. 2201–2202)
   • Improves Medicaid reimbursement rates for primary care physicians, fostering increased access for patients (Reconciliation Sec. 1202)

(Continued on next page)

Figure 15-1. The New Healthcare Reform Law Through the Cancer Lens: Key Provisions Affecting Patients With Cancer and Survivors *(Continued)*

C. Medicare
- Begins immediate reduction in Part D prescription drug coverage gap (i.e., the "donut" hole) (Sec. 3301–3315)
- Improves Medicare coverage of annual wellness visit, including a personalized prevention plan (Sec. 4103)
- Eliminates cost-sharing and deductibles in Medicare for USPSTF prevention services with "A" or "B" rating (Sec. 4104)

IV. Improving Quality of Life for Cancer Patients and Survivors
- Reauthorizes HHS's Patient Navigator program, which assists patients with maneuvering through the healthcare system, provides outreach and education for patients to encourage preventive screenings, and addresses needs that may impact compliance with screening and treatment (Sec. 3510)
- Requires commercial health insurance plans and the Federal Employee Health Benefits Plan (but not private self-insured plans) to cover the patient care costs associated with participation in clinical trials that are approved or funded by a variety of federal agencies (Sec. 10103)
- Requires the Secretary of HHS to establish national priorities and plans for improving the quality of health care, including care coordination and chronic disease management (Sec. 3011–3015)
- Authorizes Institute of Medicine conference and report on pain management and enhanced coordination of National Institutes of Health pain research, and establishes a grant program to improve health professionals' understanding and ability to assess and appropriately treat pain (Sec. 4305)
- Provides training grants in family medicine, general internal medicine, general pediatrics, physician assistantship, and geriatrics, giving priority to programs that apply team-based approaches to care (Sec. 5301)
- Expands career development awards to advanced practice nurses, clinical social workers, pharmacists, and psychologists (Sec. 5305)

Note. Reprinted with permission from Heather Eagleton, Director of Public Policy and Government Relations, American Cancer Society, September 20, 2013.

---

coverage during the time of diagnosis was problematic, as patients with cancer were considered to have a preexisting condition. Respondents cited various reasons for being uninsured, including lack of affordability (59%), waiting for coverage because of preexisting condition (16%), waiting for employment coverage (5%), waiting for coverage in general (4%), and being unemployed and lacking coverage (2%). Notably, 1% of respondents reported being dropped from their coverage because of their preexisting condition (ACS Cancer Action Network, 2011).

The increasing cost of insurance coverage creates yet another barrier for patients with cancer, survivors, and their families. For example, 4 in 10 families surveyed in 2010 reported an increase in health insurance premiums and co-payments 12 months prior to the survey (ACS Cancer

Action Network, 2011). Increases in deductibles were reported by 25%. Sadly, one in three patients diagnosed with cancer younger than 65 reported delaying health care (e.g., diagnostic and treatment services or required checkups) because of cost. Such delays in cancer screening, detection, treatment, and timely follow-up care jeopardize health outcomes and place patients at risk for delayed diagnosis, less than favorable outcomes, and increased risk for cancer recurrence (ACS Cancer Action Network, 2011).

Benefits to Patients With Cancer

While some individuals remain critical of various components outlined in the ACA, others consider it a victory for patients with cancer. This is particularly true for consumers and patients with cancer who are uninsured or underinsured or who had been insured but then were denied continuing coverage while facing a cancer diagnosis. The ACA has the potential to expand healthcare coverage to approximately 47 million nonelderly uninsured individuals nationwide (Kaiser Family Foundation, 2013). Coverage expansions through public and private insurers will ensure that more patients with cancer have access to needed care. Incentives for states to expand their Medicaid eligibility for those younger than 65 with incomes between 133% and 400% of the federal poverty level may help. However, the Supreme Court's decision to make this provision optional for states will affect the number of those insured (Kaiser Family Foundation, 2013).

The essential health benefit requirements outlined in the ACA are a plus for patients with cancer who become eligible for enrollment into health insurance exchanges. The essential benefits package is designed to emulate employer plans while ensuring consumer protections, requiring provisions for mental health parity, and stipulating cost-sharing limitations (Hutchins, Samuels, & Lively, 2013). Qualified health plans are required to provide, at a minimum, the following services (Hutchins et al., 2013).

• Ambulatory patient services
• Emergency services
• Hospitalizations
• Laboratory services
• Maternity and newborn services
• Mental health and substance use disorder services
• Behavioral health services
• Pediatric services (including oral and vision)
• Preventive and wellness care
• Chronic disease management services

- Prescription drugs
- Rehabilitative and habilitative services and devices

Provisions designed to expand access to health care are critical to eliminate cancer health disparities among the underserved. The disparities in cancer incidence, mortality, and survival among U.S. racial and ethnic populations are well documented (ACS, 2015; Millon-Underwood, Phillips, & Powe, 2008; Moy et al., 2011). These disparities are particularly prevalent among low-income individuals, regardless of ethnic or racial background. Individuals of low socioeconomic status are more likely to present with advanced cancers and are less likely to receive high-quality cancer diagnostic and treatment services, all of which influence survival (ACS, 2015). Although provisions outlined in the ACA show promise for improving cancer care and related outcomes, Moy et al. (2011) highlighted challenges related to the law's potential to reduce cancer disparities. As passed, the ACA does not require insurers to cover follow-up services for abnormalities that are noted during the screening process. Also, limited evidence exists about cancer screening strategies specific to ethnically diverse populations outlined by the U.S. Preventive Services Task Force, the leading authority offering recommendations for health screening in the ACA. Finally, these authors expressed concerns over the lack of specific recommendations for services that address the unique needs of high-risk populations, including cancer survivors (Moy et al., 2011).

In contrast, provisions calling for enhanced data collection on race and ethnicity will enable lawmakers and stakeholders to better identify and address the needs of racial and ethnic minority populations who suffer disproportionately from cancer. The elevation of the National Center on Minority Health and Health Disparities to Institute status in 2010, along with the establishment of an Office of Minority Health in various DHHS agencies, has the potential to intensify efforts focused on eradicating health disparities (Moy et al., 2011). Finally, increased funding to support federally qualified health centers (FQHCs) frequently visited by underserved populations offers another opportunity to help reduce cancer disparities (Allen et al., 2014). Continued advocacy and legislative action may still be needed to help ensure that patients with cancer receiving care at FQHCs have access to high-quality, timely, and comprehensive cancer services across the cancer continuum.

Enhancing Quality and Value

In September 2013, the Institute of Medicine released a preview of its report *Delivering High-Quality Cancer Care: Charting a New Course for a System in Crisis* (Levit, Balogh, Nass, & Ganz, 2013). To draft the report, the National Research Council established a committee to assess the quality of cancer care and address the challenges of the aging U.S. population. The committee concluded that growing demand, increasingly complex treatments, limited workforce capacity, and rising costs have led to a system in crisis. Care is often not evidence-based or coordinated, and patients often do not receive adequate education, information, or access to supportive and palliative care services. The committee established a conceptual framework for high-quality cancer care that includes engaged patients, an adequate and well-trained workforce, evidence-based care, the use of health information technology to improve the quality of care and patient outcomes, the use of evidence to quickly inform clinical practice and performance improvements, and the provision of accessible, affordable care through realigned payment models (Levit et al., 2013). The conceptual model espoused by the Institute of Medicine committee aligns well with the aims of the ACA. The ACA addresses quality, value, and performance improvement through new payment models and encourages patient-centered care and workforce capacity building.

Arguably, the single biggest challenge to quality cancer care is the misaligned payment structure, which provides incentives for the volume of services and procedures at the expense of evidence, efficiency, patient education, and patient engagement. The historical fee-for-service structure encourages healthcare spending, ignoring the impact of services delivered on health outcomes. For oncology, cost of care is a major issue for patients, providers, and the federal government. Patients with cancer can pay tens of thousands of dollars for a single course of treatment, and the cost of providing care continues to rise, sometimes exponentially for certain drug therapies (Patel & Tran, 2013). Cancer-related pharmacotherapies represented 23 of the top 55 most expensive Medicare Part B expenditures in 2010 (U.S. Government Accountability Office, 2012).

The ACA aims to improve the value, quality, and efficiency of health care while reducing costs by piloting new payment and care delivery models. The primary mechanism through which the ACA effects system change is by expanding the authority of the secretary of Health and Human Services and state Medicaid programs to pilot new models without seeking approval from Congress to do so. New models of care are intended to support integrated care, quality care, and quality improvements with a focus on value rather than number of procedures (Rosenbaum, 2011). Key payment reform models include accountable care organizations (ACOs), patient-centered medical homes (PCMHs), and bundled payment mechanisms. Other aspects of the ACA focus on reducing hospital readmissions and modifying payment to hospitals to establish value through value-based purchasing programs (Thorpe & Cascio, 2013).

The Medicare Shared Savings Program (MSSP), established through the ACA, created ACOs, which are formal groups of healthcare providers who agree to coordinate care for a certain group of patients. ACOs realign the payment structure to prioritize the quality and efficiency of care. Although ACOs were originally rolled out through the Centers for Medicare and Medicaid Services (CMS), the private sector is increasingly embracing value-based care delivery and reimbursement models, with roughly 14% of Americans receiving care from these types of organizations as of February 2013 (Oliver Wyman, 2012, 2013). According to the Oliver Wyman Health Innovation Center, if ACOs can achieve improvements in quality while reducing cost, they are positioned to force change in the healthcare delivery system at large.

The impact of ACOs on cancer care delivery could be enormous. Medicare's pioneering of ACOs is relevant to individuals 65 and older, who comprise the majority of cancer diagnoses, deaths, and survivors (Levit et al., 2013). Oncologists, as specialists, cannot start an ACO; however, they can join an unlimited number of ACOs. CMS is considering demonstration projects that would allow oncologists to lead ACOs (Wilkerson, 2012). As ACOs shift the focus to patient-centered care, accountability, and coordinated care, patients with cancer should receive proactive health care to prevent avoidable impacts of treatment and foster wellness. While the complexity of cancer care and high costs of therapy have left cancer out of early ACO configurations, considering that cancer is one of the most expensive health conditions to treat, ACOs have reason to prioritize the inclusion of oncology services to significantly lower costs (Barkley & Blau, 2013). However, Greenapple (2011) warned that oncologists might be pressured to lower costs at the expense of quality under the ACO model.

Another ACA-inspired payment model, the PCMH, focuses on the quality and accessibility of health care to ensure coordinated care. The PCMH consists of a health team that provides comprehensive health care and meets standards for performance around disease management, care transitions, and care coordination; quality, efficiency, and quality data reporting; and the Health Information Technology for Economic and Clinical Health (HITECH) Act's *meaningful use* requirements (Thorpe & Cascio, 2013). Sprandio (2010) has demonstrated the application of the PCMH for oncology care. Consultants in Medical Oncology and Hematology, the first National Committee for Quality Assurance–designated oncology PCMH, coordinated all aspects of cancer care through patient navigators, encouraged patient engagement, improved access to care through extended hours and triage services, and used data to continually improve the quality of performance and patient outcomes (Sprandio, 2010). The result was reduced emergency department referrals and visits, reduced hospital admissions, improved symptom management and palliative care, improved adherence to National Comprehensive Cancer Network clinical practice guidelines, and overall cost savings (Sprandio, 2010).

The ACA also invested in research to identify the most effective and efficient ways to serve all populations by establishing the Center for Medicare and Medicaid Innovation (CMMI) and the Patient-Centered Outcomes Research Institute (PCORI). PCORI is further discussed in the next section. CMMI is testing new models of care to improve quality and reduce cost, including the Pioneer ACO Model, which is a "high-risk, high-reward alternative to the MSSP" (Thorpe & Cascio, 2013). CMMI is also replicating the oncology PCMH model over three years starting in New Mexico (Patel & Tran, 2013). Finally, CMMI is piloting the Bundled Payments for Care Improvement (BPCI) Initiative, through which participating providers receive bundled payments—or one payment for all healthcare services related to an episode of care. An episode of care includes services related to a specific condition over a determined period of time. Through another pilot program, CMMI's Financial Alignment Initiative, health plans are given incentives to cut expenses by coordinating care for *dual eligibles*, defined as those individuals eligible for both Medicare and Medicaid (Robert Wood Johnson Foundation & George Washington University School of Public Health and Health Services, n.d.).

The full impact of these initiatives on cancer care is yet to be seen. The BPCI Initiative, rolled out by CMS on January 31, 2013, focuses on episodes of acute care and does not currently designate cancer as a qualified episode of care (CMS, n.d.). However, CMS is exploring bundled payment mechanisms for oncology care, specifically under Medicare Part B (Wilkerson, 2012). In the private sector, the largest insurer in the United States, United Healthcare, is piloting a bundled payment initiative with five oncology practices across the country, inclusive of drug and case management support but maintaining fee-for-service for other components of care (Goozner, 2011). This pilot aims to reduce costs for United Healthcare by standardizing oncology regimens that are currently highly variable, encouraging generic prescriptions, and eliminating the risk to oncology practices by paying the drug costs charged by the supplier. The plan also pays a case management fee to improve the quality of care and patient engagement in decision making, particularly toward the end of life. Payers Aetna and P4 Healthcare have also been working with oncology groups to explore clinical pathway programs (i.e., evidence-based regimens to reduce variability in care, errors, and cost) (Aetna, 2011). Blue Cross introduced a global budget with a risk-sharing alternative payment scheme in California and Massachusetts with good results (Markovitch, 2012; Song et al., 2012). The global budget provides prospective payment for anticipated costs of caring for a certain population of patients over a predefined period of time.

Finally, the ACA invests in a National Quality Strategy to improve quality, efficiency, value, and safety while enhancing health information technology to help patients get information they need about their health care and the performance of their providers (Rosenbaum, 2011). The National Quality Strategy focuses on three broad aims: better care, healthy people/healthy communities, and affordable care. Priorities include safer care, patient-centered care, effective communication, and coordination of care; effective prevention and treatment; promotion of best practices to support healthy living; and new healthcare delivery models focused on affordable, quality care. The National Quality Strategy supports the adoption and meaningful use of electronic health records, building on the HITECH Act (U.S. DHHS, 2011). The ACA also developed the Physician Feedback Program to provide CMS with quality data reports. Further, the ACA advances the Physician Quality Reporting System, which provides incentive payments for quality from 2011 to 2014 and possible reductions in payments starting in 2015 if physicians do not meet required standards (Patel & Tran, 2013).

The ACA has sparked innovation for new models of care to improve quality and reduce cost, promote value and provider accountability, encourage integration and coordination of care, and focus on the needs of patients. Much depends on the refinement and successful replication of promising models of care like the oncology PCMH, the expansion of ACOs to oncology, and the expansion of the workforce to meet growing patient needs. Looking ahead, patients, providers, and payers will need to monitor the impact of payment reform strategies on access to timely, quality oncology services for patients, especially for the most vulnerable populations. Presently, the cancer community has an opportunity to provide feedback to policy makers on issues that arise for patients during implementation of the ACA to inform health plan adjustments going forward. Attention to improved patient health outcomes, not just cost reduction, is paramount.

Advancing Oncology Research

Given the current transformation in health care, there is a need for enhanced research across the cancer continuum and across the research spectrum (from descriptive and exploratory designs to experimental and randomized clinical trials). In addition, rapid translation of science into practice is needed. An example of an organized infrastructure to direct research is PCORI, which was established by the ACA. PCORI's mission is to provide information about the best available evidence to help patients and their healthcare providers make more informed decisions. The translation of PCORI's research is intended to give patients a better understanding of the available prevention, treatment, and care options and the science that supports those options. The five initial funding areas for PCORI, all of which have implications for cancer care, are
• Assessing prevention, diagnosis, and treatment options
• Improving healthcare systems
• Improving communication and dissemination research
• Addressing disparities

- Accelerating patient-centered outcomes research and methodologic research (PCORI, 2013).

Recent discussions of comparative effectiveness research (CER) in cancer are linked to the goals of PCORI (Glasgow et al., 2013). The focus of CER is the "generation and synthesis of evidence that compares the benefits and harms of alternative methods to prevent, diagnose, treat, and monitor a clinical condition or to improve the delivery of care" (Institute of Medicine, 2009, p. 1). However, a key to the overall effectiveness of CER and, thus, the achievement of PCORI's goals, is to have a robust system for knowledge integration (Glasgow et al., 2013). Simply stated, healthcare providers and researchers must be able to translate the research into practice in a timely manner. This type of translation may mean the introduction of new and innovative practice, or it may mean moving away from traditional ways of doing things that are not evidence based. It is important for outcomes research to address the process of access to care as individuals become eligible for care and formally access insurance exchanges and healthcare systems.

Inherent with the increased access to care afforded by the ACA is the need to monitor workforce capacity and quality. With an estimated 14 million people entering the healthcare system in 2014, the president of the Association of Academic Health Centers raised the question of whether the workforce was adequately prepared (Association of Academic Health Centers, 2013). Provisions of the ACA under Title V—Health Care Workforce, Subtitle A, Purpose and Definitions, list its purpose as follows (ACA, 2010).

> To improve access to and the delivery of health care services for all individuals, particularly low income, underserved, uninsured, minority, health disparity, and rural populations by—
> (1) gathering and assessing comprehensive data in order for the health care workforce to meet the health care needs of individuals, including research on the supply, demand, distribution, diversity, and skills needs of the health care workforce;
> (2) increasing the supply of a qualified health care workforce to improve access to and the delivery of health care services for all individuals;
> (3) enhancing health care workforce education and training to improve access to and the delivery of health care services for all individuals; and
> (4) providing support to the existing health care workforce to improve access to and the delivery of health care services for all individuals. (§ 5001(1)–(4))

At the governmental level, the ACA gave the comptroller general of the United States responsibility for appointing 15 members to the National Health Care Workforce Commission (U.S. Government Accountability Office, 2012). However, as of January 2015, the commission had not met because of lack of congressional funding. The ACA also established a funding mechanism for State Healthcare Workforce Development grants and a National Center for Health Workforce Analysis (American College of Physicians, 2013). The National Center for Health Workforce Analysis focuses on supply and demand for healthcare workers and workforce investments (Health Resources and Services Administration, 2013).

While it is beyond the scope of this chapter to review the charge of the commission in detail, it is apparent that issues such as workforce training, staffing mix, and funding must be monitored at the local and community levels and that these data need clear pipelines to the data monitoring at the state and federal levels. Strategies for implementing this type of healthcare workforce surveillance are not yet clear. What is clear, however, is that this undertaking cannot be done in isolation by healthcare disciplines, healthcare facilities, or states.

The era of healthcare reform also raises questions regarding the determination, funding, and implementation of research priorities within granting agencies. While not a result of the ACA, an exemplar for "thinking outside of the box" is the Provocative Questions initiative launched by the National Cancer Institute in 2010 (http://provocativequestions .nci.nih.gov). In this initiative, investigators and others visiting the website were asked to submit questions that needed attention but might not rise to the top in traditional discussions of research priorities. Panel groups were convened, and calls for proposals were issued based on several of the questions (U.S. DHHS, 2013b). Too often, researchers look to other researchers to establish research priorities. Because research findings are intended to address population health, needs, and services, researchers must engage these populations, including healthcare providers, small business owners, marketing professionals, and technology leaders, as the solutions may be found within these groups and not from researchers in isolation.

This redefinition of how research priorities should be set brings with it the challenge of initial and sustained funding. Funders must partner to effectively identify and address synergistic research priorities (ACS, 2013). For example, partnerships to establish programs of research on common risk factors associated with cancer, diabetes, and heart disease have the potential to decrease obesity, encourage healthy nutrition, and increase physical activity. With common messaging and a common platform, risk factor reduction extends beyond one disease, and patients may see the benefit of one health behavior change on more than one disease. Another possible framework for defining research priorities could focus on the essential elements of reform as outlined within the ACA (see Table 15-1). This type of framework would encourage research across the cancer continuum while at the same time providing evaluation data for programs and interventions designed to enhance access to affordable care. These research priorities

Table 15-1. Essential Elements of Reform That Should Guide Cancer Research Priorities

Components of Reform	Examples of Potential Research Priorities
Quality health care for all Americans	Health equity and disparities across the cancer continuum Effectiveness of insurance exchanges Employer healthcare initiatives
The role of public programs	Access to community resources available to cancer survivors and caregivers Effectiveness of funding for programs
Improving the quality and efficiency of health care	Access to primary care, innovative and novel cancer therapies Genetics research Effect of premiums and co-payments on healthcare outcomes
Prevention of chronic disease and improving public health	Lifestyle and behavior modifications Nutrition and physical activity Comorbidities and cancer
Healthcare workforce	Capacity issues and ability of workforce to meet community needs Training programs for providers to meet needs of cancer survivors
Transparency and program integrity	Program implementation Program evaluation Program sustainability

Note. Based on information from U.S. Department of Health and Human Services, 2013a.

would also encourage interdisciplinary research and community engagement. The active inclusion of communities across the cancer continuum is critical because communities can better identify and define healthcare needs. Further, the inclusion of communities is critical to implement and sustain successful programs.

Lastly, more research on communication strategies is needed to ensure that everyone has realistic access to this information. For example, it may not be sufficient to place cancer information only on websites, as many population groups will continue to have issues with health and digital literacy. On the other hand, for those who are comfortable with technology (e.g., the Internet, social media), research is needed to explore the effectiveness of communicating using these type of media. Further research is needed on the best way to integrate practice change across the continuum, as well as more timely ways to disseminate these findings to the scientific and lay communities. While it is anticipated that there will be further decreases in cancer incidence and mortality rates over time with the newly insured participating in cancer prevention and early cancer detection efforts, it is critical to maintain national epidemiologic surveillance of changes in health care that may coincide with implementation of the ACA.

Conclusion

This chapter has provided a brief overview on the ACA and implications for oncology with specific emphasis on key issues, including access and quality, as well as implications for cancer research. The full impact of the ACA on improving the cancer profile of the nation remains to be seen and relies, in part, on the cancer community's active engagement and vigilant advocacy to protect the law.

References

Aetna. (2011, May 23). Aetna, P4 Healthcare expand their collaboration to Georgia, Northern Virginia and Washington, DC [Press release]. Retrieved from http://news.aetna.com/news-releases/aetna-p4-healthcare-expand-their-collaboration-to-georgia-northern-virginia-and-washington-d-c

Allen, C.L., Harris, J.R., Hannon, P.A., Parrish, A.T., Hammerback, K., Craft, J., & Gray, B. (2014). Opportunities for improving cancer prevention at federally qualified health centers. *Journal of Cancer Education, 29,* 30–37. doi:10.1007/s13187-013-0535-4

American Cancer Society. (2010). *The Affordable Care Act: How it helps people with cancer and their families.* Retrieved from http://action.acscan.org/site/DocServer/Affordable_Care_Act_Through_the_Cancer_Lens_Final.pdf?docID=18421

American Cancer Society. (2013). The Guideline Advantage. Retrieved from http://www.guidelineadvantage.org/TGA

American Cancer Society. (2015). *Cancer facts and figures 2015.* Retrieved from http://www.cancer.org/research/cancerfactsstatistics/index

American Cancer Society Cancer Action Network. (2011). *A national poll: Facing cancer in the health care system.* Retrieved from http://www.acscan.org/healthcare/cancerpoll

American College of Physicians. (2013). National Health Care Workforce Commission. Retrieved from http://www.acponline.org/advocacy/where_we_stand/assets/ii4-national-health-care-workforce.pdf

Association of Academic Health Centers. (2013, April 16). Health workforce not ready to handle the Affordable Care Act [News release]. Retrieved from http://www.aahcdc.org/Policy/PressReleases/PRView/ArticleId/118/Health-Workforce-Not-Ready-to-Handle-the-Affordable-Care-Act.aspx

Barkley, R., & Blau, M. (2013, January). Cancer costs remain a priority: Innovators apply accountable care to oncology redesigns. *Managed Healthcare Executive, 23*(1), 26–28. Retrieved from http://www.ccbdgroup.com/MHE2013.pdf

Centers for Medicare and Medicaid Services. (n.d.). Bundled Payments for Care Improvement (BPCI) Initiative: General information. Retrieved from http://innovation.cms.gov/initiatives/bundled-payments/index.html

Feldman, A.M. (2012). *Understanding health care reform: Bridging the gap between myth and reality.* Boca Raton, FL: CRC Press.

Glasgow, R.E., Doria-Rose, V.P., Khoury, M.J., Elzarrad, M., Brown, M.L., & Stange, K.C. (2013). Comparative effectiveness research in cancer: What has been funded and what knowledge gaps remain? *Journal of the National Cancer Institute, 105,* 766–773. doi:10.1093/jnci/djt066

Goozner, M. (2011). United Healthcare, five oncology practices try bundled payments. *Journal of the National Cancer Institute, 103,* 8–10. doi:10.1093/jnci/djq538

Greenapple, R. (2011). Accountable care organizations: Implications for oncologists. *Value-Based Cancer Care, 2*(3), 21. Retrieved from http://issuu.com/vbcc/docs/june_2011/21

Health Resources and Services Administration. (2013). National Center for Workforce Analysis. Retrieved from http://bhpr.hrsa.gov/healthworkforce

Hutchins, V.A., Samuels, M.B., & Lively, A.M. (2013). Analyzing the Affordable Care Act: Essential health benefits and implications for oncology. *Journal of Oncology Practice, 9,* 73–77. doi:10.1200/JOP.2012.000881

Institute of Medicine. (2009). Initial national priorities for comparative effectiveness research (Report brief). Retrieved from http://www.iom.edu/~/media/Files/Report%20Files/2009/ComparativeEffectivenessResearchPriorities/CER%20report%20brief%2008-13-09.pdf

Kaiser Family Foundation. (2013, December). *A closer look at the uninsured eligible for Medicaid and CHIP.* Retrieved from https://kaiserfamilyfoundation.files.wordpress.com/2013/12/8533-a-closer-look-at-the-uninsured-eligible-for-medicaid-and-chip.pdf

Levit, L.A., Balogh, E.P., Nass, S.J., & Ganz, P.A. (Eds.). (2013). *Delivering high-quality cancer care: Charting a new course for a system in crisis.* Retrieved from http://iom.edu/Reports/2013/Delivering-High-Quality-Cancer-Care-Charting-a-New-Course-for-a-System-in-Crisis.aspx

Markovitch, P. (2012). A global budget pilot project among provider partners and Blue Shield of California led to savings in first two years. *Health Affairs, 31,* 1969–1976. doi:10.1377/hlthaff.2012.0358

Millon-Underwood, S., Phillips, J., & Powe, B.D. (2008). Eliminating cancer-related disparities: How nurses can respond to the challenge. *Seminars in Oncology Nursing, 24,* 279–291. doi:10.1016/j.soncn.2008.08.008

Moy, B., Polite, B.N., Halpern, M.T., Stranne, S.K., Winer, E.P., Wollins, D.S., & Newman, L.A. (2011). American Society of Clinical Oncology policy statement: Opportunities in the Patient Protection and Affordable Care Act to reduce cancer care disparities. *Journal of Clinical Oncology, 29,* 3816–3824. doi:10.1200/JCO.2011.35.8903

Oliver Wyman. (2012). The ACO surprise. Retrieved from http://www.oliverwyman.com/insights/publications/2012/nov/the-aco-surprise.html#.U0hVa1VdWw0

Oliver Wyman. (2013, February 19). Accountable care organizations now serve 14% of Americans [News release]. Retrieved from http://www.oliverwyman.com/media/ACO_press_release(2).pdf

Patel, K.K., & Tran, L. (2013). Opportunities for oncology in the Patient Protection and Affordable Care Act. *American Society of Clinical Oncology Educational Book, 2013,* 436–440. doi:10.1200/EdBook_AM.2013.33.436

Patient-Centered Outcomes Research Institute. (2013). National priorities and research agenda. Retrieved from http://www.pcori.org/research-we-support/priorities-agenda

Patient Protection and Affordable Care Act, Pub. L. No. 111-148, 124 Stat. 119 (2010).

Robert Wood Johnson Foundation & George Washington University School of Public Health and Health Services. (n.d.). Health reform GPS: Navigating the Implementation Process. Retrieved from http://www.healthreformgps.org

Rosenbaum, S. (2011). The Patient Protection and Affordable Care Act: Implications for public health policy and practice. *Public Health Reports, 126,* 130–135.

Schoen, C., Collins, S.R., Kriss, J.L., & Doty, M.M. (2008). How many are underinsured? Trends among U.S. adults, 2003 and 2007. *Health Affairs, 27,* w298–w309. doi:10.1377/hlthaff.27.4.w298

Song, Z., Safran, D.G., Landon, B.E., Landrum, M.B., He, Y., Mechanic, R.E., ... Chernew, M. (2012). The 'alternative quality contract,' based on a global budget, lowered medical spending and improved quality. *Health Affairs, 31,* 1885–1894. doi:10.1377/hlthaff.2012.0327

Sprandio, J.D. (2010). Oncology patient-centered medical home and accountable cancer care. *Community Oncology, 7,* 565–572. Retrieved from http://www.d3onc.com/via_downloads/Via_Community_Oncology_Dec2010.pdf

Teitelbaum, J., & Wilensky, S. (2013). Health reform in the United States. In J. Teitelbaum & S. Wilensky (Eds.), *Essentials of health policy and law* (2nd ed., pp. 159–181). Burlington, MA: Jones & Bartlett Learning.

Thorpe, J.H., & Cascio, T. (2013, January 16). Transforming health care delivery. Retrieved from http://www.healthreformgps.org/resources/transforming-health-care-delivery

U.S. Department of Health and Human Services. (2011, March). *Report to Congress: National strategy for quality improvement in health care.* Retrieved from http://www.ahrq.gov/workingforquality/nqs/nqs2011annlrpt.pdf

U.S. Department of Health and Human Services. (2013a). Key features of the Affordable Care Act by year. Retrieved from http://www.hhs.gov/healthcare/facts/timeline/timeline-text.html

U.S. Department of Health and Human Services. (2013b). *The National Cancer Program: Managing the nation's research portfolio.* Retrieved from http://www.cancer.gov/PublishedContent/Files/aboutnci/budget_planning_leg/plan-archives/nci_plan_2013.pdf

U.S. Government Accountability Office. (2012, October 12). *Medicare: High-expenditure Part B drugs* (GAO Publication No. GAO-13-46R). Washington, DC: Author.

Wilkerson, J. (2012, December 20). CMS considers demos that would let specialists form ACOs. Daily news. Spotlight on ACOs. *InsideHealthPolicy.* Retrieved from http://www.insidehealthpolicy.com

Current Issues in Cancer Policy

CHAPTER 16

Leading Change in the Health Policy Arena

Margaret C. Wilmoth, PhD, MSS, RN, FAAN, and Alec Stone, MA, MPA

Introduction

Deciding to lead change in any arena is not for the faint of heart; this is especially true when attempting to advocate for a change in health policy. *Any* proposal to change *any* health policy causes anxiety—to the public, to the members of the professional guild who perceive they might lose something, and to those charged with leading the change. In 2009, healthcare expenditures in the United States were at 18% of the gross domestic product (Council of Economic Advisers, 2009). This statistic alone signifies the financial magnitude of the health arena, as well as the stakes of any change in the status quo related to health policy.

Those deciding to advocate for change must understand that doing so requires a long-term commitment and make a conscious decision to be in it for the long haul. This chapter will highlight the inherent complexities in the health policy advocacy system, discuss both organizational and individual attributes essential to leading change, and describe a policy process framework useful in advocating for a health policy change. The chapter will also highlight the Oncology Nursing Society (ONS) and its efforts to raise awareness for its organizational health policy agenda through volunteer and professional advocacy.

Constitutional Basis

From the beginning, the framers of the Constitution were concerned about individual freedoms and the responsibility that rests with having these freedoms. These basic rights were the foundation of the uniquely American system, and have been consistently confirmed through the legislative, executive, and judicial branches of government as the principle upon which the democracy stands. In eloquent language, the Declaration of Independence's authors accentuate their point about the rights and responsibilities of leaders and the people, with this well-known phrase:

> We hold these truths to be self-evident, that all men are created equal, that they are endowed by their creator with certain unalienable rights, that among them are life, liberty, and the pursuit of happiness—that, to secure these rights, governments are instituted among men, deriving their just powers from the consent of the governed. (Declaration of Independence, para. 2, U.S. 1776)

These powerful statements indicate the colonial leaders' understanding of government's integral role in enumerating the rights of the people, but also that the people themselves have an equal voice in those rights. Most revealing is that even after the Declaration of Independence was written and the Constitution itself stated a plan for a new country with, "We the people, in order to form a more perfect union . . . and secure the blessings of liberty to ourselves and our posterity . . ." (U.S. Const. pmbl.), a set of 10 amendments, known as the Bill of Rights, was still deemed necessary as an additional formal list of stated freedoms.

Specified in the First Amendment, adopted in 1791, shortly after the United States became a fledgling country, are those rights that many today still hold to be the most important. These include, but are not limited to, the freedoms of religion, speech, and assembly. And within the last sentence of this amendment, the framers added this remarkable concept: that citizens have the right "to petition the government for a redress of grievances" (U.S. Const. amend. I).

The guarantee of individual freedoms seems so simple, almost obvious today, but particularly after the Declaration of Independence and the creation of a never-before-seen system of government with checks and balances, these rights became the basis of democracy. That is why it was necessary to list specific rights that the framers held sacrosanct, but are often taken for granted these days, so that the stated rights could not be forgotten and taken from the intended citizens.

Redress of grievances—the right to petition, to ask one's own government to address issues of concern to its citizens—is the origin of the entire system. It is the very reason the colonists revolted in the first place. They wanted to be heard. And far from being superfluous or an evil born of necessity, having the ability, as well as responsibility, to speak up for one's interests is the cornerstone of a true democracy. It helps explain our government's peaceful transition after each election and evolution as a civil, open society. Today, we call this right *advocacy*, and it has received justifiably extensive research and commentary.

Interest Group Advocacy: Committing to Be in the Arena

The first step in successful advocacy is committing to the idea that the organization needs to be active in raising awareness of an issue. Too often, groups believe their issue is or should be apparent to others, and that immediate success in resolution of the issue would be readily attainable if only more decision makers, thought leaders, or the general public understood the importance of these concerns. In the current 24-hour news cycle, it is difficult to keep anyone's attention, and breaking through that cluttered barrier is challenging. A long-term plan with adequate funding is required for any issue to measure beyond a blip on the radar screen, and real organizational dedication is necessary to ensure that decision makers take the necessary action to change policy.

For an issue to go beyond a concern of the few to action by many, it takes personal commitment to the cause, as well as dedication of resources. This is not a new concept, but one best articulated by President Theodore Roosevelt when he delivered his now oft-quoted remarks in "The Man in the Arena," an excerpt from the speech *Citizenship in a Republic*, at the Sorbonne in Paris, April 23, 1910:

> It is not the critic who counts; not the man who points out how the strong man stumbles, or where the doer of deeds could have done them better. The credit belongs to the man who is actually in the arena, whose face is marred by dust and sweat and blood; who strives valiantly; who errs, who comes short again and again, because there is no effort without error and shortcoming; but who does actually strive to do the deeds; who knows great enthusiasms, the great devotions; who spends himself in a worthy cause; who at the best knows in the end the triumph of high achievement, and who at the worst, if he fails, at least fails while daring greatly, so that his place shall never be with those cold and timid souls who neither know victory nor defeat.

Those who seek change must be willing to advance their cause, and although Roosevelt's reference is to a boxer in the ring, politicians have used the analogy of being in the arena to demonstrate what it takes to be an activist. Applying the idea of challenging oneself for a cause, leaders, followers, professionals, and volunteers take this mantle upon themselves and attempt to change policy through a variety of mechanisms.

Nursing also has had famous champions who have advocated for policy change. From health and hygiene to evidence-based research, nurses have played an integral role in leading change. Through the years, nurses such as Elizabeth Bayley Seton, Catherine McAuley, and Gertrude Reichardt were all appalled by the conditions in health care, and, like Roosevelt's boxer, made significant individual changes in the delivery of medicine to patients; in the process, they created standards that continue today (Kalisch & Kalisch, 2004).

The pioneering nurse who radically changed the nursing profession was Florence Nightingale (Kalisch & Kalisch, 2004). Known as the "Lady with the Lamp," Nightingale trudged through a culture that put hurdles in her path at each turn. Despite these barriers, she braved war and weariness in pursuit of change. Her use of data in the reporting of her experiences did more than sensationalize her work: it lent credibility to "the heroic things that she did . . . and gave her the backing of public opinion" (Kalisch & Kalisch, 2004, p. 34). She advanced nursing, medicine, hospitals, and the treatment of patients forever.

A more recent example of advocacy that began from a single person's commitment and grew to a powerful national special interest advocacy group is Nancy G. Brinker, the founder of Susan G. Komen. In a moving tale, Brinker recounted a family history of two siblings, one of whom lost her battle to breast cancer. From that deeply personal experience, Susan's death propelled Nancy to fulfill her vow to do something—anything—to make a difference (Brinker, 2010).

Brinker revealed how, in 1982, she learned about the National Institutes of Health (NIH) and its breast cancer research funding. In a conversation with an American Cancer Society (ACS) senior officer, she mentioned her plans to hold an organizational meeting to talk about her idea of forming a foundation in her sister Suzy's memory. Upon further discussion, she was told,

> But what experience has taught us—frankly, Mrs. Brinker, it won't work. People are receptive to general messages about cancer, but breast cancer is a very private matter for the patient and not something people want to see up on a billboard. (Brinker, 2010, p. 195)

A bit put off by these comments, she thanked the man and proceeded to move forward with her plans. She confided in her husband that she was not receiving the major cancer organizational support she thought she would. He responded that she should prove her critics wrong and fulfill the promise she made to her sister. Brinker's efforts began with this note:

> I invited about two dozen ladies to the first organizational tea for what would become the Susan G. Komen Breast Cancer Foundation on July 22, 1982. Ten or twelve attended, every one of them a smart, capable, fabulous woman who has my undying gratitude. I think all of us were there because we'd lost someone we loved to breast cancer. It was personal. The conversation was committed and energized, a deep breath of fresh air after all the nay-saying I'd listened to. (Brinker, 2010, p. 196)

Thirty years later, most cancer advocates are aware of Susan G. Komen and its efforts. From fund-raising to programming, the foundation and its leaders did not listen to the naysayers. They took the challenge in stride and worked to achieve their goals. It was hard, it was labor intensive, and it was done methodically, but their advocacy continues to pay actual dividends today, investing in breast cancer research and clinical trials. Countless lives have been saved and research advances made because of their persistence. That is a testament to advocacy over adversity.

Entering the arena is essential, and so few do because they believe the challenges are too great to overcome. The profession of nursing has the potential to be powerful in leading change in the health policy arena. Nurses need to act on their altruism and commit to band together to advocate for the health policies that will lead to substantive and substantial improvements in the provision of health care for all Americans.

Complexities in the Health Policy Arena: The Iron Triangle

Achieving change in health policy, in any health policy, requires a deep appreciation of the intricacies of the specific health policy for which change is contemplated. Knowing the players and power brokers involved and understanding the economics surrounding the proposed change are critical to success. Additionally, recognizing the "iron triangle" that must be negotiated in order to change policy is essential. The iron triangle consists of special interest groups, Congress (or state legislature), and bureaucracy (see Figure 16-1) (Kingdon, 1995; McLaughlin & McLaughlin, 2008).

Special interest groups are generally considered to be a collection of individuals with similar interests who join to influence the political process (Warner, 2012). Interest groups have become increasingly sophisticated in their ability to influence policy over the years and have considerable sway over politicians. They often conduct research to support their positions, fund political action committees, hire professional lobbyists, and build temporary coalitions to expand their influence (McLaughlin & McLaughlin, 2008). For example, the "Harry and Louise" commercials paid for by the Coalition for Health Care Choices during the Clinton-era efforts on healthcare reform illustrate the power that interest groups can have on the health policy agenda. These commercials constituted an approximately $20 million year-long campaign by insurance industry groups against the Clinton healthcare plan. This ad campaign essentially turned public opinion against the proposed legislation and had a significant role in the failure of this opportunity for health system reform.

Nursing is the largest of the health professions, with 2.8 million RNs in the workforce (Health Resources and Services Administration, 2013), yet it is not the most powerful special interest group in terms of influencing health policy (Feldstein, 2006). One reason for this may be that only 6% (approximately 180,000) of the 2.8 million RNs belong to the American Nurses Association (ANA), the only full-service professional organization representing the nation's entire RN population. Another reason nursing is not viewed

Figure 16-1. The Iron Triangle of the Policy Process

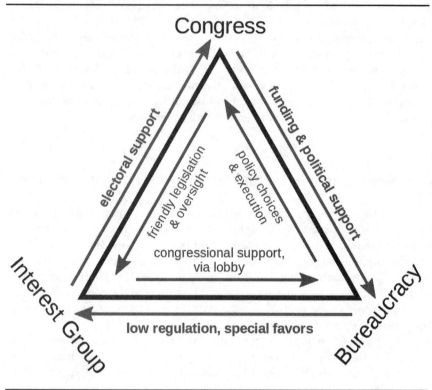

as politically powerful may be traced to the relatively small amount of money that the ANA Political Action Committee (ANA-PAC) historically raises to spend on endorsing candidates. The high-water mark of ANA-PAC's fundraising was in 1994, when it raised more than $1 million in that election cycle (Warner, 2012).

Other reasons that the profession has not been able to claim its potential political power include

- The perception by others that the work done by nurses is invisible and that it has no impact on either costs or revenues in the healthcare system
- The inability of nursing organizations to coalesce around legislative issues that represent economic interests of the profession rather than social issues (Feldstein, 2006)
- Nurses' relative lack of interest and sophistication in health policy
- Nurses' lack of active engagement in their professional organizations.

For nursing to begin to exert its potential power, and for others to view nursing as politically powerful, nurses must begin to see themselves as responsible for influencing the policy that affects their work and be personally engaged in policy activity and decisions at the national, state, local, institutional, and practice levels (Porter-O'Grady, 2011). In short, nursing as a profession has considerable coalescing to do to be recognized as an effective special interest group.

Elected officials are the second key part of the iron triangle. They are elected to do things, and their constituents expect them to act on their campaign platforms. An elected official's decision to support and act, or not to act, on a particular health policy issue is a crucial signal. Health policy is a topic that costs time, energy, and political capital; it is not an arena for half-hearted attempts (Blumenthal & Morone, 2009). Presidents wishing to make major changes in health policy must have passion, a plan, the ability to get out of the gate quickly, the skill to manage Congress, and the ability to focus on the big picture, reach the people, and know what their fallback position is if they cannot achieve it all (Blumenthal & Morone, 2009).

History is replete with examples of presidential and legislative policy failures in the health environment. The best of intentions do not translate into bills becoming law. During the 1992 presidential campaign, Democratic candidate and Arkansas governor Bill Clinton argued that with 37 million uninsured Americans, the country was in need—particularly as the only industrialized nation not operating with a social safety net—of an overhaul to healthcare coverage. After his election, President Clinton announced with great fanfare and public support a mandatory universal healthcare bill. He put his wife, Hillary Clinton, in charge of the issue, but it became apparent that balancing the goals of the Clinton plan for better coverage against a complex healthcare system that appeared to resemble socialized medicine would not pass the U.S. Congress (Oberlander, 2007).

Although the idea and many elements of the proposed legislation were positively received by the House of Representatives and Senate, both controlled by the Democrats, outside special interest groups began to publicly challenge the idea and scope of the healthcare reform legislation. Public support began to turn against the Clinton plan when Americans believed that their choices would be limited in terms of access to healthcare providers and that the economics of the enhanced coverage would be too great for the government to sustain. With the negative comments from organized insurance and business industries, there were too many political factors for the Clinton White House to overcome, and the president was not able to effectively use the bully pulpit to sway public opinion to pressure Congress to enact new healthcare legislation. Finally, the administration did not seek input from Congress before introducing the legislation, which made the task that much more challenging (Bernstein, 2008). Effective advocacy requires a coordinated plan, reliable information, and timing to be successful.

We can learn from the health care experience that large-scale, complex, and costly changes in public policy must have broad-

> scale support and be developed in close cooperation with Congress. Policy changes may be perceived as expanding benefits, but will lose support if they are seen as potentially taking away benefits from powerful constituencies. (Pfiffner, 1994, p. 71)

Similarly, when President Obama presented his healthcare reform plan, the Patient Protection and Affordable Care Act (ACA) of 2010, also commonly known as "Obamacare," it had popular support but passed with only Democratic votes in the House and only two Republican votes in the Senate. Obama's goal was the same as Clinton's, but his approach was, in fact, broader. The Obama White House had learned from the Clinton experience and coordinated its internal efforts in crafting healthcare reform with other departments and the Congress. The president also sold the essential elements of coverage and cost to the American public prior to passage of the legislation. Since then, messaging the positive effects of the law has become quite difficult because of its complexity and the rise of political hyperpartisanship.

Additionally, Obama pointed to the state of Massachusetts' plan for universal coverage. Basing much of the legislation on that state's plan, the White House extrapolated elements to create a larger pool for coverage. And, 20 years after the Clinton experiment, the country better understood the need for healthcare coverage, the cost implications of diseases on quality of life, and the role of insurance in protecting society against costs—both as an economic driver and a societal contract (Gruber, 2011). Still, even as the two sides publicly battled over the ACA, the 2010 victory was challenged in the courts. The Supreme Court finally upheld the law in a split decision in 2012 in *National Federation of Independent Business v. Sebelius*. The fight continued in the political arena during the 2014 mid-term election and candidates continued to argue that defunding the ACA is the only way to stop what they perceive to be socialized medicine.

Leveraging the bully pulpit is incumbent upon a president, and pushing controversial legislation requires effort, as it will not advance without advocates. The same is true for governors and legislators. The degree to which elected officials have passion for the health policy issue at hand is a strong indicator of their willingness to expend political capital on that issue.

A prominent example of an elected official who was willing to expend political capital on health policy was former Senator Ted Kennedy (D-MA), who wrote in his memoirs that he was a foot soldier in the war on cancer. Kennedy (2009) stated that when he was elected to the U.S. Senate, he had the opportunity to work with Dr. Sidney Farber on the Massachusetts Cancer Crusade, where he learned a great deal about the disease. He cited Farber as "the father of both modern pediatric pathology and of chemotherapy as a treatment for neoplastic (tumor-forming) disease," and as his private tutor in cancer education.

Upon learning how devastating cancer was to American families, by 1971 he had committed himself to improving health care in our country.

> Still inspired by Farber and aware that the annual death toll from cancer was at nearly 340,000 and rising, I felt the time was right for a major offensive against the disease. I wanted to pass a National Cancer Act, and bolster it with enough funding to offer realistic hope for new discoveries and breakthroughs. (Kennedy, 2009, p. 301)

Nixon signed the National Cancer Act in December of 1971, thus committing the use of the federal government's vast financial coffers as a resource to make a difference in research and treatment (National Cancer Institute, 2013). Because of Senator Ted Kennedy's national advocacy effort, "cancer research had entered a new era of federal funding and productivity," and progress would begin in earnest (Kennedy, 2009, p. 302). On the broadest of levels, cancer continues to be a disease that transcends political ideology. And because cancer transcends politics, it allows elected officials to cross party lines and to use some political capital to advocate for effective health policy.

Although they rarely set the formal public health policy agenda, career civil servants at the federal or state level, the third component of the iron triangle, have a great deal of informal power and influence and are critical to the successful implementation of any new policy. While elected officials and political appointees come and go, civil servants remain and develop extensive expertise about the topics in their portfolio. They form long-term relationships with the many power brokers and the leaders of special interest groups, and they understand the technicalities of the various policy options and which ones have a modicum of potential for success. Civil servants also know the legacy of failed policies and why they failed and thus can be helpful in modifying a policy approach that may lead to success.

The civil servants who work on Capitol Hill and are classified as congressional staff—especially committee staff—are highly knowledgeable about policy matters in their areas of expertise. They are often public health experts, economists, or lawyers with a great deal of influence on the congressional agenda because they straddle the political and technical worlds by spending long careers in and out of these positions, on and off the Hill, but still in Washington, DC, which further expands their influence (Kingdon, 1995). They arrange witnesses for congressional hearings, craft legislative language, and provide briefing materials to elected officials. Each state has legislative staff with similar expertise about state-centric policy matters and who can similarly influence the outcome of legislation. The same is true for bureaucrats at the county and even city level of policy jurisdiction. Special interest groups that see the most success in advancing their cause spend a great deal of time and energy in developing relationships with civil servants.

Another "iron triangle" that one must understand in relation to health policy is more often referred to as the triple aim: cost of care, quality of care, and access to care (Berwick, Nolan, & Whittington, 2008; Carroll, 2012). These three issues are the complex "push and pull" of issues that compete for attention in the health policy arena. The majority of health policy issues revolve around or involve one or more of these major policy buckets, each of which is grounded in the economics of health care. NIH has recognized that health economics is an underpinning of decision making for all future health policy discussions and outcomes (NIH Common Fund, 2013). A full discussion of the triple aim is beyond the scope of this chapter; additional understanding can be achieved from reviewing multiple publications from the Institute of Medicine, the Kaiser Family Foundation, and the Commonwealth Fund, among others. Healthcare professionals who wish to be involved in advocacy and politics are also advised to familiarize themselves with the types of economic philosophies that drive policy alternatives, have some awareness of the federal budget process, and be well grounded in the legislative process (Schick, 2007).

Federal Legislative Initiatives: Defining the Environment and Scope

Civics classes teach that a bill becomes law when passed by each respective chamber of Congress and signed by the President. Although this is correct, the process is more involved than it seems: a bill has to be introduced in both houses, make its way through each of the committee structures, evolve into a single, exact piece of legislation that is agreed upon by both chambers, sent to the president, and then signed into law. Traditionally, about 7,000 bills are introduced each year; more recently that number has increased to 9,000. However, the percentage of bills signed into law continues to be about 5% (Tauberer, 2011).

Additionally, Article I, Section 5, of the Constitution explicitly states that "Each House may determine the Rules of its Proceedings" (U.S. Const. art. I, § 5, cl. 2), which over time has meant that the House and Senate have adopted different sets of operating rules (Cohn, 1991). This requires an advocate to understand both chambers and how each works. Party affiliation, seniority, ideology, economics, timing, and effort are required to create a plan of political action that will result in success.

For many advocacy groups, laying out a strategy is simple, but implementing it is difficult. The complexities of transforming an idea into a campaign are challenging, particularly as the field is often a moving target, with players, goals, and components shifting at almost any turn in the process. It helps to have champions in either the House or Senate, or preferably both, who will make the issue a legislative priority and will seek to build bipartisan cosponsorship for the legislation as it makes its way from the subcommittee, to the full committee, to the floor of the chamber, and back again, before being passed and signed into law. These champions need to include both elected officials and their staff members. In many cases, advocacy groups gather their sponsorships one at a time before formally introducing the legislation. Once members of Congress see a piece of legislation and ask their staff how many of their colleagues are already on board, they may consider joining the legislation if sufficient numbers currently exist to bolster the success of said legislation.

In the House, there are rules committees, authorizing committees, and appropriations committees, to name a few. There are also committees with wide jurisdiction over massive topics, such as the Energy and Commerce, Ways and Means, and Budget committees. In addition, committees exist that have authority over specific areas, such as the Education and Workforce, Transportation, Judiciary, and Agriculture committees.

Similarly, the Senate has a committee structure with appropriations, budget, and rules committees. Navigating this rocky terrain can be treacherous. Often, an advocacy issue will be presented to members of a committee, such as the Senate Committee on Health, Education, Labor, and Pensions, with jurisdiction over healthcare issues, and its authors are told that their bill is not a healthcare bill, but in reality a finance bill because it requires the federal government to make specific allocations for funding a medical procedure. Advocates are encouraged to seek support through a different, more appropriate committee. Simultaneously, that same bill will be introduced in the Finance Committee and the sponsor will be told that it is quite obviously a health bill, as it pertains to patient care issues. The convoluted mechanisms of Congress are best negotiated by those who understand the minutia of its bylaws. "The Rules Committee's actions are neither routine nor predictable; secretive and independent, the Committee moves, like God, in mysterious ways" (Redman, 1973, p. 239), as described by the author, who spent time in the U.S. Senate as a staff member working on the creation of the National Health Services Corps in the early 1970s.

What is best to remember is that Congress is based on relationships. Those relationships among members in each chamber and between the House and Senate themselves require delicate political balances. Alliances shift, elections change the configuration of party control, and dynamics realign with changes in current events. Ultimately, each chamber is governed not just by its own rules, but also by its own style.

The House is run by the majority party, whose members choose the Speaker of the House, who controls which bills come to the floor before the Committee of the Whole (the entire House) and those that remain in a committee chair's desk drawer. With these rules, the House's majority party determines the flow of legislation. Based on population, each state has a set number of representatives, allowing larger states to have more members of the House. Presumably, the framers thought that states and regions would bind together, pitting parts of the country against one another. However, the early rise of political parties transformed the House into a partisan den, where ideology trumps geography.

The Senate is designed to provide smaller states with equal voting rights as their larger siblings. Senator Daniel Webster famously declared from the Senate floor in 1830 that he and his colleagues were a "Senate of equals, of men of individual honor and personal character, and of absolute independence. We know no masters; we acknowledge no dictators" (Cohn, 1991, p. 28). Over time, senators have developed not just collegial rights, but institutional ones that may prevent any bill from moving forward, effectively suppressing the will of the majority under the opposition of the minority. In theory, this is a magnificent safeguard, but in practice it can be frustrating.

Therefore, the procedures in each chamber are completely different today from when the founders created the Constitution. Party affiliation, seniority, and, to a certain degree, expertise determine who chairs a committee and how that gavel is wielded to advance legislation. It is important to understand the dynamics of each chamber of Congress, the motivation of the committee chairs, and the potential channels through which legislation can be passed. And, once a bill is passed, seeing it implemented as originally designed is another matter.

Federal Regulatory Efforts: Interpretation and Implementation

For years, many healthcare organizations have concentrated their advocacy efforts on the U.S. House of Representatives and the U.S. Senate. While these governing bodies are important, even essential, their mission is to legislate, to create laws. Certainly the intent of those making the laws can be traced, but a law's interpretation is not always fully understood or confirmed when the time comes for it to be enacted.

Federal regulatory agencies are derived from the 13 presidential cabinet posts. Each agency is formed by an act of Congress, their heads nominated by the president and confirmed by the Senate, and each agency has multiple divisions. In the case of the Department of Health and Human Services, originally created in 1953 as the Department of Health, Education, and Welfare, then reconfigured and renamed in 1979, several agencies exist within that cabinet that oversee issues important to health care, nursing, medicine, cancer, and ONS (Keefe et al., 1986). These subdepartments include, but are not limited to, the following.

- U.S. Food and Drug Administration: The U.S. Food and Drug Administration is responsible for protecting the public health by ensuring the safety, efficacy, and security of human and veterinary drugs, biologic products, medical devices, the nation's food supply, cosmetics, and products that emit radiation (see www.fda.gov/AboutFDA/WhatWeDo/default.htm).
- Health Resources and Services Administration (HRSA): HRSA is the primary federal agency for improving access to healthcare services for people who are uninsured, isolated, or medically vulnerable (see www.hrsa .gov/about).
- Centers for Medicare and Medicaid Services: The Centers for Medicare and Medicaid Services is charged with healthcare transformation by finding new ways to pay for and deliver care that can lower costs and improve care for seniors, the disabled, and children of families in poverty status (see http://innovation.cms.gov/About/Our-Mission).
- National Institutes of Health: NIH's mission is to seek fundamental knowledge about the nature and behavior of living systems and the application of that knowledge to enhance health, lengthen life, and reduce illness and disability (see www.nih.gov/about/mission.htm). This is the research arm of federal health care.
- Centers for Disease Control and Prevention (CDC): CDC's goal is to protect America from health, safety, and security threats, both foreign and in the United States (see www.cdc.gov/about/organization/mission.htm). Whether diseases start at home or abroad, are chronic or acute, curable or preventable, human error or deliberate attack, CDC fights disease and supports communities and citizens in doing the same.

Within each of these agencies are dedicated bureaucrats whose duties are to interpret the laws that Congress has passed and implement them through the federal government. Many are charged with oversight responsibilities for the health and well-being of the citizens. In most cases, those regulators have oversight of implementation as experts in their respective fields, with an understanding of the issues and the experience to create an environment that effectively applies the law.

These agencies, though, do have a federal mandate to interact with the general public to maintain an understanding of what the citizens need. In cases of prescription drugs, medical devices, clinical research, and other public health initiatives, agencies rely heavily on submission of public comments to expert panels and advisory boards. These suggestions are taken seriously and weighed against the interest of the whole, and then reports and guidelines are issued with policy statements that direct the agency to prioritize its agenda.

Understanding the system is an integral part of advocacy. Government has many moving parts, and the political, policy, and regulatory components all have unique roles to play in how legislation is implemented. Advocacy groups interested in advancing their own agendas need to have a clear idea of what their message is, which branch of government is best capable of implementing the policy change, and a strategy to reach the stated goals for change.

Individual Capacity for Advocacy

The individual who plans to be involved in policy advocacy should possess several characteristics, including knowledge of the process, passion, and tenacity (Blumenthal & Morone, 2009). Advocating takes time and commitment, and engaging in the political arena also requires a "suit of armor," according to Nancy Pelosi (as cited in Kornblut, 2009, p. 173), as the political (and advocacy) arena can be a brutal environment. Political skills, such as knowledge of facts and economic impact data and the ability to persuasively use these data points, are important (Leavitt, Chaffee, & Vance, 2012). Excellent advocates are skilled at having facts at their fingertips and have an elevator speech on any topic ready to roll off one's tongue at any time. The ability to craft a persuasive argument and stay on message is also important.

Political advocacy requires an awareness of one's power and how to use it, the ability to analyze the issue and strategize, and the aptitude to motivate, mobilize, and maintain interest in a collective action. Advocates need to take the time to get to know the policy issue and any previous efforts to devise a policy solution: who advocated for and against it, who worked for whom, and when and in what capacity? Knowing an issue's history may prevent needless waste of time and expenditure of political capital. While there are many routes to make an advocacy point, emotion and economics often are two sides of the same advocacy coin. Advocates can make an economic plea or an emotional one, depending on the audience. Crafting the message and creating a narrative are important and will connect with the decision maker.

In his handbook on advocacy, Christopher Kush cites Jane Weirich, former deputy director of nationwide field advocacy for ACS, with this advice:

> When we organized our national advocacy event called Celebration on the Hill, our strategy was to bring cancer survivors from every congressional district in the country, and we achieved that goal. Getting a constituent is a crucial part of getting a Congress member to pay attention, and we believed that there were great stories of cancer survival in every single congressional district in this country. We made it our challenge to find those stories and then scheduled our meetings on the Hill. (Kush, 2004, p. 25)

ACS understands that reaching its goals requires a universal approach at a very high level, but it also must be handled with precision. That is, as former Speaker of the House Tip O'Neill used to say, all politics is local. Bringing in constituents demonstrates that the organization understands how to motivate its members to engagement and mobilize them to action. ACS has a clear understanding of the legislative process and the policy implications. Most importantly, the organization was not afraid to leverage its members to make their voices heard. ACS leaders exercised their power.

Critical Attributes to Leading Change

Organizations wishing to embark on a path to advocating for a change in health policy should first undertake an organizational review to ensure they have the capacity necessary for the work ahead. Strong leadership, a strategic plan that supports the change being advocated, a solid financial base, a communications plan, and an engaged membership are the essential ingredients (International Federation of Gynecology and Obstetrics, n.d.). Unless the plan is focused on a limited and highly specific issue, no single organization is likely to muster the extended effort needed to effect the desired policy change. Therefore, it will be necessary to engage like-minded organizations to build a coalition.

Coalitions may be viewed as strategic bodies that enhance the power of a single group by leveraging the power of several organizations or individuals united around a common interest (Roberts-DeGennaro, 1986). They are becoming the most useful advocacy mechanism to reach a large internal membership and motivate them to contact their respective elected officials (Bowers-Lanier, 2012).

Once the foundation for a coalition is laid, four ingredients are essential to its effectiveness: membership, leadership, resources, and serendipity (Bowers-Lanier, 2012). Members play an important role in any organization but are critical to moving a policy issue forward. In short-term coalitions around impassioned issues, membership may be composed of each organization's members who volunteer their time advocating for politicians' votes at the last minute. Group process may not be a major concern in short-term coalitions, but those lasting longer do move through the "forming-storming-norming-performing" stages (Tuckman, 1965) and require a skilled leader to help guide the group through the rough times.

The scope of the policy issues and perceived length of the need for the coalition (short-term versus long-term) will determine the structure of the coalition, its governance, and the process by which a leader is selected, as well as a leadership succession plan. Short-term coalitions are usually focused on a single issue, election, or specific crisis situation (Roberts-DeGennaro, 1986) and may be able to function without a formal governance structure or financing (Bowers-Lanier, 2012). Long-term coalitions have the flexibility to become involved in a wider array of issues and activities; however, they are much more difficult to maintain.

Long-term coalition building begins when organizations come to a shared assessment of the policy landscape, a determination of their overlapping interests, and a shared desirable end state (Delanghe, 2007). Coalitions are vulnerable to a variety of tensions, including those from the umbrella organization and those from its member groups. Coming to an agreement on the desired outcomes for the coalition and the resources that each organization will need to contribute, including manpower and money, is an essential foundational piece for a successful coalition. Structure for meetings, a governance process, and financing the coalition's work become issues for coalitions that organize for long-term advocacy. Barriers to successful coalitions and collaborations include turf issues, lack of funding for the work to be done, and the inability to hire the staff necessary to facilitate the work (Chrislip & Larson, 1994).

A coalition requires an inspiring and skilled leader. When leading a coalition formed to create change in health policy, the leader also must have prior expertise in navigating the policy and political process and topic credibility. Expertise in collaborative leadership can be particularly helpful when working with coalitions (University of Kansas Work Group for Community Health and Development, 2013).

Use of a collaborative leadership model is helpful when inclusiveness and empowerment are needed to build the coalition, when there are complex problems to be addressed by several groups, or when an issue affects a whole community or profession (Chrislip & Larson, 1994). Collaborative leaders should have good facilitation skills, be adept in dealing with conflict, understand group processes, and be trusted and respected by all the groups and individuals with whom they must interact. Leaders manage three levels of an organization simultaneously: keeping the group moving toward action, maintaining internal relations among coalition members, and developing trust among all members (Mizrahi & Rosenthal, 2001). The leader's role in achieving the coalition's goals cannot be overemphasized.

An example of a coalition that has been in existence in several forms for about a dozen years is the Nursing Community (www.thenursingcommunity.org), of which ONS is a member. This coalition, currently with a membership of 61 national nursing organizations, was formed to advocate at the national level on three primary issues: healthcare reform to improve quality, reduce cost, and increase access; federal funding for nursing education, practice, and retention; and federal legislation that improves and advances nursing practice, education, and research (Nursing Community, n.d.). Members engage in monthly meetings to craft policy priorities, action plans, and ways to engage with leaders on Capitol Hill, such as hosting receptions, nominating nurse leaders for federal committee positions, and coordinating Hill visits.

The Nursing Community evolved from early efforts to support the Nurse Reinvestment Act in 2002 at the suggestion of several members of Congress.

These members urged the formation of a mechanism that would allow the profession to prioritize policy issues and then present a more cohesive and consistent message on these issues. Coalitions take time to develop and mature, and by 2008, members of the Nursing Community had developed enough mutual trust to successfully work with congressional committee staff during the crafting stage of what became the ACA.

There are pitfalls in building and leading coalitions that need to be considered by those advocating for a group. Determining the purpose of the coalition, the policy issues around which the coalition will focus, and how success will be measured is important (Mizrahi & Rosenthal, 2001). Crafting a succession plan for leadership is critical, as is having a dues structure to support the policy work that must take place. Failure to have the right groups at the table or to collaborate with larger groups (e.g., AARP) may lead to being irrelevant, at best, or at worst, sabotage (Bowers-Lanier, 2012). Trust in the leaders and trust in each other are critical to the success of a coalition. Trust is only built by having all members attend all scheduled meetings and by valuing the perspectives of all members. Persistent distrust among coalition members and turf issues among members can undermine coalitions (Bowers-Lanier, 2012). Coalitions are formed for action; failure to act generally revolves around poor leadership or the inability to agree on a policy solution. However, coalitions also must be savvy about knowing when to advocate and when not to move forward with their plans.

Setting and Moving the Agenda

Knowing when to move forward on an agenda or when to pull back and wait for another opportunity involves a risk based on careful analysis of both the policy and the politics. This decision point applies to individuals, organizations, or coalitions. Kingdon (1995) asserted that

> predecision processes remain relatively uncharted territory . . . we know more about how issues are disposed of than we know about how they came to be issues on the governmental agenda in the first place, how the alternatives from which decision makers chose were generated, and why some potential issues and some likely alternatives never came to be the focus of serious attention. (p. 1)

A savvy leader is tuned into the discussions taking place across the various components of the iron triangle and knows when a piece of legislation might move. Patience is a key virtue, as it is common for many policy solutions to be introduced and float around the "policy primeval soup" for years before they make it to the floor for a vote (Kingdon, 1995).

Kingdon (1995) proposed a model asserting that it is only when three different streams come together that a policy solution moves to the level of legislative action. The three streams are the problem stream, the policy stream, and the political stream. The *problem stream* refers to the policy makers who are confronted with numerous problems and issues requiring their attention and the complexities involved with getting them to focus enough on an issue to raise it to a high level of awareness and intent for action (Berkowitz, 2012; Kingdon, 1995). What is often missed at this point of the process is clearly identifying the policy problem that needs attention so an adequate policy solution can be devised.

Second is the *policy stream*, referring to the multiple ideas and approaches to solving a problem that then need to coalesce into a viable policy among several alternatives (Kingdon, 1995). Questions that need to be considered in crafting policy solutions include the technical feasibility, value acceptability, and consideration of future constraints, such as budgetary and public acceptability (Kingdon, 1995). It is not unusual for multiple policy solutions to be proposed for the same problem. One recent example is the content of the House and Senate bills that ultimately became the ACA. The two chambers were lobbied by many of the same interest groups, yet H.R. 3962, the Affordable Health Care for America Act, passed by the House of Representatives on November 7, 2009, proposed different policy solutions to the same problems that were addressed in the Senate bill that was passed on December 24, 2009, and which ultimately became the law.

Finally, the politics need to line up so that the proverbial needle can be threaded through the political constraints in the *political stream.* This stream tends to be somewhat independent of the problem and policy streams, with its own dynamics (Kingdon, 1995). Factors that comprise the political stream include election results, ideologic distributions in the legislative body, timing of elections, and public advocacy campaigns (Kingdon, 1995). Consensus building and bargaining take place as the time comes to move on an issue. Bargaining can take place between the administration and interest groups, between the administration and a member of Congress or with a committee, or within Congress among elected officials. The savvy policy advocate will have developed sources that can shed some light on the prevailing mood and the politics surrounding a specific issue.

Once the timing is right, then the Problem-Centered Public Policymaking Process Model (also known as the 6 Ps Model) provides a framework that describes the various factors that will influence movement of the chosen policy solution in the form of a legislative bill through to passage to become law (see Table 16-1) (Porche, 2012). Nursing organizations or coalitions of organizations wishing to influence the policy process about an identified policy problem need to strategize their activities and consider each of these components as they plan their activities. They need to consider each component of the 6 Ps and determine whether they have done enough homework and

Table 16-1. The 6 Ps Model

Components of the Model	Factors to Consider
Policy	What is current law? What are policy solutions and alternatives?
Process	What are the legislative processes, rules of each legislative body, and timing? What are Congressional Budget Office scoring conventions? Other rules and regulations?
Players	Who are the legislators? Which party is in the majority in each legislative body? What legislative committees and staff are involved? Who are the stakeholders on both sides of the issue?
Politics	Who is in political power and for how much longer? When is the next election? Who are the relevant political interest groups?
Press	How is the message being primed and framed? By whom? How to best use the 24/7 news cycle?
Public and the Polls	What is public opinion on the issue? Who is doing the polling? What do focus groups have to say? What does our internal polling show about support for this policy issue and proposed solution?

relationship building before deciding to publicly take a stance and advocate for a specific policy solution.

Case Study: Oncology Nursing and Symptom Management

Like other national membership societies, ONS has had a government affairs professional on staff for many years. In this case, the ONS Health Policy department oversees these kinds of issues and activities. Working with other divisions—Research, Education, Communication, and Membership—Health Policy leads a small team of internal staff and outside consultants to raise awareness of the field of oncology nursing with what is broadly referred to as decision makers. These are people both within and outside the organization, elected officials, media representatives, coalition partners, thought leaders, and others who have an interest in the issues affecting ONS, as well as others who can have some part in helping to change that policy through their advocacy.

Since its inception in 1975, ONS has had the traditional evolutionary arc regarding public policy and government affairs. While based in Pittsburgh, Pennsylvania, ONS has always kept an eye toward Washington, DC, and on how the legislative and regulatory environment affected its members and the field of nursing generally. Beginning with staff simply tracking issues from Pittsburgh in the early years, the organization finally committed to hiring professional staff with policy experience who live and work in the greater DC area. Along with staff came an office, resources, materials, and, on occasion, an intern. In 2006, after years of tracking and analyzing a variety of bills and following policies emanating from federal regulatory agencies, ONS decided to introduce a piece of legislation of its own. That issue was education reimbursement.

Reimbursement is both a simple idea and a complicated process to explain, but one that needed to be formally addressed, according to ONS, to assist the field of oncology nursing. Oncology nurses, like other healthcare professionals, provide education about cancer care to their patients. However, unlike other healthcare professionals, nurses are not reimbursed for their time and hence cannot bill Medicare for their expertise. ONS thought that this should be rectified and sought congressional leadership to introduce the issue. As the most trusted healthcare providers, nurses have a seminal role in patient education. The connections nurses have to patients are visceral, and having nurses understand their role in educating patients is a transformational process. Such legislation would enable oncology nurses to have dedicated time with patients with cancer, much like patients with diabetes and kidney disease have with their educators, and ONS believes the health and financial aspects of this dedicated and reimbursed time would positively change patient treatment and care for cancer survivors.

The latest iteration of the legislation was introduced in April 2013 as the Improving Cancer Education Treatment Act, H.R. 1661. Its only objective, stripped down from previous editions that had included unspecified increased funding for the NIH and a financial request for an Institute of Medicine report on the impact of symptom management education, was to merely reimburse an oncology nurse for one hour of time to speak with a patient. ONS's position was clearly stated in language that legislators expect (ONS, n.d.-b, n.d.-c).

To be fair, the bill—like so much healthcare legislation—has a cost associated with it. ONS estimated in 2009 that educating patients with cancer through Medicare would cost approximately $45 million a year. That figure becomes $680 million between the years of 2009 and 2018. However, ONS predicts that the cost savings for that education would more than pay for the hour of reimbursed nursing time.

Initial efforts were successful. Outreach to two U.S. Representatives' offices yielded bipartisan cosponsorship in Congressmen Steve Israel (D-NY) and Pat Tiberi (R-OH). Israel was interested in the cancer treatment aspects of the bill, and Tiberi had a strong relationship with a constituent who is an oncology nurse. He toured a cancer institute in his district, at her urging, and was convinced that more needed to be done for patients. These two House members became ONS's congressional champions.

In addition, considerable efforts were made at the grasstops level, which is the complementing approach to grassroots. When dealing with the tops, or actual decision makers and elected officials, ONS put dedicated staff to work, literally walking the halls of the U.S. Capitol building and taking copies of the bill to different offices, meeting with congressional health staffers, and requesting that the representative join a list of cosponsors.

Grassroots work is motivating and mobilizing the organizational membership in their home districts to contact their respective elected officials for a cause. ONS asked its chapters, more than 250 across the country, to reach out to their members of Congress and urge them to cosponsor this legislation. Originally introducing the legislation in 2006, ONS sought to have one hour of time spent by a certified oncology nurse reimbursed through Medicare for educating patients with cancer about their treatment. At its height, in 2010, the legislation received 41 bipartisan cosponsors. Grasstops and grassroots initiatives continue today to increase that number in hopes of generating a large enough list of cosponsors to bring the bill to a committee vote and eventually pass the House.

Over the years, ONS has transformed its internal grassroots initiative many times. Like other organizations, branding for the organization, its mission, and its legislative priorities is ever-changing. Keeping the membership interested and engaged is itself a constant challenge. ONS initially had two to four state health policy liaisons per state who were to lead the effort in their respective congressional districts. From state-based leaders, who emphasized their local oncology nurses, to eventually growing into a single national ONS voice for advocacy, the grassroots activities have been honed to reflect a single ONS message that can be translated within each congressional district.

The ONS Health Policy department thought it best to synthesize the different elements of advocacy into a single subgroup of those members interested in government relations. Now, more than 2,500 members receive monthly emails and correspondence that relate to the ONS health policy agenda. Members of this group can keep up to date with advocacy efforts and are able to reach out to their elected officials on behalf of ONS regularly.

To fully connect with elected officials, ONS had to define its message, create an engaging narrative, and first explain who it was and what its membership did:

> The Oncology Nursing Society (ONS) is a professional association of more than 35,000 members committed to promoting excellence in oncology nursing and the transformation of cancer care. . . . ONS members are a diverse group of professionals who represent a variety of professional roles, practice settings, and subspecialty practice areas. Registered nurses, including staff nurses, advanced practice nurses, case managers, educators, re-

searchers, and consultants, and other healthcare professionals, benefit from membership. The society offers useful information and opportunities for nurses at all levels, in all practice settings, and in all subspecialties. (ONS, n.d.-a)

This powerful definition, and the goodwill that nurses, especially oncology nurses, continue to have in health care, allows ONS to cultivate a wide audience of support. Coalition work is essential in advocacy, and no group can be completely successful without the help of its broader community. ONS is no exception to this rule and has spent years reaching out to potential partners, in the nursing, cancer, and general health advocacy areas.

"The power of coalitions lies in their ability to bring people together from diverse perspectives around clearly defined purposes to achieve common goals" (Bowers-Lanier, 2012, p. 626), and forming those groups around issues is often more difficult than originally imagined. ONS has an internal grid used to assess its relationships with more than 110 coalition partners that have various degrees of commitment to and from ONS. The grid allows ONS to rank and organize its constituent relationships, which enables ONS to be active in a variety of issues that, if tackled alone, its voice could either not be heard or would require considerably more effort to penetrate the cacophony of voices. But together with other organizations, ONS adds value, strengthening an issue that is a public policy priority for oncology nurses.

Successful efforts of ONS coalition partnerships include

- ANA
- Association of Community Cancer Centers
- Campaign for Tobacco-Free Kids
- Health Professions and Nursing Education Coalition
- National Coalition for Cancer Survivorship
- National Comprehensive Cancer Network
- National Patient Advocate Foundation
- Nursing Community
- One Voice Against Cancer
- Pain Care Forum.

That so many organizations seek the support of ONS is a testament to the commitment of its members' efforts to advocate for nursing, cancer, and healthcare issues. Not every initiative is successful, but playing nicely in the sandbox is a long-term strategy that reaps future dividends. Leveraging support for a cause requires constant attention. Using the constantly changing world of technology to reach both internal and external targeted audiences is a key component to advocacy.

These days, social media has taken over as a wonderful way to issue support or opposition through people's personal networks. Organizations— ONS included—use Facebook, Twitter, email updates, action alerts, YouTube, LinkedIn, its own RSS feed, and other devices to motivate and mobilize their membership to action. Using social media to raise awareness for issues, engage members in a dialogue of support, and educate a specific audience is now a cornerstone to building a network of activists. Many ONS members participate in the ONS Connect Blog, retweet messages, and circulate articles from the organization's quarterly news magazine, *ONS Connect*, to spread the word. It seems that these days anyone can be an activist from the palm of their hand, and ONS is teaching its members that they too can weigh in on the hot topics of the day with just the push of the button. The easier advocacy becomes technologically, the more oncology nurses will consume the space.

ONS's efforts to gain recognition for the work that oncology nurses do in educating patients with cancer on symptom management still continue. Various legislative and regulatory avenues are available to ONS as it champions the cause for professional reimbursement for time spent on patient education. As with most advocacy work, ONS hopes to use its members' expertise in passing legislation that will change the professional nature of its field, but also recognizes that having a dedicated piece of legislation is an excellent tool with which to impress upon decision makers the many issues important to nurses and the field of oncology.

Conclusion

Leading change in the health policy arena is challenging, complicated, invigorating, and rewarding. It may take a suit of armor at times. Leading change requires an advocate who cares about and has a commitment to the cause. Advocacy comes from two Latin words, *ad* and *vocare*, meaning "to" and "summon"; it implies movement and words. Advocates lead change and have a dedication to shift attitudes on an issue and form a new course of action. An advocate asks, "How can I make a difference?", then, individually or in partnership, attempts to strategize to an endpoint, reevaluating to accommodate shifts in the environment to continue to achieve that goal (Walls, 1993).

Advocacy takes many forms and comes from a single source, small groups, and large coalitions. Nonprofit organizations and membership societies have played an integral role in positioning change in America, dating back to Alexis de Tocqueville's journey across the young nation (Bass, Arons, Guinane, & Carter, 2007). He described a country that relied on the relationships formed by Americans who were interested in addressing problems through joint resolution.

During the past two centuries, civic and volunteer activism has yielded professionalized advocacy. Nurses are advocates not only by occupation, but personality, and their efforts on behalf of patients, peers, and the field have helped to create significant change in public policy (Priest, 2012). The work is never done; the agenda never complete. It evolves, expands, and enlightens. Nurses hold a uniquely trusted place in the hearts of the public and must seize their place as the trusted professionals with the patient in mind as health policy is crafted and enacted. Their advocacy is perceived as pure, and in politics, perception is reality. It is time for all nurses to suit up, enter the arena, and lead the necessary improvements in health care through policy advocacy.

References

Bass, G.D., Arons, D.F., Guinane, K., & Carter, M.F. (2007). *Seen but not heard: Strengthening nonprofit advocacy*. Washington, DC: Aspen Institute.

Berkowitz, B. (2012). The policy process. In D.J. Mason, J.K. Leavitt, & M.W. Chaffee (Eds.), *Policy and politics in nursing and health care* (6th ed., pp. 49–64). St. Louis, MO: Elsevier Saunders.

Bernstein, C. (2008). *A woman in charge: The life of Hillary Rodham Clinton*. New York, NY: Vintage.

Berwick, D.M., Nolan, T.W., & Whittington, J. (2008). The Triple Aim: Care, health, and cost. *Health Affairs, 27*, 759–769. doi:10.1377/hlthaff.27.3.759

Blumenthal, D., & Morone, J.A. (2009). *The heart of power: Health and politics in the Oval Office*. Berkeley, CA: University of California Press.

Bowers-Lanier, R. (2012). Coalitions: A powerful political strategy. In D.J. Mason, J.K. Leavitt, & M.W. Chaffee (Eds.), *Policy and politics in nursing and health care* (6th ed., pp. 626–632). St. Louis, MO: Elsevier Saunders.

Brinker, N.G. (2010). *Promise me: How a sister's love launched the global movement to end breast cancer*. New York, NY: Crown Archetype.

Carroll, A. (2012, October 3). The "iron triangle" of health care: Access, cost, and quality. *JAMA Forum*. Retrieved from http://newsatjama.jama.com/2012/10/03/jama-forum-the-iron-triangle-of-health-care-access-cost-and-quality

Chrislip, D.D., & Larson, C.E. (1994). *Collaborative leadership: How citizens and civic leaders can make a difference*. San Francisco, CA: Jossey-Bass.

Cohn, M.S. (Ed.). (1991). *How Congress works* (2nd ed.). Washington, DC: Congressional Quarterly.

Council of Economic Advisers. (2009, June). *The economic case for health care reform*. Retrieved from http://www.whitehouse.gov/administration/eop/cea/TheEconomicCaseforHealthCareReform

Declaration of Independence para. 2 (U.S. 1776).

Delanghe, C. (2007). Panel II: Coalition building. In J.R. Martin (Ed.), *Conference report: A nation at war. Seventeenth Annual Strategy Conference* (pp. 53–59). Carlisle, PA: Strategic Studies Institute.

Feldstein, P.J. (2006). *The politics of health legislation: An economic perspective* (3rd ed.). Chicago, IL: Health Administration Press.

Gruber, J. (with Newquist, H.P.). (2011). *Health care reform: What it is, why it's necessary, how it works*. New York, NY: Hill and Wang.

Health Resources and Services Administration. (2013, April). *The U.S. nursing workforce: Trends in supply and education*. Retrieved from http://bhpr.hrsa.gov/healthworkforce/reports/nursingworkforce/nursingworkforcefullreport.pdf

Improving Cancer Education Treatment Act of 2013, H.R. 1661, 113th Cong.

International Federation of Gynecology and Obstetrics. (n.d.). Strengthening organisational capacity and health professional associations: Toolkit. Retrieved from http://figo-toolkit.org

Kalisch, P.A., & Kalisch, B.J. (2004). *American nursing: A history* (4th ed.). Philadelphia, PA: Lippincott Williams & Wilkins.

Keefe, W.J., Abraham, H.J., Flanigan, W.H., Jones, C.O., Ogul, M.S., & Spanier, J.W. (1986). *American democracy: Institutions, politics, and policies* (2nd ed.). Chicago, IL: Dorsey Press.

Kennedy, E.M. (2009). *True compass: A memoir.* New York, NY: Twelve/Hachette Book Group.

Kingdon, J.W. (1995). *Agendas, alternatives, and public policies* (2nd ed.). New York, NY: Harper-Collins.

Kornblut, A.E. (2009). *Notes from the cracked ceiling: Hillary Clinton, Sarah Palin, and what it will take for a woman to win.* New York, NY: Crown.

Kush, C. (2004). *The one-hour activist: The 15 most powerful actions you can take to fight for the issues and candidates you care about.* San Francisco, CA: Jossey-Bass.

Leavitt, J.K., Chaffee, M.W., & Vance, C. (2012). Learning the ropes of policy, politics, and advocacy. In D.J. Mason, J.K. Leavitt, & M.W. Chaffee (Eds.), *Policy and politics in nursing and health care* (6th ed., pp. 19–28). St. Louis, MO: Elsevier Saunders.

McLaughlin, C.P., & McLaughlin, C.D. (2008). *Health policy analysis: An interdisciplinary approach.* Burlington, MA: Jones & Bartlett Learning.

Mizrahi, T., & Rosenthal, B.B. (2001). Complexities of coalition building: Leaders' successes, strategies, struggles, and solutions. *Social Work, 46,* 63–78. doi:10.1093/sw/46.1.63

National Cancer Institute. (2013, August 5). NIH almanac. Retrieved from http://www.nih.gov/about/almanac/organization/NCI.htm

National Federation of Independent Business v. Sebelius, 132 S. Ct. 2566 (2012).

National Institutes of Health Common Fund. (2013, December 2). Health economics: Overview. Retrieved from http://commonfund.nih.gov/Healtheconomics/overview

Nursing Community. (n.d.). Core principles. Retrieved from http://www.thenursingcommunity.org/#!core-principles/cel2

Oberlander, J. (2007). Learning from failure in health care reform. *New England Journal of Medicine, 357,* 1677–1679. doi:10.1056/NEJMp078201

Oncology Nursing Society. (n.d.-a). About ONS. Retrieved from https://www.ons.org/about-ons

Oncology Nursing Society. (n.d.-b). *Groundbreaking cancer treatment education legislation authored by Representative Israel and ONS introduced in Congress.* Pittsburgh, PA: Author.

Oncology Nursing Society. (n.d.-c). *Medicare payment for cancer patient treatment education issue brief.* Pittsburgh, PA: Author.

Patient Protection and Affordable Care Act, Pub. L. No. 111–148, 124 Stat. 119 (2010).

Pfiffner, J.P. (1994). President Clinton's health care reform proposals of 1994. Retrieved from http://cspc.nonprofitsoapbox.com/storage/documents/President_Clintons_Health_Care_Reform_Proposals.pdf

Porche, D.J. (2012). *Health policy: Application for nurses and other healthcare professionals.* Burlington, MA: Jones & Bartlett Learning.

Porter-O'Grady, T. (2011). Leadership at all levels. *Nursing Management, 42*(5), 32–37. doi:10.1097/01.NUMA.0000396347.49552.86

Priest, C. (2012). Advocacy in nursing and health care. In D.J. Mason, J.K. Leavitt, & M.W. Chaffee (Eds.), *Policy and politics in nursing and health care* (6th ed., pp. 31–38). St. Louis, MO: Elsevier Saunders.

Redman, E. (1973). *The dance of legislation.* New York, NY: Simon & Schuster.

Roberts-DeGennaro, M. (1986). Building coalitions for political advocacy. *Social Work, 31,* 308–311. Retrieved from http://sw.oxfordjournals.org/content/31/4/308.full.pdf+html

Roosevelt, T. (1910). The man in the arena. Excerpt from the speech *Citizenship in a Republic,* delivered at the Sorbonne, in Paris, France, on April 23, 1910. Retrieved from http://www.theodore-roosevelt.com/trsorbonnespeech.html

Schick, A. (2007). *The federal budget: Politics, policy, process* (3rd ed.). Washington, DC: Brookings Institution Press.

Tauberer, J. (2011). Kill bill: How many bills are there? How many are enacted? *Govtrack.us Blog.* Retrieved from https://www.govtrack.us/blog/2011/08/04/kill-bill-how-many-bills -are-there-how-many-are-enacted

Tuckman, B.W. (1965). Developmental sequence in small groups. *Psychological Bulletin, 63,* 384– 399. doi:10.1037/h0022100

U.S. Const. amend. I.

U.S. Const. art. I, § 5, cl. 2.

U.S. Const. pmbl.

University of Kansas Work Group for Community Health and Development. (2013). Section 11. Collaborative leadership. In *Community Tool Box.* Retrieved from http://ctb.ku.edu/en/ table-of-contents/leadership/leadership-ideas/collaborative-leadership/main

Walls, D. (1993). *The activist's almanac: The concerned citizen's guide to the leading advocacy organizations in America.* New York, NY: Simon & Schuster.

Warner, J.R. (2012). Interest groups in health care policy and politics. In D.J. Mason, J.K. Leavitt, & M.W. Chaffee (Eds.), *Policy and politics in nursing and health care* (6th ed., pp. 594– 601). St. Louis, MO: Elsevier Saunders.

CHAPTER 17

Using Research to Influence Policy

Gail Mallory, PhD, NEA-BC, and Barbara Given, PhD, RN, FAAN

Introduction

It is important for research teams to establish a goal to influence policy as a part of their research programs. In an ideal world, all research would have implications for practice and be easily translated for patient care and policy. The majority of clinical and health services research is designed to answer important healthcare questions, such as "why" and "what if," through rigorous methods (Clancy, Glied, & Lurie, 2012). Clarke (2012) described the conservative nature of healthcare practices. Health care often is based on what has appeared to work in the past, rather than on what the research evidence has shown to be effective. Practice, and subsequently healthcare policy, that is built on research evidence is increasingly being recognized as essential to quality cancer care.

Currently, research outcomes are infrequently translated into meaningful governmental policies or directly into practice. Healthcare providers focus on the science and generally think about research to generate knowledge to improve the quality of cancer care delivered in oncology practices. It is not easy to influence policy, even with the most rigorously generated research outcomes. Clinical and health services research is only one of numerous factors that influence health policy. Others include opinions, federal legislators, policy makers, media, advocacy groups, professional organizations, and other pressure groups. Stakeholder engagement in knowledge generation is critical if the outcomes are to be translated. There are often several stakeholder groups with varying ideas, opinions, and evidence sources regarding a specific health policy (e.g., the Patient Protection and Affordable Care Act, stem cell research); all have to be considered.

Proactive steps to influence policy can only be accomplished by combining well-documented research with strong, ongoing relationships and partnerships with elected officials; legislative, policy, and regulatory processes; and relevant stakeholders. Healthcare reform, quality of care, safety, equitable care, workforce issues, and access to care are all issues from a policy perspective that provide opportunities for researchers. Findings then can be used to shape policy. The focus of this chapter will be on strategies to develop and use research to influence policy creation and implementation.

Research and Health Policy

Research outcomes that reflect a systematic, rigorous process for generating new knowledge can act as a powerful tool for providing information needed for policy formation (Walt & Gilson, 1994). A major stated outcome of clinical and health services research is to guide health policy. Scientific research reports often have a section on policy implication. A prerequisite for evidence-based policy formation is the timely provision of scientifically sound, up-to-date information to policy makers (World Health Organization, 2012) in a form that is understandable and applicable to the practice and policy arena—the healthcare system. The extent to which such research is translated into policy action, however, is dependent on the success of communicating understandable research results and products effectively among researchers, relevant stakeholders, and policy makers.

Health policies are most often laws (but can also be rules, regulations, or judicial decisions) that define strategies, actions, or programs to reach desired health conditions for society (Grimshaw, Eccles, Lavis, Hill, & Squires, 2012). After a law is signed by the president or governor, it is assigned to a regulatory agency (usually within the U.S. Department of Health and Human Services for health policies at the federal level), which develops the rules and regulations pertaining to that law (another opportunity to influence policy making). Although this chapter will focus on strategies to influence governmental health policy, it is important to note that these strategies can also apply to organizations, agencies, or health systems.

Health policy does not come only from research. Science is just one source that influences policy. Much of the focus of cancer healthcare policy in the United States is on the organization of care for patients, the economics of care (health equity, selection of cost-effective care), and the efficient and equitable allocation of resources (Niessen, Grijseels, & Rutten, 2000). To overcome some of the problems with cost, quality, safety, access, patient outcomes, workforce issues, and medication availability, healthcare providers need to build strong, interactive, ongoing relationships among researchers, stakeholders, and policy makers.

Several frameworks to guide the integration of research into policy have been developed and refined during the years since rigorous scientific methods were developed (Florence Nightingale was most likely the first nurse to use research evidence to influence healthcare policy) (Hinshaw, 2011; Lavis, Lomas, Hamid, & Sewankambo, 2006; Lavis, Robertson, Woodside, McLeod, & Abelson, 2003; Richmond & Kotelchuck, 1983; Shamian & Shamian-Ellen, 2011; Tabak, Khoong, Chambers, & Brownson, 2012; Weiss, 1979). Richmond and Kotelchuck (1983) identified the three major components of the research-to-policy process: (a) knowledge and information, (b) political will, and (c) social action. These will provide the structure for this chapter. Other models and frameworks provide more detail, but most are encompassed by these broad components.

In 2013, the Agency for Healthcare Research and Quality (AHRQ) published a summary report titled *Closing the Quality Gap: Revisiting the State of the Science* (McDonald, Chang, & Schultz, 2013), which also will be used throughout this chapter to demonstrate some of the recommended strategies for using research to influence cancer care policy. The report provided a critical assessment of the evidence for eight topics related to the quality of health care, which were

- Bundled payments
- Effectiveness of the patient-centered medical home
- Quality improvement strategies to address health disparities
- Effectiveness of medication adherence interventions
- Effectiveness of public reporting
- Prevention of healthcare-associated infections
- Quality improvement measurement of outcomes for people with disabilities
- Health care and palliative care for patients with advanced and serious illnesses.

The report also included key messages by audience, such as patient/consumer/caregiver, healthcare professional, healthcare delivery organization, policy maker, and research community. Effectiveness of medication adherence interventions and health care and palliative care for patients with advanced and serious illnesses are frequent topics of research for clinical and health services researchers and will be used for strategy examples.

Knowledge and Information

Policy is derived from an understanding that if a health problem exists, a broad, generalizable, and widespread approach will be used to find the solution. What is needed is a clear perspective on the problem, as well as engagement and consensus among the stakeholders that a solution is possible and that the research provides the information needed for the solution (Ridenour & Trautman, 2009). To effectively influence policy, research results have to be relevant and timely for the problem and translated into understandable messages. Good science is vital to help move from problem into action, both for the knowledge base and for effective implementation of policies. Clinical and health services researchers need to identify key health problems as they develop their research programs so that outcomes have the potential to influence health policy that will have a positive effect on health care.

A clear definition of the health-related problem is needed, including the cause, extent of the problem, and anything that affects the problem. When considering influencing health policy, ask: What is the healthcare need (problem) or cancer care issue we are trying to influence with the research? When considering the topic of adherence to oral chemotherapy, there is a need for research on effective treatment outcomes that can be impacted by nursing interventions. The cost of the medication as it affects adherence has also raised policy issues. AHRQ identified the following messages to the *research community* related to *medication adherence*:

- Medication adherence interventions are a "black box."
- Greater consistency in outcomes would strengthen the evidence base.
- Mechanisms of effectiveness should be examined.
- Additional outcomes beyond medication adherence should be included in evaluations. (McDonald et al., 2013, p. 11)

AHRQ messages to the *research community* related to *palliative care* (including symptom management and quality of life) were as follows:

- Broader populations should be included.
- There should be a focus on key research gaps.
- Quality improvement should be integrated into palliative care interventions. (McDonald et al., 2013, p. 12)

Stakeholders, policy makers, and researchers need to agree on the problems. AHRQ's identification of medication adherence and palliative care as research topics with gaps increases the potential that clinical and health services research can influence policy development in these areas.

One of the major issues in healthcare delivery in the United States today is the cost of care. It is essential to understand the economic value of healthcare interventions at all levels of care—primary, secondary, and tertiary prevention. Without that understanding, it is difficult to get policy makers' attention in today's healthcare system. Cost variables need to be included in all research programs that could lead to policy; therefore, they should be included in all research.

Clinical researchers traditionally have not included cost variables in their research. They are a vital consideration, and economists should be included as a part of research teams. If changes in practice and policy are to occur, the costs to patients and to the healthcare system are always relevant.

Other questions that researchers need to answer in developing their research programs include

- Would this research find the solution?
- Is the evidence solid and credible enough to address the need, or are there enough research findings to solve the problem?
- What are the facilitators and barriers, costs and disruptions?

This might pose a dilemma for researchers, as the priorities of the funding agency might not be in sync with these policy-related questions. Researchers have to keep both dimensions in mind. Furthermore, one study (even if it is a large randomized clinical trial) should not be used in discussion of research findings with policy makers. It is essential for the policy-making process (and for evidence-based practice changes) that the process of conducting systematic reviews and meta-analyses be taught and valued in graduate education and that funding be made available for this important component of using research to influence policy. Newhouse et al. (2012) provided an excellent example of a systematic review that can be used to develop messages for policy makers regarding optimizing the use of advanced practice nurses.

Accessing research in usable forms is one of the greatest difficulties faced by policy makers in using research findings. Research results often do not reach government officials or health practitioners; they are disseminated in academic circles, not in the policy realm. Published manuscripts seldom get to decision makers, and if they do, the policy makers are not likely to read a scientific publication. Thus, policy implications at the end of manuscripts seldom reach policy makers. A high impact score of a journal does not lead to policy changes. Policy makers seldom access the same sources as researchers, and do not go to PubMed to do a search to answer a question. The use of aggregated studies, systematic reviews, and Cochrane reviews are frequently powerful sources for informing policy. It is the researchers who can bring these aggregated reviews to policy makers in understandable terms. Organizations such as the Institute of Medicine (IOM), the Robert Wood Johnson Foundation (RWJF), and the Kaiser Family Foundation often provide a neutral forum for experts, and increasingly consumers, to come together to reach consensus regarding the state of the science and gaps that need to be addressed through research and policy (Adler & Page, 2008; Altman, 2014; IOM, 2010; Kaiser Family Foundation, n.d.; Pew Charitable Trusts, n.d.; RWJF, n.d., 2009, 2013).

It is not always easy to establish a consensus on the importance of policy topics, including the AHRQ topics of adherence and palliative care, as well as other topics that could be affected by research led by clinical and health services researchers. Once the importance is agreed upon, the actual definition of the extent of the problem and its impact on quality of life and cost of care from enough stakeholders is needed to move the topics forward toward healthcare policy.

Political Will

Political will refers to the researcher's readiness to undertake active efforts to influence policy makers, after completing research outcomes and assessing the current political environment. Shamian and Shamian-Ellen (2011) described this as the first phase of the policy development process. It is essential to assess the political and cultural values and beliefs of both policy makers and other stakeholders. Even if policy makers have similar values and beliefs, they may not agree on the importance of the topic because of other priorities and limited resources. Political environments change over time and can be influenced by various factors. It is important to assess, plan, reassess, and continue to plan strategies and ongoing building of stakeholder partnerships throughout the development of the research program to effectively influence policy makers. This ongoing assessment of the political environment also will increase the chances that the researcher will be "ready" with research outcomes when the environment is open to or needs those agenda items. A prerequisite for evidence-based policy formulation is *timely provision* of scientifically rigorous information to policy makers. Research often takes years to complete and publish, so results might not be available when needed. If it is not the correct time, no one will be interested. Davis, Gross, and Clancy (2012) described this as disparate time frames (deliberate versus opportunistic). These disparate time frames can lead to frustration with the health policy process and need to be recognized as a part of the process. Questions to consider during this component of influencing policy using research include
• Who would support the solution? Who would oppose it?
• What will be the approach to the opposition?
• Who cares? Who is interested?
• What resources are available?

Social Action

Researchers (and stakeholders and partners) need to agree on the message and then communicate the science to multiple disciplines and to multiple levels of decision makers and stakeholders in a variety of ways. Each group may use a different language; most probably will not use research language (format and style). Therefore, learning the language of the group, whether it be legislators, regulators, or insurers, is vital. Researchers have to establish the linkage with stakeholders and then stay involved (medium, message, and messenger). Policy makers have little time and many sources for information, so researchers' messages need to stand out—they should be clear, short, and not in research form. The work needs to be available in easy-to-digest sound bites. Policy makers often believe that research makes few contributions to decision making; they do not understand how to use the data, or the data may not be in the format that they can use.

One of the challenges to the use of research by policy makers is that the incentives in each environment (academia and policy arenas) are very different. The policy maker and researcher may have conflicting incentives for the cancer-related problem to be addressed. Policy makers require brief, nontechnical, definitive answers and statements. Researchers are concerned with preparing technical papers that will be critiqued by peers and published in scientific journals that meet vigorous methodologic standards. Scientific papers are seldom useful to policy makers (Given, 1993) as written. Thus, researchers must prepare documents in a usable and understandable format to meet the need. Policy makers may need assistance on how to interpret and use the data, and they seldom want complex statistical analysis; they want interpreted data. To do this, the researcher needs to collaborate with the stakeholders.

The following are examples of messages to *policy makers* from the AHRQ report related to *adherence to medications*:

- Decreasing out-of-pocket costs can improve medication adherence for patients with cardiovascular disease and diabetes.
- Improved medication adherence does not necessarily mean improvement in other outcomes. (McDonald et al., 2013, p. 10)

This information related to medication adherence for cardiovascular disease and diabetes needs to be correlated with adherence to expensive oral chemotherapy medications and for all populations.

The following were messages to *policy makers* from the AHRQ report related to *palliative care*:

- Few intervention targets decrease healthcare utilization.
- The effectiveness of policy-focused interventions is unknown. (McDonald et al., 2013, p. 11)

The lack of formal communication channels is a barrier to effective translation, dissemination, and uptake of research results. Policy makers find it difficult to identify researchers, while researchers face problems in identifying policy makers, so nothing happens. Research results can have the greatest impact on policy when effective communication exists among researchers, policy makers, and the community, including people affected by the health problem being addressed (Porter & Prysor-Jones, 1997).

Clinical and health services researchers often are not a part of communication networks designed to help pass on messages, so they need to make and maintain the contact needed for collaboration early. Researchers need to understand not only the role of congressional staff members, but also how these staff members may be affected by the media. When they are opposed to a measure, pressure groups and interest groups can impede policy advancement. Thus, when researchers have relevant research that can and should affect policy, they need to find partners who support the findings and will join in the effort to advance the policy or implications for the policy. It is vital to know which legislators are likely to sponsor health legislation and which agency (and which people within the agency) is responsible for developing the regulations needed to implement the policies. Researchers should ask

• Who are the stakeholders and what other groups are interested in solving the health problem?
• What is the gap in knowledge that the research results could fill?
• What will make the policy work?
• Can the research be translated to enable utilization in practice if the policy is accepted?

Outcomes observed in research studies may not be easily adopted or results stated the same way as outcomes as in real-world practice; this is a challenge. Researchers have to consider and present results in the terms and outcomes of the users/stakeholders. For example, researchers may use some measure or tool or a number of tools that are psychometrically sound but are not usable in practice because of time or capacity restraints. Researchers need to translate this type of information prior to approaching policy makers.

Partners from other disciplines might bring power, visibility, and additional resources to the issue at hand. For oncology clinicians and researchers, this might be the American Society of Clinical Oncology, American Nurses Association, Association of Community Cancer Centers, Cancer Support Community, or advocacy groups. These are important organizations to involve in formulating the research base for a policy issue. Most health professional associations have policy priorities and agendas (AcademyHealth, 2012; American Society of Clinical Oncology, n.d.; Field, Plager, Baranowski, Healy, & Longacre, 2003; Kelley & Papa, n.d.; Oncology Nursing Society, 2013) that they use to guide their strategies and partnerships. They will ask the following questions (Grady, 2011).

• Who would benefit from the evidence if policy were influenced?
• Is the focus of the research related to the priorities for oncology care?
• Who/which groups want the solution of the problem for care?
• Who wants or needs the results of the science?
• Of those interested in the solution, who is willing to be a partner?

Oncology researchers must establish access to those responsible for policy formulation. Being involved as they focus on issues such as guidelines or standards is important for healthcare professionals. An excellent example of collaboration and opportunities to influence an important quality and safety issue is the publication *American Society of Clinical Oncology/Oncology Nursing Society Chemotherapy Administration Safety Standards Including Standards for the Safe Administration and Management of Oral Chemotherapy* (Neuss et al., 2013).

This chapter identifies only a few examples of opportunities to influence patient care quality and safety. Patient safety, shortage of cancer drugs, and workforce issues are all examples that can be used to capture the attention of policy makers and consumers through the media. Other issues relevant to safety for patients and healthcare professionals, such as falls, adverse events, coordination of care, and care transitions (especially to survivorship or end-of-life care), are also important areas for research to influence both policy and regulation development and implementation.

Researchers often have difficulty in disseminating research findings to policy audiences and other nonacademic circles in formats that are useful. They are uncertain as to whom they should communicate research findings and have difficulties in identifying and accessing policy makers. They express concern about what to distribute and how to propagate their research results. It is essential for graduate programs to require a health policy course and experiences that focus on the use of research to influence policy and include assignments to develop policy briefs. Examples of policy briefs can be found in the literature (Betz, Smith, Melnyk, & Rickey, 2011).

Strategies to Facilitate Influencing Policy

Knowledge and Information

If healthcare professionals are to do a better job of affecting health policies, they will need preparation in policy transfer as part of their research education. The ability to produce brief research summaries with key bullet points, clear policy recommendations, and simple language is essential (Betz et al., 2011). An example of a policy brief from the American Association of Colleges of Nursing about the nursing workforce demonstrates these principles (see American Association of Colleges of Nursing, 2011). To influence the health policy process, it is vital to design and implement research with policy in mind. Considering translation and implementation funding will be critical. Can findings be translated and easily implemented in practice? The data must also be usable. Are the findings important enough to have a major impact if scaled up?

To be useful for policy, research findings must be presented in clear terms for the lay audience with data that are simple to understand and recommendations for actions (Hinshaw, 2011). Research results need to be communicated differently to each policy audience and according to the type of policy, decision, or program being influenced. The language should not be research jargon; it must be understandable to the stakeholder. The presentation should be clear, concise, bulleted, and short.

To make research powerful, researchers should focus on politically important topics, problems, and issues; work with those who have personal authority; and publish in a wide variety of media, formats, and journals. Researchers must learn how to get on legislative agendas and be asked to testify. In the current era, oncology researchers need to get involved with healthcare systems and large data sets, and the Medicare and Medicaid Minimum Data Set, OASIS (the Outcome and Assessment Information Set), and the Surveillance, Epidemiology, and End Results (SEER) Program of the National Cancer Institute should be considered.

It is also important to develop a consistent research program around an important cancer care problem and ongoing collaborative relationships among the potential stakeholders. If researchers and stakeholders are truly collaborating on a regular basis, the stakeholders will call the researcher when they need expertise, and it will be easier for the researcher to contact them (and be heard) with important findings. A consistent research program and relationships with stakeholders will increase the researcher's visibility as an expert (or a developing expert) in that field. The recognition of that expertise will lead to appointments to key panels, opportunities to testify, and invitations from the media for comment.

Identifying and working with a health policy research mentor will be invaluable to learn the skills needed to influence policy with research throughout the researcher's career. This needs to be done as a career is developed so that skills and contacts are available when needed. Being active in professional associations such as the Oncology Nursing Society and the American Society of Clinical Oncology also provides opportunities for involvement on national expert panels and mentoring.

What makes oncology research relevant to policy makers? The oncology community needs a consistent message on the topic showing it has a shared professional perspective. The community must maintain visibility if it is to influence the policy process (Ridenour & Trautman, 2009).

Political Will

Oncology researchers need to be known and visible to be asked to participate. Researchers need to involve the information's end users throughout the research process so that interaction becomes a continual process. Effective communication between researchers and policy makers at each stage of the research fosters a sense of ownership and familiarity. Collaboration would enable decision makers to develop a greater understanding of how to use research to support policy development and to translate substantive research findings into policy.

Oncology researchers should identify, on a regular basis, individuals within the local, state (including the state health department and the governor's office), and national levels who are focused on implementing policies on the relevant health issue. It is important to understand that changes in regulations and policies occur. Spend time noting government reports and looking at who introduces or sponsors legislation and what they say, and align with them. When political leadership changes, look at health-related committees and their staff members. It is essential to develop a working relationship with local legislators (policy makers) and their staff prior to critical issues arising. Inviting legislators and their staff to visit the research office or clinical setting or meet with research staff members is an effective method of facilitating connections and establishing legitimacy and credibility. Visits to clinical research sites offer visual reinforcement of the clientele served, as well as a need for services or solutions.

When working on specific research projects, researchers should include policy staff members. If policy makers are interested and involved in ongoing research projects, they will stay informed of the progress. Researchers need to keep them informed of new findings as they occur.

It is useful to establish links and dealings with legislative staff members and legislators. Meeting annually is helpful to review the two or three areas of research that are important to legislation. Some researchers and universities invite state and federal policy makers to campus and do a "show and tell" about their research. In this way, legislators and staff members get brief information and may recall the topics when needed for policy. Getting evidence into the hands of individuals who have a stake in findings and can act on them or push them forward is vital. Oncology researchers need to maintain an up-to-date and accurate contact list that includes relevant policy individuals to contact and need to keep in touch with those contacts. They also should work with legislators and fund-raisers to understand their positions and platforms.

Social Action

Strong supportive networks and connections with important stakeholders, as well as the ability to make research visible through press releases, public relation departments, government relations departments, media attention, and marketing, are crucial. Watch for these opportunities. Articulate how the research will work in the real world and that it will not add a burden, be disruptive, or have negative unintended consequences.

It is essential for healthcare providers to use multiple approaches to make their science heard, such as consulting with policy-related and regulatory agencies and providing congressional testimony, often in collaboration with advocacy groups. Providing testimony to IOM when they are developing their reports is essential.

Oncology researchers need to write editorials and use the op-ed process to make their case and maintain interest in the research. Working with public relations and marketing networks can help in systematically disseminating information about the research.

An often-overlooked opportunity for social action for researchers to influence policy is the regulatory component of policy making. After a law is signed by the president (federal) or governor (state), then the law is ready for implementation. Government agencies, such as the Department of Health and Human Services (DHHS), are responsible for developing the rules for implementing the law. All divisions of DHHS are required to publish draft rules and regulations for public comment prior to implementation and on a regular basis thereafter. The current top DHHS regulations include the Patient Protection and Affordable Care Act, Health Insurance Portability and Accountability Act, human research protections, and health information technology (U.S. DHHS, 2014). Monitoring these opportunities for feedback and providing research-based comments is an essential aspect of how research can affect health policy (Feetham, 2011; U.S. DHHS, 2014).

Conclusion

Oncology researchers and their research outcomes have much to contribute to health policy. It is through usable reports and continued collaborations that the contributions will be noted and applied. With the new healthcare law, it will be important for oncology researchers to move beyond merely reporting their results in professional scientific journals; they must provide reports and other communications in the relevant form and language useful to stakeholders and policy makers who need the evidence. Oncology clinical and health services research has much to offer to create needed healthcare policy.

References

AcademyHealth. (2012). 2012–2014 strategic priority areas. Retrieved from http://www.academyhealth.org/About/About.cfm?ItemNumber=9078

Adler, N.E., & Page, E.K. (Eds.). (2008). *Cancer care for the whole patient: Meeting psychosocial health needs.* Retrieved from http://www.nap.edu/openbook.php?record_id=11993

Altman, D.E. (2014, August). President's message: The Kaiser Family Foundation's role in today's health care system. Retrieved from http://kff.org/presidents-message

American Association of Colleges of Nursing. (2011). Example of a health policy brief: Ensuring access to safe, quality, and affordable healthcare through a robust nursing workforce.

In B.M. Melnyk & E. Fineout-Overholt (Eds.), *Evidence-based practice in nursing and healthcare: A guide to best practice* (2nd ed., pp. 534–537). Philadelphia, PA: Wolters Kluwer Health/Lippincott Williams & Wilkins.

American Society of Clinical Oncology. (n.d.). Policy priorities. Retrieved from http://ascoaction.asco.org/PolicyPriorities.aspx

Betz, C.L., Smith, K.A., Melnyk, B.M., & Rickey, T. (2011). Disseminating evidence through publications, presentations, health policy briefs, and the media. In B.M. Melnyk & E. Fineout-Overholt (Eds.), *Evidence-based practice in nursing and healthcare: A guide to best practice* (2nd ed., pp. 355–393). Philadelphia, PA: Wolters Kluwer Health/Lippincott Williams & Wilkins.

Clancy, C.M., Glied, S.A., & Lurie, N. (2012). From research to health policy impact. *Health Services Research, 47*, 337–343. doi:10.1111/j.1475-6773.2011.01374.x

Clarke, S.P. (2012). Politics and evidence-based practice and policy. In D.J. Mason, J.K. Leavitt, & M.W. Chaffee (Eds.), *Policy and politics in nursing and health care* (6th ed., pp. 329–335). St. Louis, MO: Elsevier Saunders.

Davis, M.M., Gross, G.P., & Clancy, C.M. (2012). Building a bridge to somewhere better: Linking health care research and health policy. *Health Services Research, 47*, 329–336. doi:10.1111/j.1475-6773.2011.01373.x

Feetham, S.L. (2011). The role of science policy in programs of research and scholarship. In A.S. Hinshaw & P.A. Grady (Eds.), *Shaping health policy through nursing research* (pp. 53–71). New York, NY: Springer.

Field, R.I., Plager, B.J., Baranowski, R.A., Healy, M.A., & Longacre, M.L. (2003). Toward a policy agenda on medical research funding: Results of a symposium. *Health Affairs, 22*, 224–230. doi:10.1377/hlthaff.22.3.224

Given, B. (1993). Researchers: Where has all the policy gone? *Puget Sound Quarterly, 16*(5), 3, 10.

Grady, P.A. (2011). Research: A foundation for health policy. In A.S. Hinshaw & P.A. Grady (Eds.), *Shaping health policy through nursing research* (pp. 17–33). New York, NY: Springer.

Grimshaw, J.M., Eccles, M.P., Lavis, J., Hill, S.J., & Squires, J.E. (2012). Knowledge translation of research findings. *Implementation Science, 7*, 50. doi:10.1186/1748-5908-7-50

Hinshaw, A.S. (2011). Science shaping health policy: How is nursing research evident in such policy changes? In A.S. Hinshaw & P.A. Grady (Eds.), *Shaping health policy through nursing research* (pp. 1–15). New York, NY: Springer.

Institute of Medicine. (2010, March 19). About the IOM: Making a difference. Retrieved from http://www.iom.edu/About-IOM/Making-a-Difference.aspx

Kaiser Family Foundation. (n.d.). About us: History and mission. Retrieved from http://kff.org/history-and-mission

Kelley, B., & Papa, K. (n.d.). *Research insights: Using HSR to influence policy change and population health improvement*. Retrieved from http://www.academyhealth.org/files/RI2013PopHealth.pdf

Lavis, J.N., Lomas, J., Hamid, M., & Sewankambo, N.K. (2006). Assessing country-level efforts to link research to action. *Bulletin of the World Health Organization, 84*, 620–628. doi:10.2471/BLT.06.030312

Lavis, J.N., Robertson, D., Woodside, J.M., McLeod, C.B., & Abelson, J. (2003). How can research organizations more effectively transfer research knowledge to decision makers? *Milbank Quarterly, 81*, 221–248. doi:10.1111/1468-0009.t01-1-00052

McDonald, K.M., Chang, C., & Schultz, E. (2013, January). *Closing the quality gap: Revisiting the State of the Science—Summary report* (Prepared by Stanford-UCSF Evidence-based Practice Center under Contract No. 290-2007-10062-I; AHRQ Publication No. 12(13)-E017). Retrieved from http://www.ahrq.gov/research/findings/evidence-based-reports/gapsumtp.html

Neuss, M.N., Polovich, M., McNiff, K., Esper, P., Gilmore, T.R., LeFebvre, K.B., ... Jacobson, J.O. (2013). 2013 updated American Society of Clinical Oncology/Oncology Nursing Society chemotherapy administration safety standards including standards for the safe administration and management of oral chemotherapy. *Oncology Nursing Forum, 40,* 225–233. doi:10.1188/13.ONF.40-03AP2

Newhouse, R.P., Weiner, J.P., Stanik-Hutt, J., White, K.M., Johantgen, M., Steinwachs, D., ... Bass, E.B. (2012). Policy implications for optimizing advanced practice registered nurse use nationally. *Policy, Politics, and Nursing Practice, 13,* 81–89. doi:10.1177/1527154412456299

Niessen, L.W., Grijseels, E.W.M., & Rutten, F.F.H. (2000). The evidence-based approach in health policy and health care delivery. *Social Science and Medicine, 51,* 859–869. doi:10.1016/S0277-9536(00)00066-6

Oncology Nursing Society. (2013, January). *Health policy agenda, 113th Congress, 1st session.* Pittsburgh, PA: Author.

Pew Charitable Trusts. (n.d.). About: Mission and values. Retrieved from http://www.pewtrusts.org/en/about/mission-and-values

Porter, R.W., & Prysor-Jones, S. (1997). *Making a difference to policies and programs: A guide for researchers.* Washington, DC: Support for Analysis and Research in Africa (SARA) Project.

Richmond, J.B., & Kotelchuck, M. (1983). Political influences: Rethinking national health policy. In C.H. McGuire, R.P. Foley, A. Gorr, R.W. Richards, & Associates (Eds.), *Handbook of health professions education* (pp. 386–404). San Francisco, CA: Jossey-Bass.

Ridenour, N., & Trautman, D. (2009). A primer for nurses on advancing health reform policy. *Journal of Professional Nursing, 25,* 358–362. doi:10.1016/j.profnurs.2009.10.003

Robert Wood Johnson Foundation. (n.d.). About RWJF: Our mission. Retrieved from http://www.rwjf.org/en/about-rwjf.html

Robert Wood Johnson Foundation. (2009, July). Addressing the quality and safety gap—part I: Case studies in transforming hospital nursing and building cultures of safety. *Charting Nursing's Future, 10.* Retrieved from http://www.rwjf.org/content/dam/farm/reports/issue_briefs/2009/rwjf43263

Robert Wood Johnson Foundation. (2013, June). Improving patient access to high-quality care: How to fully utilize the skills, knowledge, and experience of advanced practice registered nurses. *Charting Nursing's Future, 20.* Retrieved from http://www.rwjf.org/content/dam/farm/reports/issue_briefs/2013/rwjf405378

Shamian, J., & Shamian-Ellen, M. (2011). Shaping health policy: The role of nursing research—Three frameworks and their application to policy development. In A.S. Hinshaw & P.A. Grady (Eds.), *Shaping health policy through nursing research* (pp. 35–51). New York, NY: Springer.

Tabak, R.G., Khoong, E.C., Chambers, D.A., & Brownson, R.C. (2012). Bridging research and practice: Models for dissemination and implementation research. *American Journal of Preventive Medicine, 43,* 337–350. doi:10.1016/j.amepre.2012.05.024

U.S. Department of Health and Human Services. (2014, June 30). Regulations. Retrieved from http://www.hhs.gov/regulations/index.html

Walt, G., & Gilson, L. (1994). Reforming the health sector in developing countries: The central role of policy analysis. *Health Policy and Planning, 9,* 353–370. doi:10.1093/heapol/9.4.353

Weiss, C.H. (1979). The many meanings of research utilization. *Public Administration Review, 39,* 426–431. doi:10.2307/3109916

World Health Organization. (2012). *The WHO strategy on research for health.* Retrieved from http://www.who.int/phi/WHO_Strategy_on_research_for_health.pdf

CHAPTER 18

Legislative Topics in Cancer Research and Practice

Barbara Holmes Damron, PhD, RN, FAAN, and Carolyn Phillips, ACNP-BC, MSN, AOCNP®

Introduction

Through the millennia, governments have had a convoluted relationship with the advancement of science and the prevention, diagnosis, and treatment of diseases, including cancer. The issues regarding health and science are becoming more complex, as is the allocation of scarce resources. The overarching goal of preventing and treating cancer is further complicated by the increase in competition for the limited resources, including financial and human, needed to achieve the goal. The decisions made at all levels of government—federal, tribal, state, county, and municipal—directly influence the rate of progress made in the fight against cancer. Competing philosophical ideologies, which are a cornerstone of the checks and balances in the U.S. political system and can result in productive compromise, can halt progress when played out in a climate of political polarization. At times it appears that the polarization in Washington, DC, produces nothing but paralysis. Yet, scientists and clinicians must move forward to prevent and treat cancer. What are the high-priority policy issues in science, medicine, health care, and public health affecting cancer in the second decade of the 21st century?

The future of oncology holds great opportunity to build upon the significant progress that has been made against cancer. This progress would not have been possible without the robust basic, biomedical, and behavioral research enterprises funded by the federal government, philanthropic individuals and organizations, and the public sector. As a result of these scientific advancements, more than 13 million cancer survivors are alive in the United States and 1,024,000 fewer cancer deaths have occurred since 1990 and 1991 for men and women, respectively, as a result of declining death rates (Howlader et al., 2012). However, without improved funding provided by the U.S. Congress to the National Institutes of Health (NIH) and the National Cancer Institute (NCI), this progress will decline, with serious implications for the United States and the world. Furthermore, the barriers to promoting a culture of health and reducing healthcare disparities must be addressed.

Previous chapters in this book have provided a thorough review of the historical role policy has played in the advancement of the prevention, diagnosis, and treatment of cancer and cancer survivorship. This chapter will address key current legislative issues and provide an overview of the policy issues related to cancer research funding. It will then discuss select policy issues related to the cancer trajectory, starting with access to quality cancer care issues and moving to policy issues inherent in cancer prevention, screening, treatment, and survivorship. It concludes with a brief outlook into future legislative issues.

Current Legislative Themes

Numerous cancer agencies and organizations monitor governmental issues related to cancer at both the state and federal levels and advocate for select cancer policy issues. Table 18-1 summarizes the main cancer organizations and selected current legislative themes they are monitoring; this is not an all-inclusive table. These organizations include nonprofit voluntary health organizations, professional membership organizations, government agencies, and disease-specific advocacy groups. While each of these organizations addresses specific issues, many of them overlap.

Of utmost concern among all stakeholders is the most serious funding crisis in cancer in decades. Since 2003, the amount of annual funding provided to NIH and NCI by Congress has been significantly less than what is needed to simply keep pace with inflation, with the result being shrinking budgets and essentially a 20% reduction in these agencies' ability to support lifesaving research. This was compounded by the March 2013 sequestration, during which NIH was forced to absorb $1.6 billion in direct budget cuts and NCI suffered a budget cut of $293 million. As a result of these factors, NIH is now funding the lowest number of research projects since 2001 (Sawyers et al., 2013). Therefore, the funding of cancer research, including the entire trajectory of translational research—which transforms scientific discovery from laboratory, clinical, or population studies into clinical applications that reduce cancer incidence, morbidity, and mortality (President's Cancer Panel, 2007)—is at the core of the majority of the current legislative themes related to cancer.

Table 18-1. Cancer Organizations and Current Legislative Topics

Theme	Advocating Agencies and Organizations
Funding of federal agencies (National Institutes of Health, National Cancer Institute [NCI]) for cancer research	American Association for Cancer Research (AACR) (www.aacr.org) American Cancer Society Cancer Advocacy Network (ACS CAN) (www.acscan.org) American Society of Clinical Oncology (ASCO) (www.asco.org) Livestrong Foundation (www.livestrong.org) Leukemia & Lymphoma Society (LLS) (www.lls.org)
Access to quality care	AACR ACS CAN American College of Surgeons (ACoS) Commission on Cancer (CoC) (www.facs.org) ASCO Association of Community Cancer Centers (ACCC) (www.accc-cancer.org) Livestrong Foundation National Coalition for Cancer Survivorship (NCCS) (www.canceradvocacy.org) Oncology Nursing Society (ONS) (www.ons.org) Susan G. Komen Advocacy Alliance (www.komen.org)
Payment/reimbursement	ACCC Livestrong Foundation (Iatrogenic infertility) NCCS
Screening and prevention	AACR ACS CAN ACoS CoC American Institute for Cancer Research (www.aicr.org) ONS Susan G. Komen Advocacy Alliance
Cancer research policy	AACR
Health disparities	AACR ACS CAN Friends of Cancer Research—advocate for NCI (www.focr.org)
U.S. Food and Drug Administration	AACR LLS National Comprehensive Cancer Network (NCCN) (www.nccn.org) NCCS ONS

(Continued on next page)

Table 18-1. Cancer Organizations and Current Legislative Topics *(Continued)*

Theme	Advocating Agencies and Organizations
Tobacco control	AACR ACS CAN Livestrong Foundation ONS
Health insurance coverage Affordable Care Act	Livestrong Foundation LLS NCCS ONS Susan G. Komen Advocacy Alliance

Oncology practice reimbursement
• Meaningful quality reporting and
  practice improvement
• Physician fee schedule
• Medicare physician fee sched-
  ule—innovative models for can-
  cer care delivery
	ACCC
	ASCO
	NCCS
	ONS

Breakthrough therapies	Friends of Cancer Research NCCN
Comparative effectiveness research	Friends of Cancer Research NCCN
Risk evaluation and mitigation strategies	NCCN ONS
Nursing shortage	ONS
Clinical trials	NCCS ONS
Patient and survivor quality of life	ACS CAN
Cancer survivorship	ACoS CoC Livestrong Foundation NCCS

Another seismic impact on legislative issues facing the cancer community is the Patient Protection and Affordable Care Act (ACA) of 2010. Chapter 15 in this book provides an excellent overview of the sections of the ACA that are pertinent to oncology. It is important for healthcare professionals to understand current and emerging legislative issues in the context of the ACA.

Funding Cancer Research

As recently as five decades ago, only a few cancer treatments existed, and the side effects of these treatments were extremely difficult for patients to tolerate. The dramatic improvements in the ability to prevent, detect, and treat cancer are due to the investment in cancer research.

National Institutes of Health Appropriations

NIH is the world's leading supporter of biomedical research. Today, it comprises 21 institutes and 6 centers. Legislative activity related to NIH actually dates back to an act passed on July 16, 1798, which established the Marine Hospital Service, the forerunner of the present-day Public Health Service. This was also the first prepaid medical care plan in the United States, as a monthly hospital tax of 20 cents was deducted from the pay of merchant seamen (NIH, 2013). After an amending act in 1799 to the original legislation, multiple laws and acts ensued for nearly 150 years until NCI was established on August 5, 1937. It was not until July 1, 1944, that the Public Health Service Act consolidated and revised laws and created the National Institute of Health (singular at this time), making NCI a division of it (NIH, 2013). Subsequently, it was not until 1948, when the National Heart Act (Public Law 80-655) created the National Heart Institute (now the National Heart, Lung, and Blood Institute), that the agency was renamed the National Institutes of Health (NIH Office of History, 2013).

Within NIH, the Office of Budget advises and supports the NIH director on budget policy issues affecting NIH, the medical research community, and the public. The Office of Budget participates in the development of all NIH's budget projections; maintains active and efficient communications with the U.S. Department of Health and Human Services (DHHS), the Office of Management and Budget, and Congress; and monitors and coordinates budget activities of the 27 NIH institutes and centers (NIH Office of Budget, n.d.).

Table 18-2 summarizes the specific U.S. congressional committees that pertain to NCI, along with the names of the chairs and ranking members for the 113th Congress (2013–2014). These committees appropriate funds, authorize programs, or oversee activities of NCI (NCI Office of Government and Congressional Relations, n.d.-a).

What is now referred to as *authorizing* legislation was originally simply called legislation. Authorizing legislation exemplifies the legislative power that the Constitution bestows upon Congress. This legislation provides for authority over federal agencies and can prescribe what an agency can and cannot do in implementing its assigned responsibilities. Authorizing legislation can give an agency broad authority or can restrict its implementation freedom by legislating in minute detail (Schick, 2007).

Table 18-2. U.S. Congressional Committees of Interest to the National Cancer Institute, 114th Congress, 2015–2016

Committee/ Subcommittee	House	Senate
Appropriations		
Committee	Committee on Appropriations • Chair: Harold Rogers (R-KY) • Ranking: Nita Lowey (D-NY)	Committee on Appropriations • Chair: Thad Cochran (R-MS) • Ranking: Barbara Mikulski (D-MD)
Subcommittee	Subcommittee on Labor, Health and Human Services, Education and Related Agencies • Chair: Jack Kingston (R-GA) • Ranking: Rosa DeLauro (D-CT)	Subcommittee on Labor, Health and Human Services, Education and Related Agencies • Chair: Roy Blunt (R-MO) • Ranking: Patty Murray (D-WA)
Authorizing		
Committee	Committee on Energy and Commerce • Chair: Fred Upton (R-MI) • Ranking: Frank Pallone, Jr. (D-NJ)	Committee on Health, Education, Labor, and Pensions • Chair: Lamar Alexander (R-TN) • Ranking: Patty Murray (D-WA)
Subcommittee	Subcommittee on Health • Chair: Joe Pitts (R-PA) • Ranking: Gene Green (D-TX)	–
Oversight		
Committee	Committee on Oversight and Government Reform • Chair: Jason Chaffetz (R-UT) • Ranking: Elijah Cummings (D-MD)	Committee on Homeland Security and Governmental Affairs • Chair: Ron Johnson (R-WI) • Ranking: Tom Carper (D-DE)
Subcommittee	Committee on Energy and Commerce Subcommittee on Oversight and Investigations • Chair: Tim Murphy (R-PA) • Ranking: Diana DeGette (D-CO)	Subcommittee on Federal Spending Oversight and Emergency Management • Chair: Rand Paul (R-KY) • Ranking: Tammy Baldwin (D-WI) Subcommittee on Regulatory Affairs and Federal Management • Chair: James Lankford (R-OK) • Ranking: Heidi Heitkamp (D-ND)

(Continued on next page)

Table 18-2. U.S. Congressional Committees of Interest to the National Cancer Institute, 114th Congress, 2015–2016 *(Continued)*

Committee/ Subcommittee	House	Senate
	Cancer Groups	
Committee	House Cancer Caucus • Steve Israel (D-NY) and Lois Capps (D-CA) Childhood Cancer Caucus • Cochairs: Michael McCaul (R-TX) and Chris Van Hollen (D-MD)	Senate Cancer Coalition • Cochair: Dianne Feinstein (D-CA)

Note. From "Committees of Interest: Committees of Interest to NCI, 114th Congress, 2015–2016," by National Cancer Institute, n.d. Retrieved from http://legislative.cancer.gov/committees.

Authorization laws have two basic purposes. They establish, continue, or modify federal programs, and they are a prerequisite under House and Senate rules (and sometimes under statutes) for Congress to appropriate budget authority for programs (U.S. Senate Committee on Appropriations, n.d.).

Congress and the president establish programs through the authorization process. Congressional committees with jurisdiction over specific subject areas write the legislation. The term *authorization* is used because this type of legislation authorizes the expenditure of funds from the federal budget. It may specify how much money should be spent on a program, but it does not actually set aside the money. Many programs are authorized for a specific amount of time. The committees are supposed to review the programs before their expiration to determine how well they are working (NCI Office of Government and Congressional Relations, n.d.-a).

The term *authorization* causes confusion because of the broad scope and types of authorizing measures, as well as the term's various meanings in federal budgeting. In addition to licensing federal agencies, authorization laws also license the House and Senate to consider appropriations. Furthermore, it is necessary to distinguish between discretionary authorizations and direct spending, and between substantive legislation and authorization of appropriations. Essentially, discretionary authorizations do not provide budget resources, but provide authority to appropriate, whereas direct spending legislation provides budgetary resources. Appropriations acts provide the amount of discretionary authorizations that may be spent, and authorizing legislation specifies how direct spending may be spent (Schick, 2007).

Authorizing committees have the lead role in determining the amount of direct spending for a federal agency. Appropriations committees control discretionary spending. Enabling federal agencies to incur obligations prior to receiving appropriations moves the legislative power from the appropriations committees to authorizing committees.

Appropriations acts are laws passed by Congress that allow federal agencies to incur obligations and for the Treasury to make payments for specific purposes. Appropriations have also evolved as mandates that require agencies to carry out prescribed activities by spending all of the funds that are appropriated to them (Schick, 2007). Appropriations can be inserted into any law, but practice that actually predates the Constitution involves appropriating in acts that are distinct from other types of legislation (Schick, 2007).

In appropriations bills, Congress and the president state the amount of money that will be spent on federal programs during the next fiscal year. Each house of Congress has 12 appropriations subcommittees. They are divided among broad subject areas, and each is supposed to write an annual appropriations measure (NCI Office of Government and Congressional Relations, n.d.-b). It is possible to have programs authorized but not funded.

For purposes of this chapter, authorizing committees either create new or renew existing federal programs, and appropriations committees provide the funding for federal programs. A third category of committees, oversight committees, conduct audits on federal programs to ensure that the public trust is not misused or betrayed (NCI Office of Government and Congressional Relations, n.d.-a).

NIH provides the Senate and House appropriations committees with estimates, rationale, and justifications for the requested funding at the president's budget request level for research (intramural and extramural) and research support activities (infrastructure, administration). This is called the NIH Congressional Justification. NIH has 27 separate appropriations for which documentation is prepared (NIH Office of Budget, n.d.). The Congressional Justification for the NIH fiscal year 2015 budget request was $30.362 billion (U.S. DHHS, 2014). However, since enactment of the National Cancer Act of 1971, NCI is required to prepare a plan and corresponding budget and submit this directly to the president for consideration with the congressional budget (NCI Office of Budget and Finance, n.d.). Because NCI *bypasses* the NIH process, this report is referred to as the *bypass budget*. It is imperative that funding for the overall NIH, as well as for NCI, continues at levels necessary to maintain the country's leadership in the biomedical sciences.

Patient-Centered Outcomes Research Institute

The authorizing legislation for the Patient-Centered Outcomes Research Institute (PCORI) was established in the ACA under Title VI, Part III, Subtitle D—Patient-Centered Outcomes Research, Section 6301. PCORI is a U.S.-

based nongovernmental institute created to examine the clinical effectiveness and appropriateness of different medical treatments. It is based on comparative effectiveness research, which provides evidence on the effectiveness, benefits, and harms of different treatment options. Ultimately, PCORI aims to help people make informed healthcare decisions and to improve healthcare delivery and outcomes (PCORI, 2014a). The engagement of people from within the community, including patients, is a major strength of PCORI.

The Patient-Centered Outcomes Research Trust Fund (PCORTF) was also authorized by Congress as part of the ACA. PCORI is funded through PCORTF, which receives income from the General Fund of the Treasury and from a fee assessed on Medicare, private health insurance, and self-insured plans. PCORTF received $210 million total in appropriations for fiscal years 2010–2012. For fiscal years 2013–2019, PCORTF received $150 million from the general funding appropriation plus an annual $2 fee per individual assessed on Medicare, private health insurance, and self-insured plans, as well as an adjustment for increases in healthcare spending. The law mandates that each year, 20% of PCORTF funding is to be transferred to DHHS to support dissemination and research capacity building efforts. Of that 20%, 80% is transferred to the Agency for Healthcare Research and Quality for these purposes (PCORI, 2013).

Efforts by bipartisan staff in the U.S. Senate have succeeded in working with PCORI to move to successful governance. Initially plagued by problems between the Board of Governors and the Methodology Committee, these two entities have settled into a productive working relationship. The 21-member Board of Governors represents "a broad range of perspectives and collective expertise in clinical health services research," while the 17-member Methodology Committee works "to define methodological standards for research and develop and regularly update a translation table to guide health care stakeholders towards the best methods for patient-centered outcomes research" (PCORI, 2014b).

The main goal of comparative effectiveness research is to identify which intervention will deliver the best treatment to the right patient. As dictated by the ACA, research findings are prohibited from being construed as guidance for payment, coverage, or treatment. The work of PCORI, through comparative effectiveness research, can decrease the use of medical care that is unnecessary and potentially harmful.

Access to Quality Cancer Care

Of the many factors that influence an individual's access to quality cancer care, several are currently in the forefront of legislative activity. These include workforce issues, drug shortages, access to new drugs, and risk evaluation and mitigation strategies (REMS).

Workforce Issues

One of the major barriers to accessing quality care is the shortage of healthcare providers. Health Professional Shortage Areas (HPSAs), as defined by the Health Resources and Services Administration (HRSA), may be designated as having a shortage of primary medical care, dental, or mental health providers and may be urban or rural areas, population groups, or medical or other public facilities (HRSA, 2014). At the start of 2014, HRSA reported approximately 6,000 designated primary care HPSAs, 4,800 dental HPSAs, and 3,900 mental health HPSAs (HRSA, 2014). According to the American Society of Clinical Oncology (ASCO), by 2025, there could be a shortage of more than 1,487 oncologists, based on a predicted growth in demand of 42% with only 28% growth in supply (ASCO, 2014).

Multiple factors are converging to contribute to the increased need for a larger healthcare workforce. One major factor is the ACA's goal to enable more individuals to obtain health insurance coverage, thereby creating more need for providers without a comparable increase in the number of providers trained and entering the workforce. The ACA is projected to increase the demand for medical oncologists by an additional 130 full-time clinical care oncologists per year by 2025 as a result of more individuals having health insurance (Yang et al., 2014). A worsening nursing shortage is expected as well, with the most intense shortage seen in the South and the West (Juraschek, Zhang, Ranganathan, & Lin, 2012), and projections estimate a deficit of 260,000 by 2025 (Buerhaus, Auerbach, & Staiger, 2009). Schools and colleges of nursing are having difficulty expanding capacity (American Association of Colleges of Nursing, 2014), and the nursing workforce is aging. The aging of baby boomers, accompanied by their increased need for health care, intensifies the nursing shortage.

Complicating the workforce shortage are the scope-of-practice debates that are ongoing, mainly between advanced practice registered nurses (APRNs) and certain medical specialties, including family practice medicine, anesthesiology, pediatrics, and obstetrics. A pivotal force in this debate was the Institute of Medicine (IOM) landmark report *The Future of Nursing: Leading Change, Advancing Health* (IOM Committee on the Robert Wood Johnson Foundation Initiative on the Future of Nursing, 2011). Physicians are highly trained and skilled providers, and certain services should only be provided by physicians who have received more extensive and specialized education and training than APRNs. However, the education and roles of APRNs have evolved such that APRNs enter the workplace trained and qualified to provide more services than had previously been conducted by RNs in general. APRNs are not physician extenders or physician substitutes, although some of their services include activities that were formerly associated only with physicians, such as assessing and diagnosing patient conditions, prescribing medications, and ordering and evaluating tests. More importantly, APRNs work from a different philosophical and theoretical base, with emphasis on health promotion, disease prevention, and early diagnosis, and incorporate multiple services from other disciplines, including nutrition, social work, and psychology.

The tension between states' rights and federal power is evident in the scope-of-practice laws, as these are state based and vary widely from state to state. The 50 states and the District of Columbia have practice and licensure laws that range from full to restricted practice for APRNs. *Full practice* includes state practice and licensure laws that provide for nurse practitioners to evaluate and diagnose patients; order and interpret diagnostic tests; and initiate and manage treatments (including prescribing medications) under the exclusive licensure authority of the state board of nursing. This is the model recommended by IOM and the National Council of State Boards of Nursing. Nineteen states and the District of Columbia allow this full practice of APRNs without oversight by physicians. *Reduced practice* is state practice and licensure laws that limit APRNs' ability to engage in at least one element of nurse practitioner practice. In this situation, the state requires a collaborative agreement with an outside health discipline, such as a physician, for the APRN to provide patient care. Nineteen states authorize this kind of practice. *Restricted practice* is state practice and licensure laws that restrict the ability of nurse practitioners to engage in at least one element of nurse practitioner practice. The state requires supervision, delegation, or team management by an outside health discipline for APRNs to provide patient care. Twelve states currently restrict the practice of APRNs by requiring collaboration, oversight, and supervision by physicians through these restricted practice laws. Figure 18-1 shows the 50 states and the District of Columbia and their respective practice laws. The workforce shortage issues and the ACA will require states to reexamine their current scope-of-practice laws (American Association of Nurse Practitioners, 2014).

Drug Shortages

The number of prescription drug shortages in the United States nearly tripled between 2005 and 2010, with shortages becoming more severe as well as more frequent (White House Office of the Press Secretary, 2011). This has resulted in disruption of access to care, which in turn has threatened patients' response to treatment and overall health (Stefanik, 2011). In 2011, President Obama signed Executive Order No. 13588 on U.S. Food and Drug Administration [FDA] oversight of prescription medication supplies and prevention of shortages (Oncology Nursing Society [ONS], n.d.-a). This order directs FDA to take steps that will help prevent and reduce current and future disruptions in the supply of lifesaving medicines (White House Office of the Press Secretary, 2011).

Figure 18-1. Advanced Practice Registered Nurse Practice Laws

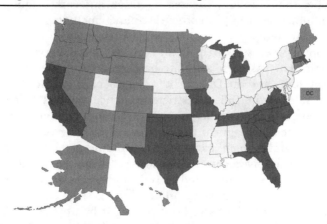

■ **Full Practice:** State practice and licensure laws provide for nurse practitioners (NPs) to evaluate patients, diagnose, order and interpret diagnostic tests, initiate and manage treatments—including prescribe medications—under the exclusive licensure authority of the state board of nursing. This is the model recommended by the Institute of Medicine and National Council of State Boards of Nursing.

☐ **Reduced Practice:** State practice and licensure laws reduce the ability of NPs to engage in at least one element of NP practice. State requires a regulated collaborative agreement with an outside health discipline in order for the NP to provide patient care.

■ **Restricted Practice:** State practice and licensure laws restrict the ability of an NP to engage in at least one element of NP practice. State requires supervision, delegation or team-management by an outside health discipline in order for the NP to provide patient care.

Note. From "2014 Nurse Practitioner State Practice Environment," by American Association of Nurse Practitioners, 2014. Retrieved from http://www.aanp.org/legislation-regulation/state-legislation-regulation/state-practice-environment. Copyright 2014 by American Association of Nurse Practitioners. Reprinted with permission.

Additional consequences of drug shortages include limitations placed on clinical trials, thereby decreasing researchers' ability to test new treatments and protocols (ONS, n.d.-a). Providers are forced to alter patients' current drug regimens by omitting or decreasing full dosages, which deviates from the standard of care. This deviation can result in higher costs, less convenient regimens for patients, and the risk of poorer clinical outcomes (ASCO, 2014). Further complicating the issue is the shortage of other important medications, such as antinausea medications, IV fluids, and pain medications (ASCO, 2014). At times, treatment protocols must be modified to less effective therapies that may have worse side effect profiles, which in turn opens the possibility of the patient not tolerating the new drug therapy and resulting in decreased quality of life (Stefanik, 2011). Although shortages of new drugs have declined, overall shortages, including new and existing drugs, have increased since 2007 (U.S. Government Accountability Office [GAO], 2014). Figure 18-2 shows the number of active drug shortages.

Drug shortages are generally due to two overarching issues: quality problems and economics (U.S. GAO, 2014). An immediate cause involves the manufacturer halting or slowing production to focus on quality problems. This decrease in production triggers a supply disruption. Other manufacturers are restricted in responding to this disruption because of constrained manufacturing capacity. Second, the free market both promotes and hinders drug manufacturing. The competitive free market stimulates and motivates effective and profitable drug manufacturing. At the same time, because profit margins are a major outcome measurement for a drug manufacturer's success, decisions to enter or leave the market, as well as decisions regarding infrastructure investments, are made based on profit margins. An example of this is the economics of the generic sterile injectable drug market. Low profit margins in this area have led some manufacturers to exit the market.

There have been criticisms and shortcomings of FDA's management of drug shortages. For example, specific policies or procedures governing data management were not created, and routine quality checks on the data were not performed. These discrepancies are inconsistent with internal control standards. These shortcomings ultimately make it difficult to analyze the

Figure 18-2. Active Drug Shortages

Number of Active Drug Shortages from January 2007 through June 2013

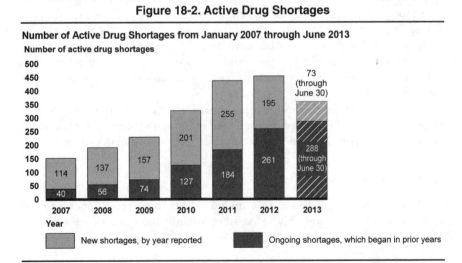

Note. From Drug Shortages: Public Health Threat Continues, Despite Efforts to Help Ensure Product Availability, by U.S. Government Accountability Office, 2014. Retrieved from http://www.gao.gov/products/GAO-14-194.

data to understand the full cause of the drug shortage and what can be done to prevent future shortages.

FDA has become more responsive to the drug shortage problem within the past few years, and consequently, more potential shortages have been prevented. FDA implemented the Food and Drug Administration Safety and Innovation Act (FDASIA) in 2012, which has resulted in FDA developing procedures to enhance coordination between FDA headquarters and field staff. However, it was still in need of policies and procedures to govern its data management and the resources to perform routine quality checks on its data (U.S. GAO, 2014).

Subsequently, President Obama signed the FDASIA into law on July 9, 2012. This new law reauthorized, for the fifth time, the Prescription Drug User Fee Act (PDUFA). Through this law, FDA is provided with "the necessary resources to maintain a predictable and efficient review process for human drug and biologic products" (U.S. FDA, 2013a, para. 1). The intent of this law was to ensure that FDA would continue to receive consistent, stable funding during fiscal years 2013–2017 that would allow the agency to fulfill its mission (U.S. FDA, 2013a), and it directed FDA to establish a task force on drug shortages that would develop and submit to Congress a strategic plan to enhance FDA's efforts in preventing and minimizing drug shortages. In October 2013, FDA issued its *Strategic Plan for Preventing and Mitigating Drug Shortages*. This plan provided direction to attain two goals: (a) strengthen FDA's mitigation response, and (b) develop long-term prevention strategies (U.S. FDA, 2013b).

Many organizations and agencies continue to work with Congress, FDA, and other stakeholders to pass legislation on this matter. For example, H.R. 6611, which would alter Medicare reimbursement for injectable generics with three or fewer manufacturers, would help ensure that people with cancer have access to timely, comprehensive, quality care and was supported by numerous cancer advocacy organizations (Association of Community Cancer Centers [ACCC], 2014).

Within Congress and among the general public, however, questions remain regarding the need for more resources for FDA versus the need for increased accountability from FDA on the efficiency of its resource management.

Access to New Drugs

Other barriers to access to care include those that prevent access to specific types of new drugs. These barriers include the costs of cancer drug treatment and the difficulty of getting new drugs to market.

Cost

The annual cost of cancer care is expected to rise from $104 billion in 2006 to $173 billion in 2020. Part of this increase is caused by the cost of new novel drug therapies (ASCO, 2014). The cost of cancer care, even for those with insurance, may be prohibitive; some of the newly approved cancer therapies cost as much as $100,000 per course of treatment (ASCO, 2014). Additionally, new cancer treatments often require significant patient cost sharing (ACCC, 2014).

A full discussion regarding strategies to address the increasing cost of cancer care is beyond the scope of this chapter. However, it must be emphasized that continuation of the traditional volume-based, fee-for-service model will not result in healthcare cost reduction in general, much less in oncology. Furthermore, until payment models exist that adequately reimburse healthcare providers for delivering comprehensive care, neither a reduction in cost nor improvement in quality will occur. It is imperative for Congress to consider three main aspects of healthcare delivery in order to lower costs: (a) the broad range of healthcare providers, including community health workers, APRNs, specialized physicians, and others, (b) what services are best provided by which type of provider (in terms of quality and cost-effectiveness), and (c) the full range of approaches to care for patients before, during, and after a cancer diagnosis, including preventive interventions, supportive services, palliative care, and team coordination. In the short term, a realistic and reasonable solution to the problem of the Medicare Sustainable Growth Rate—the method used by the Centers for Medicare and Medicaid Services to control spending by Medicare on physician and other healthcare provider services—must be developed.

Breakthrough Therapies

An example of the tension between the free-market philosophy and a more socialistic approach to drug discovery is seen in the area of breakthrough therapies. Although the cost of cancer drugs is a barrier to quality, evidence-based care, we as a society continue to demand that more and newer drugs be developed to treat not only cancer but numerous other acute and chronic conditions. Until a solution arises that will be embraced by both liberal and conservative philosophies, the allocation of scarce resources will continue to pose policy and political challenges. While we want the costs of drugs to decrease, we also want new drugs to be developed more quickly and to be made available more quickly to the general public, all of which bears the burden of additional costs. FDA created a special track that was given the designation *breakthrough therapy* to help accelerate the development and review of new drugs for serious and life-threatening conditions such as cancer. The FDA Center for Drug Evaluation and Research and Center for Biologics Evaluation and Research were part of the FDASIA. For a drug to be designated as a breakthrough therapy, documented preliminary clinical evidence must demonstrate that the drug may show substantial improvement over existing therapy on at least one clinically significant endpoint (U.S. FDA, 2014e). Table 18-3 summarizes the number of requests for breakthrough therapy designation since passage of the law.

Oral Parities

Another barrier limiting patients from receiving appropriate cancer drug therapy is that patients often have to bear considerably higher out-of-pocket expenses for oral cancer drugs than for IV therapy or other injected medications (ACCC, 2014). Twenty states have enacted oral parity laws that require insurers to provide coverage for orally administered drugs that is no less favorable than coverage for IV infusions; however, these laws are inconsistent from state to state, and most states do not have oral parity laws in place.

The Cancer Drug Coverage Parity Act of 2013 (H.R. 1801) was introduced in April 2013 and referred in July 2013 to the Subcommittee on Health, Employment, Labor, and Pensions. This bill is a reintroduction of H.R. 2746 and would ensure affordable access to treatment for patients regardless of how the treatment is administered.

Biosimilars

A biosimilar drug is a biologic product that is highly similar to an already U.S.-licensed reference biologic product and has "no clinically meaningful differences" in safety, purity, or potency to the reference product. There can be "minor differences in clinically inactive components" (U.S. FDA, 2014b, para 2). The term *interchangeability* is also used in this setting and means that the biologic product is biosimilar to the U.S.-licensed reference biolog-

Table 18-3. Breakthrough Therapy Requests

Year	Requests Received	Granted	Denied	Performance*
Center for Drug Evaluation and Research				
2012	2	1	1	100%
2013	92	31	52	96.74%
2014 (through 11/5/14)	97	29	48	99%
Center for Biologics Evaluation and Research				
2012	0	0	0	–
2013	11	1	10	100%
2014 (through 11/5/14)	26	6	17	91%

*Percent where action was taken within 60 days of receipt of the request for breakthrough therapy designation.
Note. Based on information from U.S. Food and Drug Administration, 2014e.

ic product and is expected to produce, in any given patient, the same clinical result as the reference product. Pharmacies may substitute interchangeable biologic products for a reference product without intervention from a healthcare provider. This is predicated upon the understanding that, for biologic products that are administered more than once to an individual, "the risk in terms of safety or diminished efficacy of alternating or switching between use of the biological product and the reference product will not be greater than the risk of using the reference product without such alternation or switch" (U.S. FDA, 2014b, para. 3).

An abbreviated licensure pathway for biologic products that are demonstrated to be biosimilar to or interchangeable with an FDA-licensed biologic product was included in the ACA. The Biologics Price Competition and Innovation Act of the ACA allows for a biologic product to be considered biosimilar if data, among other criteria, show that the product is highly similar to an already approved biologic product (U.S. FDA, 2014b). The use of biosimilars can be cost-saving to patients.

Risk Evaluation and Mitigation Strategies

To ensure that the benefits of certain prescription drugs or biologic agents outweigh their risks, FDA can require risk minimization strategies. This risk evaluation and mitigation strategy, or REMS, was authorized by Title IX of the 2007 Food and Drug Administration Amendments Act. This act authorized FDA to require pharmaceutical and biologic sponsors to develop a risk management program for certain drugs (U.S. FDA, 2014a).

Typically, drug manufacturers or sponsors develop a REMS for a particular drug, and FDA reviews and approves the REMS. However, FDA can require a REMS from a manufacturer if it determines that additional safety measures beyond the professional labeling are needed to ensure that a drug's benefits outweigh its risks. FDA can require this before or after a drug is approved. No two REMS are exactly alike, as there are specific safety measures that are unique to a particular drug or class of drugs. A REMS can be required for a single drug or a class of drugs, and each has its own specific safety measures. A REMS for a new drug application or a biologic license application may contain one or more of the following: (a) a medication guide or patient package insert, (b) a communication plan, (c) elements to assure safe use (ETASU), and (d) an implementation system. A REMS for an abbreviated new drug application, which is used for generic products, may contain all except the communication plan (U.S. FDA, n.d.). In September 2008, FDA required 16 products to have a REMS (Vogel & Haas, 2011). U.S. FDA (2015) maintains a list of products requiring a REMS.

Although manufacturers are financially responsible for the development of a REMS, healthcare providers who prescribe the medication are also affected. For example, both healthcare professionals and distributors may need to follow specific safety directions and procedures prior to shipping, prescribing, or dispensing the drug. Through the ETASU, FDA may require the drug manufacturer to develop education and training certification for prescribers who distribute the drug, patient and prescriber education, and medication guides. Additionally, registries for the prescriber, patient, and pharmacy may be required by the ETASU, with restricted access to the medication (only for specialty pharmacies) (ONS, n.d.-b).

An increasing number of drugs and biologic agents are being regulated by FDA through REMS programs, which is creating a significant effect on the oncology community and other specialties. In February 2009, FDA instituted a classwide REMS for controlled-release opioids (such as fentanyl, hydromorphone, methadone, morphine, oxycodone, and oxymorphone), citing risks of misuse, abuse, and accidental overdose (American Academy of Pain Medicine, 2009). Beginning in February 2010, REMS programs are required for erythropoietin-stimulating agents (Vogel & Haas, 2011).

The impact of REMS programs on patients is both positive and negative. The potential positive effects include better communication with healthcare providers, improved informed consent with better understanding of the drug risks, and enhanced patient, caregiver, and family education. The potential negative effects on patients include decreased or delayed access to certain medications, a complicated process to fill a prescription, increased drug cost, and difficulty interpreting information because of the higher reading levels of many medication guides and language barriers (Vogel & Haas, 2011).

Cancer Prevention, Screening, Treatment, and Survivorship

NCI estimated that in 2012 approximately 13.7 million Americans were living with a history of cancer; they projected that this number will increase to 18 million by 2022 (Sawyers et al., 2013). By 2030, cancer will become the leading cause of death in the United States (ASCO, 2014). Approximately one-third of cancer cases are attributed to poor nutrition, lack of physical activity, and overweight and obesity (Sawyers et al., 2013). As the number of cancer survivors increases, so does the need for better care for cancer survivors and prevention of primary and secondary cancers.

Tobacco Cessation and Control

The American Cancer Society estimated that, in 2015, almost 171,000 cancer deaths will be caused by tobacco use (American Cancer Society, 2015). About 70% of the lung cancer burden can be attributed to smoking alone (World Health Organization, n.d.). However, tobacco use can also cause cancers of the esophagus, larynx, oral cavity, pharynx, kidney, bladder, pancreas, stomach, and cervix. This is a very preventable cause of death.

In 1964, the U.S. Surgeon General released the first report on tobacco and health. At that point, cigarette consumption in the United States began to decline. However, lung cancer death rates in men did not begin to decrease until 1990. The lung cancer death rate among U.S. women, who both began and quit smoking in large numbers later than men, began to decrease in the early 2000s after increasing for many decades.

On January 17, 2014, the U.S. Surgeon General released a report titled *The Health Consequences of Smoking—50 Years of Progress* highlighting the significant progress that has occurred in tobacco control and prevention. In addition, the new report also provided additional recommendations about ending the epidemic of tobacco use in the United States, as well as new data about the health consequences of tobacco use (U.S. Surgeon General, 2014).

The past 50 years have seen the implementation of significant policy initiatives, including comprehensive tobacco control programs at the federal, state, and local levels; smoke-free workplace laws; restrictions on advertising and promotion to teenagers; and cigarette excise tax increases that discourage tobacco use among teens (ASCO, 2014; U.S. Surgeon General, 2014). Senator Richard Durbin (D-IL), with cosponsors Senators Richard Blumenthal (D-CT) and Frank Lautenberg (D-NJ), introduced the Tobacco Tax Equity Act in 2013, which seeks to amend the Internal Revenue Code of 1986 to provide tax rate parity among all tobacco products (NCI Office of Government and Congressional Relations, 2013). The bill seeks to impose the same tax rate upon all forms of tobacco (i.e., the tax rate on all tobacco products would be the same per unit level as cigarettes). Previously, cigars, smokeless tobacco, and pipe tobacco had been taxed at a dramatically lower rate than cigarettes, while small cigars and roll-your-own tobacco products were taxed at the same level (NCI Office of Government and Congressional Relations, 2013).

Electronic cigarettes, also known as e-cigarettes, are battery-operated products designed to deliver nicotine, flavor, and other chemicals (U.S. FDA, 2014c). The potential risks of e-cigarettes, whether used as intended or not, are not known, nor is it known how much nicotine or other potentially harmful chemicals are being inhaled during use because e-cigarettes have not been fully studied. Consumers are being led to believe that these are harmless products, but this is not based on scientific evidence. It is also not known whether e-cigarettes are a gateway to other tobacco products, which are known to cause disease and lead to premature death.

Currently, the FDA Center for Drug Evaluation and Research regulates only e-cigarettes that are marketed for therapeutic purposes. The FDA Center for Tobacco Products currently regulates cigarettes, cigarette tobacco, roll-your-own tobacco, and smokeless tobacco.

Laws seeking to control the sale of and the amount of tax placed upon e-cigarettes are being proposed at state and municipal levels. FDA intends to issue a proposed rule extending its authority over tobacco products to include other products such as e-cigarettes.

Obesity

The World Cancer Research Fund International estimates that about one-quarter to one-third of the new cancer cases expected to occur in the United States in 2013 will be related to overweight or obesity, lack of physical inactivity, and poor nutrition, and thus could also be prevented. Obesity has reached epidemic proportions, as more than two-thirds of Americans are either overweight or obese. Specifically, the obesity rates more than doubled in adults ages 20–74 between 1976–1980 and 1999–2002, increasing from 15.1% to 31%. These increases occurred in all race, ethnicity, and gender groups. During the past decade, obesity trends in women have remained relatively stable, whereas among men, prevalence increased from 28% during 1999–2002 to 36% during 2009–2010 (American Cancer Society, 2013; World Cancer Research Fund International, n.d.). Figure 18-3 reflects the obesity trends in adults ages 20–74 from 1976 to 2012.

The Healthy Lifestyles and Prevention America (HeLP America) Act is a bill that includes various wellness provisions: expanded access to fresh fruits and vegetables for all low-income elementary schools, tax incentives for businesses that offer comprehensive workplace wellness programs to their employees, improved physical activity and athletic opportunities for individuals with disabilities, and greater oversight with regard to food and tobacco marketing. This bill has moved through the Senate Committee on Health, Education, Labor, and Pensions, but as of this writing has not been heard in a House committee (NCI Office of Government and Congressional Relations, 2013).

Human Papillomavirus Vaccination

With approximately 14 million new cases of human papillomavirus (HPV) each year, more than 79 million people in the United States are now infected (Centers for Disease Control and Prevention [CDC], 2014b). There currently is no cure for HPV, only treatment for some of the related health problems, and most strains of HPV are asymptomatic (National Conference of State Legislatures, 2014).

Of the 40 different types of genital HPV, some cause genital warts in both males and females, and others cause cancer, including cancers of the uterine cervix, vulva, vagina, penis, anus, and oropharynx (CDC, 2014b). Nearly 70% of cervical cancers and 90% of genital warts are caused by one of four strains of HPV: 6, 11, 16, and 18. FDA approved two commercially available vaccines in 2006 and 2009, respectively: Gardasil® and Cervarix®. Most

Figure 18-3. Obesity* Trends, Adults Ages 20–74 by Gender and Race/Ethnicity†, United States, 1976–2012

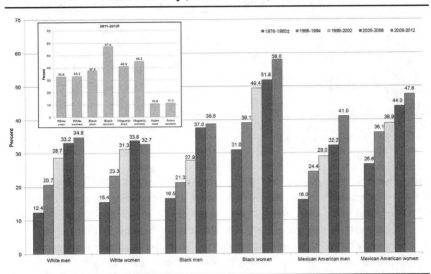

* Body mass index of 30.0 kg/m² or greater. † Persons of Mexican origins may be of any race. Whites, blacks, and Asians are all non-Hispanic (NH). Data estimates for NH white and NH black races starting in 1999 data may not be strictly comparable with estimates for earlier years because of changes in Standards for Federal Data on Race and Ethnicity. Hispanic includes all Hispanics, not just Mexican American Hispanic persons. ‡ Data for Mexican Americans are for 1982–84. § NH Asian persons and all Hispanic persons were over-sampled in the 2011–12 National Health and Nutrition Examination Survey sample, NH Asian persons for the first time. *Note:* Rates are age-adjusted.

Source: National Center for Health Statistics. *Health, United States, 2013: With Special Feature on Prescription Drugs.* Hyattsville, MD. 2014. Complete trend data available at http://www.cdc.gov/nchs/hus/contents2013.htm#069. Accessed May 20, 2014. Insert: National Health and Nutrition Examination Survey Public Use Data File, 2011–2012. National Center for Health Statistics, Centers for Disease Control and Prevention, 2014.

Note. From *Cancer Prevention and Early Detection Facts and Figures: Tables and Figures 2014,* by American Cancer Society, 2014. Retrieved from http://www.cancer.org/acs/groups/content/@research/documents/document/acspc-042924.pdf. Copyright 2014 by American Cancer Society. Reprinted with permission.

recently, in December 2014, FDA approved Gardasil 9, which covers nine strains of HPV (6, 11, 16, 18, 31, 33, 45, 52, and 58). These five additional strains count for approximately 20% of cervical cancers (U.S. FDA, 2014d). Table 18-4 summarizes information about the two vaccines.

It is estimated that 21,000 HPV-associated cancers can be prevented each year by vaccination. The major female cancers caused by HPV are cervical, anal, vaginal, vulvar, and oropharyngeal, while oropharyngeal cancers are the most common male HPV-caused cancer (CDC, 2014a).

CDC recommends that all 11- or 12-year-old girls receive the three doses of either brand of HPV vaccine to protect against cervical cancer. Girls and

Table 18-4. Human Papillomavirus (HPV) Vaccines

Vaccine	HPV Strain Protection	Current Indications
Cervarix® (GlaxoSmithKline)	16, 18	Females ages 9–25
Gardasil® (Merck & Co., Inc.)	6, 11, 16, 18	Females ages 9–26 Males ages 9–26
Gardasil 9	6, 11, 16, 18, 31, 33, 45, 52, 58	Females ages 9–26 Males ages 9–15

Note. Based on information from GlaxoSmithKline Inc., n.d.; Merck Sharp & Dohme Corp., 2014; U.S. Food and Drug Administration, 2014d.

young women ages 13–26 who had not received any or all doses when they were younger also are recommended to receive the vaccine (CDC, 2014b). CDC recommends Gardasil for all boys age 11 or 12 and for males ages 13–21 who did not get any or all of the three recommended doses when they were younger. All men may receive the Gardasil vaccine through age 26 (CDC, 2014b). As of 2014, Cervarix is not indicated for males.

In general, vaccinations continue to be controversial; the debate over HPV vaccination has added to this national discussion. HPV vaccination can get folded into the school vaccination debate, which is decided mainly by state legislatures. Again, the tension between federal and state authority arises. Vaccination recommendations, along with most health-related guidelines, are made at the national level, usually through professional organizations or a federal agency. In this case, the CDC's Advisory Committee on Immunization Practices (ACIP), a group of public health and medical experts, develops recommendations on how to use vaccines to control diseases in the United States. ACIP was established under Section 222 of the Public Health Service Act and is governed by its charter. However, even after ACIP makes recommendations, school vaccination requirements are then decided mostly by state legislatures. Some state legislatures delegate this authority to a regulatory body, such as the state health department, but the legislature is still needed to provide the funding (National Conference of State Legislatures, 2014).

Controversy around HPV vaccinations include issues related to school mandates, as well as moral objectives. Some individuals support the availability of the vaccine but do not support school mandates, as they feel this should be a parental decision. Others question specific drugs' costs and safety. Furthermore, some parents, as well as those without children, have voiced moral objections about having a vaccine mandated for a sexually transmitted infection, which they feel interferes with their teaching of sexual abstinence prior to marriage.

Financing further complicates the HPV vaccine controversy. If states make the vaccine mandatory, then they must also address the funding stream, including Medicaid and State Children's Health Insurance Program coverage, youth who are uninsured, and whether to require HPV vaccination coverage by insurance plans. The latter has caused circling back to the question of whether the vaccine should be required (National Conference of State Legislatures, 2014).

Currently, the HPV vaccine is available through the federal Vaccines for Children Program in all 50 states. This program provides vaccines for children ages 9–18 who are covered by Medicaid, children who are Alaska Native or Native American, and some children who are underinsured or uninsured (National Conference of State Legislatures, 2014).

Sadly, while the debate and controversy over HPV vaccination proceeds, women who are underinsured or uninsured continue to have a disproportionate number of deaths from the diseases that are prevented by vaccines. Just as mammography and Pap tests are underused by women who have no regular source of health care or who are without health insurance or who have immigrated to the United States within the past 10 years, the same picture is evolving with HPV vaccinations (CDC, 2012). Although the ACA seeks to prevent these disparities, the challenges of obtaining insurance coverage for low-income individuals, whether through insurance exchanges or Medicaid, coupled with the increased problems of access to care, have not been overcome, and vulnerable populations continue to have poorer health outcomes.

Treatment: Clinical Trials

A robust clinical trials system is imperative in the development of efficient approaches to the prevention, diagnosis, and treatment of cancer. While essentially 100% of children with cancer are treated through clinical trials, fewer than 5% of adults with cancer each year will participate in a clinical trial (Sawyers et al., 2013). NCI has launched a new clinical trials research network with the intent of improving treatment. The National Clinical Trials Network (NCTN) is replacing the previous national clinical trials program, the Clinical Trials Cooperative Group Program. IOM's 2010 report *A National Cancer Clinical Trials System for the 21st Century: Reinvigorating the NCI Cooperative Group Program* identified four goals for modernizing the then-existing clinical trials system, which were to

• Improve speed and efficiency of trial development and activation
• Incorporate innovative science and trial design
• Improve prioritization, selection, support, and completion of trials
• Offer incentives for participation of patients and physicians.

Prompted by this report, NCI reorganized the clinical trials system by consolidating the groups that conduct clinical trials in adult patients with cancer from nine to four groups. The Cancer and Leukemia Group B Cooperative Group, the North Central Cancer Treatment Group, and the American College of Surgeons Oncology Group merged to form the Alliance for Clinical Trials in Oncology. The Eastern Cooperative Oncology

Group (ECOG) and the American College of Radiology Imaging Network (ACRIN) merged to become ECOG-ACRIN. The National Surgical Adjuvant Breast and Bowel Project, the Radiation Therapy Oncology Group, and the Gynecologic Oncology Group formed into NRG Oncology. The Southwest Oncology Group remains independent. Ten years previously, the Children's Oncology Group was consolidated from four groups into one and will not merge with any other group (Printz, 2013). Figure 18-4 demonstrates the consolidation of the groups.

After many state-level battles with insurance companies to prevent individuals from being dropped by insurance plans if they were on a clinical trial, or to get insurers to cover the costs of routine patient care associated with participation in clinical trials, the ACA put into law, beginning January 2014, the requirement that private insurers cover routine patient costs associated with participation in approved clinical trials (ASCO, 2012). Section 2709 of the ACA, now codified at 42 U.S.C. § 300gg-8, provides three guarantees and protections:

• A qualified individual may not be prevented from participating in an approved clinical trial.
• A clinical trial participant cannot be discriminated against by a payer.
• The payer must cover qualified individuals' routine patient costs for services delivered in-network.

This statute applies to all third-party payers of health benefit or insurance claims, including group health plans, self-insured employers' health benefit plans, health insurance issuers, and federal employee health benefit plans. Section 2709 does not preempt state laws relating to clinical trials that have more stringent requirements or provide greater protection to patients (ASCO, 2012).

Even with these improvements through the ACA and with the reorganization at NCI, investigators must still deal with many barriers when they are developing clinical trials. The enormous amount of paperwork, the required but sometimes unnecessary procedures, the development of inclusion and exclusion criteria that can limit trial populations, and the approval of often dozens of institutional review boards all contribute to the difficulty of patient recruitment and increase costs. Furthermore, the trial populations do not always reflect the many diverse patient populations in this country or, at times, the populations for whom the treatment was originally intended (Leaf, 2013).

Survivorship Care

While surviving cancer is cause for celebration, the process of surviving cancer comes at high cost to patients and the system. Patients must face the ongoing possibility of a recurrence, as well as an increased risk for the development of other morbidities, such as diabetes, cardiovascular disease,

Figure 18-4. Consolidation of Clinical Trials Groups

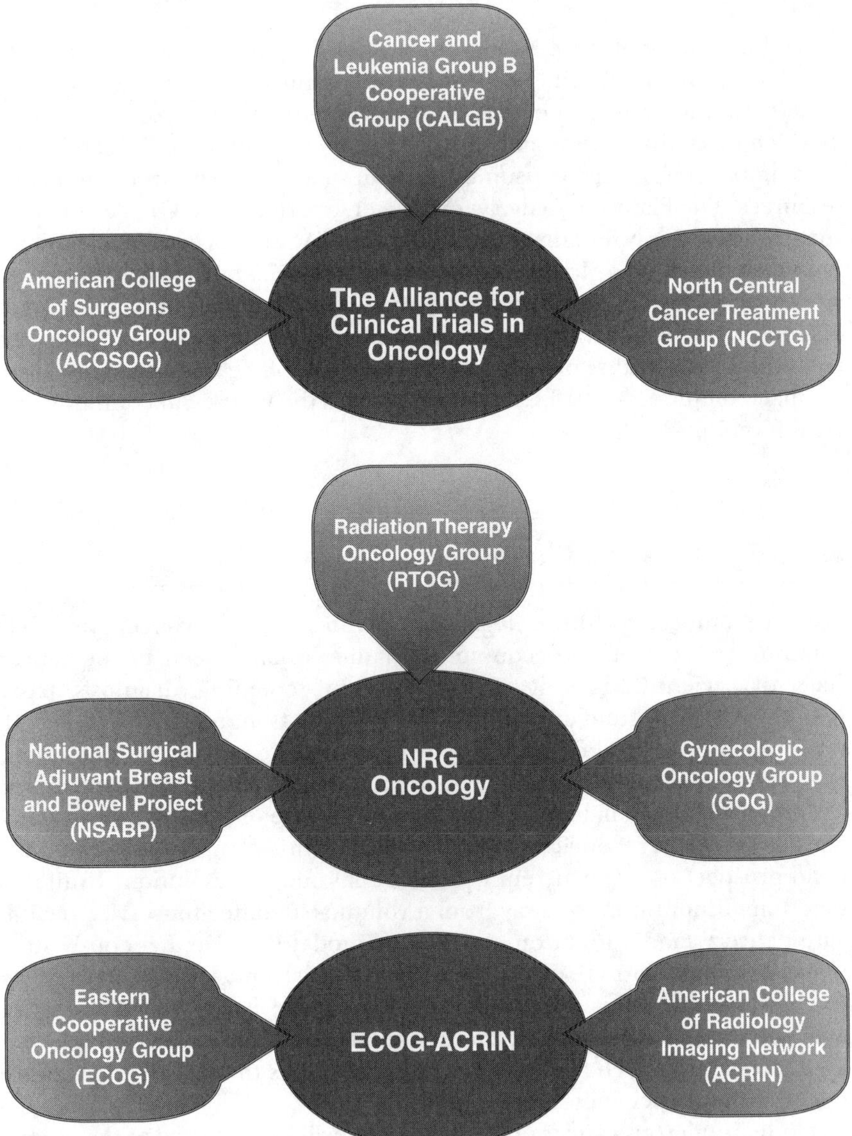

Cancer and Leukemia Group B Cooperative Group (CALGB)

American College of Surgeons Oncology Group (ACOSOG)

The Alliance for Clinical Trials in Oncology

North Central Cancer Treatment Group (NCCTG)

Radiation Therapy Oncology Group (RTOG)

National Surgical Adjuvant Breast and Bowel Project (NSABP)

NRG Oncology

Gynecologic Oncology Group (GOG)

Eastern Cooperative Oncology Group (ECOG)

ECOG-ACRIN

American College of Radiology Imaging Network (ACRIN)

osteoporosis, and altered functional status. To best serve cancer survivors, multiple healthcare providers are needed in addition to oncologists (ASCO, 2014).

As the number of people diagnosed and living with cancer continues to increase exponentially, the healthcare community is tasked to not only better address the long-term effects of cancer treatment, but also to find ways in which this information can be communicated to survivors. This endeavor, while important, is time consuming and taps already taxed and unavailable resources. The Planning Actively for Cancer Treatment (PACT) Act of 2013, sponsored by Representatives Lois Capps (D-CA) and Charles Boustany (R-LA), proposes a new Medicare cancer care planning and coordination service to facilitate a shared decision-making process available to patients upon diagnosis that would include the development of a written care plan and communication of that plan during an in-person office visit. The bill was introduced on June 25, 2013, and was referred to the House Subcommittee on Health on July 23, 2013.

Future Legislative Themes

In the immediate future, legislative action related to cancer will likely continue to focus on the economic dynamics of all aspects of the cancer trajectory: scientific investigation, prevention, screening, diagnosis, treatment, survivorship, and end-of-life care. With the Congressional Budget Office projecting federal deficits of $6.6 trillion in the coming decade under the president's budget plan (Congressional Budget Office, 2014), coupled with the lack of a Senate budget plan and a House of Representatives budget plan that is irreconcilable with the president's plan, there is essentially no prospect of a concurrent congressional budget resolution. Until it is determined how to move away from a volume-based, fee-for-service healthcare delivery model to an outcome-based model that simultaneously stimulates discovery and creativity, economics will continue to be the driving force. Folded into this overarching discussion and framework is the ACA, with the numerous improvements *and* negative unintended consequences that accompany it. The driving question continues to be, Can we improve health while reducing costs?

Of the numerous cancer policy topics that will be discussed at the municipal, state, tribal, and federal levels, a select few will be discussed here. With the current system of health care in the United States still largely based on volume rather than quality, unsustainable growth in cancer costs will continue because of the increasingly complex nature of cancer diagnosis and treatment coupled with the rapidly growing population of individuals requiring cancer care services. Ironically, as diagnostic and treatment technologies advance, progress has been slow in halting the disparities in access to this high-quality care. The dichotomy of the excitement surrounding unprecedented scientific progress juxtaposed with the concern about increased health disparities is a thoughtful reminder of the challenges of creating effective and operational policy.

Research Funding

Of utmost concern is the need for continued funding for the scientific advancement of knowledge about all aspects of oncology, from basic cell biology to innovative ways to prevent and halt this group of diseases, including the incorporation of genomic sequencing throughout the spectrum. Budget pressures have been forcing NIH to reject increasing numbers of valid, important research proposals. This puts scientific progress at risk and leads many of the country's brightest new investigators to consider careers outside of science or scientific careers in other countries. NIH once funded one in three research proposals. However, for the past 10 years, it has only funded an average of one in six (Collins, 2013). The NIH budget was at its height in fiscal year 2010 at $31.2 billion, falling to $30.15 billion for fiscal year 2014 (NIH, 2014). While this is of grave concern, the oversight of NIH, as with all federal agencies, must continue to include the ongoing review, monitoring, and supervision of all programs, activities, and policy implementation.

Payment Systems

The development of new payment systems that will create incentives for high-value, outcome-driven, patient-centered care is being examined by the U.S. Congress, the federal administration, and the oncology community (ASCO, 2014). Both political parties and chambers of Congress showed increased interest in piloting alternative payment models under Medicare during the recent Medicare Sustainable Growth Rate debates (ASCO, 2014). The historical dominance of fee-for-service and medicine/treatment-driven forms of payment is shifting toward prospective payment models, clinical pathways, and patient-centered medical homes (ASCO, 2014). Included in this must be payment models for prevention and screening services with emphasis not only on diagnosis and treatment. Also necessary is the evaluation of the difficult question of who is needed to provide what types of care. Although the advanced and highly specialized training of physicians and surgeons is necessary for many procedures, the broad and comprehensive training of other professionals, such as APRNs, is necessary for the successful incorporation of the preventive and patient-centered aspects. Furthermore, the role of community health workers (also referred to as lay advisers and community health representatives) in the continuum is showing evidence of effectiveness in the management of several diseases (Meade et al., 2014). Breaking out of the physician-led pyramid team will be challenging and difficult.

Genetics and Genomics

Genomic research is expected to make a huge impact on the practice of health care. As healthcare providers move from examining just a few genes at a time, whole genomic sequencing will allow practitioners to diagnose and treat cancers in a targeted manner unlike any preceding treatments, thereby greatly changing the practice of health care (National Human Genome Research Institute, 2014). However, this exciting and necessary approach involves numerous new legal, ethical, social, and regulatory challenges. Preeminent among these concerns are the issues of how risk is defined and how healthcare providers address incidental findings (i.e., genetic information discovered unintentionally) (Michalek & Wicher, 2011). Policies and procedures must also be in place to prevent misuse of genetic technologies and information. Underserved and underprivileged populations have legitimate concerns about the advancement of these technologies, specifically in light of past atrocities (e.g., the Tuskegee syphilis study in African Americans and the unauthorized use of genetic material of the Havasupai Tribe) (Katz et al., 2006; Mello & Wolf, 2010). The need for policies and legislation that protect and promote has never been greater.

Quality in Cancer Care

While many healthcare providers and patients view the U.S. cancer care system as the best in the world, the quality of care throughout the cancer trajectory continues to be difficult to define and measure. This results in inconsistency, contributing to disparities in outcomes for different populations and unnecessary costs (ASCO, 2014). The oncology community must be integrally involved with the legislature and federal agencies as quality is defined and measures are developed. The establishment of benchmarks that include benefits and services essential to the care of all patients with cancer is a consideration for the current system of health insurers, as well as for the crafting of the future system.

Looking to the Future

The advancements and opportunities in cancer health policy are vast and dynamic. From the oldest descriptions of cancer discovered in Egypt that date back to about 3000 BCE, the Edwin Smith Papyrus (American Cancer

Society, 2012), to the rapid discoveries and changes in the prevention, diagnosis, and treatment of cancer today, this group of diseases called cancer continues to challenge technologic advances and the necessary policies needed to maintain progress. Cancer research is advancing extremely quickly and on many fronts. Concurrently, the U.S. healthcare system continues its dynamic evolution. Looking to the future in cancer policy, it can be helpful to consider trends in health care in general. Emanuel (2014) proposed six megatrends for the future of health care, which were

1. End of insurance companies as we know them
2. VIP care for the chronically and mentally ill
3. The emergence of digital medicine and closure of hospitals
4. End of employer-sponsored health insurance
5. End of health care inflation
6. Transformation of medical education. (p. 319)

Although one can identify numerous other megatrends, the fact that the country is in the midst of the most pivotal healthcare changes since the 1960s will clearly influence the development of both useful and wasteful policies.

Conclusion

As the nation moves forward with the enormous challenge of providing improved health care at reduced cost, many promising approaches are emerging. However, emphasis must be directed toward improving population health and restraining growth in spending, the classic source of bipartisan friction. Policies that consistently address these two factors must be identified, evaluated, implemented, and reinforced.

References

American Academy of Pain Medicine. (2009). *Risk evaluation and mitigation strategies (REMS) for opioids; Request for comments* (Docket No. FDA-2009-N-0143) [Communication to U.S. Food and Drug Administration]. Chicago, IL: Author.

American Association of Colleges of Nursing. (2014). Nursing shortage. Retrieved from http://www.aacn.nche.edu/media-relations/fact-sheets/nursing-shortage

American Association of Nurse Practitioners. (2014). State practice environment. Retrieved from http://www.aanp.org/legislation-regulation/state-legislation-regulation/state-practice-environment

American Cancer Society. (2012). *The history of cancer.* Atlanta, GA: Author.

American Cancer Society. (2013). *Cancer prevention and early detection facts and figures 2013.* Retrieved from http://www.cancer.org/acs/groups/content/@epidemiologysurveilance/documents/document/acspc-037535.pdf

American Cancer Society. (2015). *Cancer facts and figures 2015.* Retrieved from http://www.cancer.org/research/cancerfactsstatistics/index

American Society of Clinical Oncology. (2012). Summary [of] the Affordable Care Act statute regarding insurance coverage for individuals participating in approved clinical trials. Retrieved from http://www.asco.org/sites/default/files/aca_summary_clinical_trials.pdf

American Society of Clinical Oncology. (2014). The state of cancer care in America, 2014: A report by the American Society of Clinical Oncology. *Journal of Oncology Practice, 10,* 119–142. doi:10.1200/JOP.2014.001386

Association of Community Cancer Centers. (2014). Ensuring quality cancer care. Retrieved from http://www.accc-cancer.org/advocacy/QualityCare-Guidelines.asp

Buerhaus, P.I., Auerbach, D.I., & Staiger, D.O. (2009). The recent surge in nurse employment: Causes and implications. *Health Affairs, 28,* w657–w668. doi:10.1377/hlthaff.28.4.w657

Cancer Drug Coverage Parity Act of 2013, H.R. 1801, 113th Cong.

Centers for Disease Control and Prevention. (2012). Cancer screening—United States, 2010. *Morbidity and Mortality Weekly Report, 61,* 41–45. Retrieved from http://www.cdc.gov/mmwr/preview/mmwrhtml/mm6103a1.htm

Centers for Disease Control and Prevention. (2014a). Genital HPV infection—Fact sheet. Retrieved from http://www.cdc.gov/std/HPV/STDFact-HPV.htm

Centers for Disease Control and Prevention. (2014b). Vaccines and immunizations: HPV vaccination. Retrieved from http://www.cdc.gov/vaccines/VPD-VAC/hpv/default.htm

Collins, F.S. (2013, March 5). *NIH Congressional Testimony.* Committee on Appropriations Subcommittee on Labor, Health and Human Services, Education and Related Agencies.

Congressional Budget Office. (2014, April 17). *An analysis of the president's 2015 budget.* Retrieved from http://www.cbo.gov/publication/45230

Emanuel, E.J. (2014). *Reinventing American health care: How the Affordable Care Act will improve our terribly complex, blatantly unjust, outrageously expensive, grossly inefficient, error prone system.* New York, NY: PublicAffairs.

Food and Drug Administration Amendments Act of 2007, Pub. L. No. 110-85, 121 Stat. 823.

Food and Drug Administration Safety and Innovation Act, Pub. L. No. 112-144, 126 Stat. 993 (2012).

GlaxoSmithKline Inc. (n.d.). Cervarix. Retrieved from http://www.cervarix.ca

Health Resources and Services Administration. (2014). Shortage designation: Health professional shortage areas and medically underserved areas/populations. Retrieved from http://www.hrsa.gov/shortage

Healthy Lifestyles and Prevention America Act, S. 39, 113 Cong. (2013).

Howlader, N., Noone, A.M., Krapcho, M., Neyman, N., Aminou, R., Waldron, W., ... Cronin, K.A. (Eds.). (2012, April). *SEER cancer statistics review, 1975–2009 (vintage 2009 populations).* Retrieved from http://seer.cancer.gov/csr/1975_2009_pops09

Institute of Medicine. (2010). *A national cancer clinical trials system for the 21st century: Reinvigorating the NCI Cooperative Group Program.* Retrieved from http://iom.edu/Reports/2010/A-National-Cancer-Clinical-Trials-System-for-the-21st-Century-Reinvigorating-the-NCI-Cooperative.aspx

Institute of Medicine Committee on the Robert Wood Johnson Foundation Initiative on the Future of Nursing. (2011). *The future of nursing: Leading change, advancing health.* Retrieved from http://www.nap.edu/catalog.php?record_id=12956

Juraschek, S.P., Zhang, X., Ranganathan, V., & Lin, V.W. (2012). United States registered nurse workforce report card and shortage forecast. *American Journal of Medical Quality, 27,* 241–249. doi:10.1177/1062860611416634

Katz, R.V., Kegeles, S.S., Kressin, N.R., Green, B.L., Wang, M.Q., James, S.A., ... Claudio, C. (2006). The Tuskegee Legacy Project: Willingness of minorities to participate in biomedical research. *Journal of Health Care for the Poor and Underserved, 17,* 698–715. doi:10.1353/hpu.2006.0126

Leaf, C. (2013). *The truth in small doses: Why we're losing the war on cancer—and how to win it.* New York, NY: Simon & Schuster.

Meade, C.D., Wells, K.J., Arevalo, M., Calcano, E.R., Rivera, M., Sarmiento, Y., ... Roetzheim, R.G. (2014). Lay navigator model for impacting cancer health disparities. *Journal of Cancer Education, 29,* 449–457. doi:10.1007/s13187-014-0640-z

Mello, M.M., & Wolf, L.E. (2010). The Havasupai Indian tribe case—Lessons for research involving stored biologic samples. *New England Journal of Medicine, 363,* 204–207.

Merck Sharp & Dohme Corp. (2014). About Gardasil. Retrieved from http://www.gardasil.com/about-gardasil/about-gardasil/

Michalek, A.M., & Wicher, C.C. (2011). Ethics corner—Biospecimen banking: Poetry of the flesh. *Journal of Cancer Education, 26,* 212–214. doi:10.1007/s13187-011-0206-2

National Cancer Institute Office of Budget and Finance. (n.d.). Plan and budget proposal: The nation's investment in cancer research. Retrieved from http://obf.cancer.gov/financial/plan.htm

National Cancer Institute Office of Government and Congressional Relations. (n.d.-a). Committees of interest. Retrieved from http://legislative.cancer.gov/committees

National Cancer Institute Office of Government and Congressional Relations. (n.d.-b). The U.S. House of Representatives Committee on Appropriations: About the committee. Retrieved from http://appropriations.house.gov/about

National Cancer Institute Office of Government and Congressional Relations. (2013, March 13). *Legislative update for the Clinical and Translation Research Advisory Committee: Activities of the 113th Congress—first session.* Retrieved from http://deainfo.nci.nih.gov/advisory/ctac/0313/LegislativeReport.pdf

National Conference of State Legislatures. (2014). HPV vaccine policies. Retrieved from http://www.ncsl.org/research/health/hpv-vaccine-state-legislation-and-statutes.aspx

National Human Genome Research Institute. (2014). Health issues in genetics. Retrieved from http://www.genome.gov/10001872

National Institutes of Health. (2013). The NIH Almanac: Legislative chronology. Retrieved from http://www.nih.gov/about/almanac/historical/legislative_chronology.htm

National Institutes of Health. (2014). Research Portfolio Online Reporting Tools (RePORT): NIH Data Book. Retrieved from http://report.nih.gov/nihdatabook

National Institutes of Health Office of Budget. (n.d.). History. Retrieved from http://officeofbudget.od.nih.gov/history.html

National Institutes of Health Office of History. (2013, April 11). About: Timelines: NIH institutes, centers, and offices. Retrieved from http://history.nih.gov/about/timelines_institutes.html

Oncology Nursing Society. (n.d.-a). Public health issues: Drug shortages. Retrieved from http://www.ons.org/advocacy-policy/public-health

Oncology Nursing Society. (n.d.-b). *Risk evaluation and mitigation strategies (REMS) overview.* Pittsburgh, PA: Author.

Patient-Centered Outcomes Research Institute. (2013). How we're funded. Retrieved from http://www.pcori.org/content/how-were-funded

Patient-Centered Outcomes Research Institute. (2014a). About us. Retrieved from http://www.pcori.org/about-us/mission-and-vision

Patient-Centered Outcomes Research Institute. (2014b). Governance. Retrieved from http://www.pcori.org/content/governance

Patient Protection and Affordable Care Act, Pub. L. No. 111-148, 124 Stat. 119 (2010).

Planning Actively for Cancer Treatment (PACT) Act of 2013, H.R. 2477, 113th Cong.

President's Cancer Panel. (2007). *Transforming translation: Harnessing discovery for patient and public benefit.* Washington, DC: National Cancer Institute.

Printz, C. (2013). NCI cooperative clinical trials groups proceed with reorganization: New system aims to improve efficiency and address changing research needs. *Cancer, 119,* 3423–3424. Retrieved from http://onlinelibrary.wiley.com/doi/10.1002/cncr.28360/full

Public Health Service Act, 42 § U.S.C. 217a (1944).

Sawyers, C.L., Abate-Shen, C., Anderson, K.C., Barker, A., Baselga, J., Berger, N.A., ... Weiner, G.J. (2013). AACR cancer progress report 2013. *Clinical Cancer Research, 19*(Suppl. 20), S1–S98. doi:10.1158/1078-0432.CCR-13-2107

Schick, A. (2007). *The federal budget: Politics, policy, process* (3rd ed.). Washington, DC: Brookings Institution Press.

Stefanik, D. (2011, September 26). Draft: Oncology Nursing Society oral statement before the Food and Drug Administration (FDA) Center for Drug Evaluation and Research (CDER) Public Workshop to Address Drug Shortages. Retrieved from http://www2.ons .org/LAC/Issues/media/ons/docs/LAC/issues/drugshortages/draft-of-drug-shortage -statement-2011.pdf

Tobacco Tax Equity Act, S. 194, 113th Cong. (2013).

U.S. Department of Health and Human Services. (2014). *Fiscal year 2015: Budget in brief. Strengthening health and opportunity for all Americans.* Retrieved from http://www.hhs.gov/budget/ fy2015/fy-2015-budget-in-brief.pdf

U.S. Food and Drug Administration. (n.d.). A brief overview of risk evaluation and mitigation strategies (REMS). Retrieved from http://www.fda.gov/downloads/aboutfda/ transparency/basics/ucm328784.pdf

U.S. Food and Drug Administration. (2013a). Prescription Drug User Fee Act (PDUFA): PDUFA V: Fiscal years 2013–2017. Retrieved from http://www.fda.gov/forindustry/userfees/ prescriptiondruguserfee/ucm272170.htm

U.S. Food and Drug Administration. (2013b). *Strategic plan for preventing and mitigating drug shortages.* Retrieved from http://www.fda.gov/downloads/drugs/drugsafety/drugshortages/ ucm372566.pdf

U.S. Food and Drug Administration. (2014a). Drugs: Approved risk evaluation and mitigation strategies (REMS). Retrieved from http://www.fda.gov/drugs/drugsafety/postmarketdrug safetyinformationforpatientsandproviders/ucm111350.htm

U.S. Food and Drug Administration. (2014b). Drugs: Information for healthcare professionals (biosimilars). Retrieved from http://www.fda.gov/Drugs/DevelopmentApprovalProcess/ HowDrugsareDevelopedandApproved/ApprovalApplications/TherapeuticBiologic Applications/Biosimilars/ucm241719.htm

U.S. Food and Drug Administration. (2014c). Electronic cigarettes (e-cigarettes). Retrieved from http://www.fda.gov/newsevents/publichealthfocus/ucm172906.htm

U.S. Food and Drug Administration. (2014d). FDA news release: FDA approves Gardasil 9 for prevention of certain cancers caused by five additional types of HPV. Retrieved from http:// www.fda.gov/NewsEvents/Newsroom/PressAnnouncements/ucm426485.htm

U.S. Food and Drug Administration. (2014e). Frequently asked questions: Breakthrough therapies. Retrieved from http://www.fda.gov/regulatoryinformation/legislation/federalfood drugandcosmeticactfdcact/significantamendmentstothefdcact/fdasia/ucm341027.htm

U.S. Food and Drug Administration. (2015). Approved Risk Evaluation and Management Strategies (REMS). Retrieved from http://www.fda.gov/Drugs/DrugSafety/PostmarketDrug SafetyInformationforPatientsandProviders/ucm111350.htm#Shared

U.S. Government Accountability Office. (2014, February 10). *Drug shortages: Public health threat continues, despite efforts to help ensure product availability* (Publication No. GAO-14-194). Retrieved from http://www.gao.gov/products/GAO-14-194

U.S. Senate Committee on Appropriations. (n.d.). Budget process: Authorization vs appropriation. Retrieved from http://www.appropriations.senate.gov/content/budget-process

U.S. Surgeon General. (2014). *The health consequences of smoking—50 years of progress: A report of the Surgeon General.* Retrieved from http://www.surgeongeneral.gov/library/reports/50-years -of-progress/index.html

Vogel, W.H., & Haas, M. (2011). REMS: Application for the advanced practitioner in oncology. *Journal of the Advanced Practitioner in Oncology, 2,* 51–57. Retrieved from http://www .advancedpractitioner.com/media/118635/jadpro_051.pdf

White House Office of the Press Secretary. (2011, October 31). Fact sheet: Obama administration takes action to reduce prescription drug shortages in the U.S. Retrieved from http://www.whitehouse.gov/the-press-office/2011/10/31/fact-sheet-obama-administration-takes-action-reduce-prescription-drug-sh

World Cancer Research Fund International. (n.d.). *Cancer facts and figures.* Retrieved from http://www.wcrf.org/int/cancer-facts-and-figures

World Health Organization. (n.d.). Cancer prevention. Retrieved from http://www.who.int/cancer/prevention/en

Yang, W., Williams, J.H., Hogan, P.F., Bruinooge, S.S., Rodriguez, G.I., Kosty, M.P., ... Goldstein, M. (2014). Projected supply of and demand for oncologists and radiation oncologists through 2025: An aging, better-insured population will result in shortage. *Journal of Oncology Practice, 10,* 39–45. doi:10.1200/JOP.2013.001319

EPILOGUE:

Looking Toward the Future

Otis W. Brawley, MD, FACP, Chief Medical Officer for the American Cancer Society

Policy is a principle, a strategy, or an approach adopted to achieve a goal. Good, thoughtful policy is realistic and is aimed at the greater good. It can be adopted at multiple levels. Most commonly we think of local, state, and federal government policy, but policies are also adopted by political parties, businesses, other organizations, or even individuals. As it relates to health, the goal of good policy is better health for the population.

As related to cancer, the goal of policy is cancer control. Thus, cancer policy involves interventions aimed at reducing cancer risk, incidence, morbidity, and mortality. It translates into efforts to prevent, screen for, and treat cancer, as well as attempts to develop knowledge about how to prevent, screen for, or treat cancer. Elements of cancer control policy include support for research to identify useful interventions, decision making to determine that an intervention should be employed, and implementation of that intervention. Public education can also be an element of cancer control policy; this is especially important in areas of disease prevention.

There is need to formulate thoughtful, informed policy. *Thoughtful* and *informed* are key characteristics, as there is the potential for waste of resources and diversion of efforts from things that are actually good and effective.

As this book demonstrates, a number of groups can influence the development and adoption of policy. This is especially true of government policy. Numerous interest groups influence policy making. Some of the loudest, most influential voices are often voluntary and professional organizations. Some of these organizations are well meaning and well informed. Some are well meaning and misinformed. They can support policy that may be inefficient and even harmful in the long term. The interests of advocates in a certain policy should always be studied. Much attention has been placed on financial conflict of interest, but more attention needs to be placed on emotional conflict of interest and ideology.

Let us look at the current state of health care in a succinct attempt to identify the needs for good policy and some of the failures of policy to adequately address issues related to cancer.

The National Cancer Act was signed in 1971. It was the result of the devastation that cancer had caused in the United States. Per one study, there was a 70-year rise in age-adjusted death rates from 64 per 100,000 in 1900 to 163 per 100,000 in 1970 (age adjusted to the 2000 U.S. Census) (U.S. Census Bureau, 2003). The goal was to create a National Cancer Program, an organization centered on the National Cancer Institute, to battle cancer. This organization would have the resources and authority to track cancer incidence and mortality and develop prevention, screening, and treatment technologies.

The year 1991 was the peak of cancer age-adjusted mortality. By 2011, the last year for which data are available, the cancer death rate had declined by greater than 20%. Much of the decline is due to smoking cessation that began among men in the mid-1950s and among women in the mid-1960s. There has been a 35% decline in the breast cancer death rate and a near 40% decline in colorectal cancer death rate (Howlader et al., 2013).

While this decline indicates that a significant number of cancer deaths are being prevented in the United States, it is also evidence that some policies, such as tobacco control policies beginning in the 1950s and 1960s, are starting to work. It is important to note that the United States was the 31st country to have a 20% decline in cancer mortality (American Cancer Society, 2011).

It is commonly said that the United States has the best healthcare system in the world. Although the United States developed a number of new anticancer technologies through the National Cancer Act, many other countries have been better at broadly implementing these research findings.

The United States is especially poor at disseminating lifesaving technologies to the entire population, despite the fact that is has the most expensive healthcare system in the world. Health care in the United States cost $2.7 billion in 2011. That is more than $8,000 in one year for every man, woman, and child in the country. The second-most expensive nation in the world in 2011 was Norway. It spent nearly half as much, $4,100 for every man, woman, and child (Brawley & Virgo, 2010; Virgo et al., 2013).

Much of the inefficiency in American medicine involves a lack of focus on good, proven preventive health care and an irrational overconsumption of unnecessary screening and treatment technologies. It is interesting that, in the healthcare reform debate, many policy makers talk about the threat of the rationing of health care. In reality, we should be discussing the irrational use of health care and the need for its rational use. This is a policy issue.

It is a fact that healthcare providers commonly perform screening tests of little or no proven value, while many Americans do not get tests of clear proven value. We overtreat many patients with expensive and sometimes inferior treatments and often ignore the harm that overtreatment causes.

Such misuse of resources actually diverts these resources from those who need them. This perpetuates an underserved population with disparate outcomes.

While every country has populations with disparate outcomes, disparities are particularly severe in the United States (Jemal et al., 2008). The United States has a significant disenfranchised underclass. These people are medically underserved and have significantly worse outcomes compared to the general population. The disparate U.S. population is best defined as those who do not get the medical services commonly accepted as services people should get. There is a tendency to describe the underserved using racial categorization and focus on African Americans or Hispanics, but the underserved Caucasian population is the largest underserved cohort in the country. Socioeconomic status and rural residency are better indicators of those who receive poor health care than is ethnicity.

One example of socioeconomic status as an identifier of those at risk for poor outcomes involves health insurance and colon cancer. In a landmark study published in 2008, Ward et al. showed that, among Americans with colorectal cancer, those who were diagnosed at stage II (Dukes B) with insurance or Medicare at diagnosis had a superior five-year survival rate compared to those who did not have insurance or Medicare when diagnosed with stage I (Dukes A) disease. Insurance is a powerful determinant of survival among American patients with cancer. Insurance is a key element in cancer survival, and availability of insurance is, of course, a policy issue.

Tobacco is the cause of about one-third of all cancers in the United States (Glynn, Seffrin, Brawley, Grey, & Ross, 2010). Even so, one might consider the country's public health policy as it relates to tobacco as somewhat successful. In 1955, 55% of men smoked cigarettes (U.S. Department of Agriculture Economic Research Service, 2007). Today, 21% of adult men smoke. In 1965, 35% of women smoked cigarettes. Today, 16% smoke. There are large differences in the prevalence of smokers by state. A quarter of the residents of West Virginia and Kentucky smoke. This compares to about 10%–12% of residents of Utah and California. These differences are directly linked to the strength of tobacco control policies in these states (Centers for Disease Control and Prevention, 2010). This serves as evidence that we can do better in tobacco control policy.

Good scientific study has demonstrated that the combination of obesity, high caloric intake, and lack of physical activity causes cancer (Thun, DeLancey, Center, Jemal, & Ward, 2010). Indeed, the combination of the three is destined to surpass tobacco as the leading cause of cancer in the next decade or so (Colditz, Wolin, & Gehlert, 2012). This brings into question our policies on nutrition and physical activity. In this area, more so than any other, there is a need to develop good policy at multiple levels. Governments, schools, the food and restaurant industry, health insurers, and even employers will have to be involved.

As we look to the future, attention to policy and efficiency in medicine will be an even more pressing issue. Increased development of imaging and screening technology is forcing the definition of cancer to evolve from a mid–19th-century histologic diagnosis to a 21st-century diagnosis involving genomics and histology (Virchow, 1859; Welch & Black, 2010). Cancer prevention and treatment is entering an era of targeted diagnosis and precision medicine (Roychowdhury & Chinnaiyan, 2014). Some cancers will be best observed, whereas others will require expensive therapy.

While I have discussed prevention, screening, and treatment, it is important to note that the most pertinent question that should guide policy development is, "How can we provide adequate high-quality care, including preventive care, to all?"

References

American Cancer Society. (2011). *Global cancer facts and figures* (2nd ed.). Retrieved from http://www.cancer.org/research/cancerfactsstatistics/global

Brawley, O.W., & Virgo, K.S. (2010). From the guest editors: Introduction for the impact of health care reform on cancer patients. *Cancer Journal, 16,* 551–553. doi:10.1097/PPO.0b013e3182031591

Centers for Disease Control and Prevention. (2010). State-specific prevalence of cigarette smoking and smokeless tobacco use among adults United States, 2009. *Morbidity and Mortality Weekly Report, 59,* 1400–1406. Retrieved from http://www.cdc.gov/mmwr/preview/mmwrhtml/mm5943a2.htm

Colditz, G.A., Wolin, K.Y., & Gehlert, S. (2012). Applying what we know to accelerate cancer prevention. *Science Translational Medicine, 4,* 127rv4. doi:10.1126/scitranslmed.3003218

Glynn, T., Seffrin, J.R., Brawley, O.W., Grey, N., & Ross, H. (2010). The globalization of tobacco use: 21 challenges for the 21st century. *CA: A Cancer Journal for Clinicians, 60,* 50–61. doi:10.3322/caac.20052

Howlader, N., Noone, A.M., Krapcho, M., Garshell, J., Neyman, N., Altekruse, S.F., ... Cronin, K.A. (Eds.). (2013, April). SEER cancer statistics review, 1975–2010 [Based on November 2012 SEER data submission]. Retrieved from http://seer.cancer.gov/archive/csr/1975_2010/

Jemal, A., Thun, M.J., Ward, E.E., Henley, S.J., Cokkinides, V.E., & Murray, T.E. (2008). Mortality from leading causes by education and race in the United States, 2001. *American Journal of Preventive Medicine, 34,* 1–8.e7. doi:10.1016/j.amepre.2007.09.017

National Cancer Act of 1971, Pub. L. No. 92-218, 85 Stat. 778.

Roychowdhury, S., & Chinnaiyan, A.M. (2014). Translating genomics for precision cancer medicine. *Annual Review of Genomics and Human Genetics, 15,* 395–415. doi:10.1146/annurev-genom-090413-025552

Thun, M.J., DeLancey, J.O., Center, M.M., Jemal, A., & Ward, E.M. (2010). The global burden of cancer: Priorities for prevention. *Carcinogenesis, 31,* 100–110. doi:10.1093/carcin/bgp263

U.S. Census Bureau. (2003). Mini-historical statistics: No. HS-13. Live births, deaths, infant deaths, and maternal deaths: 1900 to 2001. In *Statistical abstract of the United States: 2003* (pp. 21–22). Retrieved from https://www.census.gov/statab/hist/HS-13.pdf

U.S. Department of Agriculture Economic Research Service. (2007). Cigarette consumption, United States, 1900–2007. In *Tobacco outlook report.* Washington, DC: Author.

Virchow, R. (1859). *Die cellularpathologie in ihrer begründung auf physiologische und pathologische gewebelehre.* Berlin, Germany: Verlag von August Hirschwald.

Virgo, K.S., Bromberek, J.L., Glaser, A., Horgan, D., Maher, J., & Brawley, O.W. (2013). Health care policy and cancer survivorship. *Cancer, 119,* 2187–2199. doi:10.1002/cncr.28066

Ward, E., Halpern, M., Schrag, N., Cokkinides, V., DeSantis, C., Bandi, P., ... Jemal, A. (2008). Association of insurance with cancer care utilization and outcomes. *CA: A Cancer Journal for Clinicians, 58,* 9–31. doi:10.3322/CA.2007.0011

Welch, H.G., & Black, W.C. (2010). Overdiagnosis in cancer. *Journal of the National Cancer Institute, 102,* 605–613. doi:10.1093/jnci/djq099

Index

The letter f *after a page number indicates that relevant content appears in a figure; the letter* t, *in a table.*